State-of-Art in Innate Immunity

Editors

Silvia Fischer
Elisabeth Deindl

MDPI • Basel • Beijing • Wuhan • Barcelona • Belgrade • Manchester • Tokyo • Cluj • Tianjin

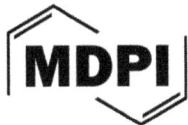

Editors
Silvia Fischer
Justus Liebig University Giessen
Germany

Elisabeth Deindl
Ludwig-Maximilians-Universität München
Germany

Editorial Office
MDPI
St. Alban-Anlage 66
4052 Basel, Switzerland

This is a reprint of articles from the Special Issue published online in the open access journal *Cells* (ISSN 2073-4409) (available at: https://www.mdpi.com/journal/cells/special_issues/Cells_Innate_Immune).

For citation purposes, cite each article independently as indicated on the article page online and as indicated below:

LastName, A.A.; LastName, B.B.; LastName, C.C. Article Title. *Journal Name* **Year**, *Volume Number*, Page Range.

ISBN 978-3-0365-5323-8 (Hbk)
ISBN 978-3-0365-5324-5 (PDF)

Cover image courtesy of Silvia Fischer

© 2022 by the authors. Articles in this book are Open Access and distributed under the Creative Commons Attribution (CC BY) license, which allows users to download, copy and build upon published articles, as long as the author and publisher are properly credited, which ensures maximum dissemination and a wider impact of our publications.
The book as a whole is distributed by MDPI under the terms and conditions of the Creative Commons license CC BY-NC-ND.

Contents

About the Editors vii

Silvia Fischer and Elisabeth Deindl
State of the Art of Innate Immunity—An Overview
Reprinted from: *Metals* **2022**, *11*, 2705, doi:10.3390/cells11172705 1

Ulf Andersson, Kevin J. Tracey and Huan Yang
Post-Translational Modification of HMGB1 Disulfide Bonds in Stimulating
and Inhibiting Inflammation
Reprinted from: *Metals* **2021**, *10*, 3323, doi:10.3390/cells10123323 3

**Karsten Grote, Marina Nicolai, Uwe Schubert, Bernhard Schieffer, Christian Troidl,
Klaus T. Preissner, Stefan Bauer and Silvia Fischer**
Extracellular Ribosomal RNA Acts Synergistically with Toll-like Receptor 2 Agonists to
Promote Inflammation
Reprinted from: *Metals* **2022**, *11*, 1440, doi:10.3390/cells11091440 21

**Christoph Arnholdt, Konda Kumaraswami, Philipp Götz, Matthias Kübler, Manuel Lasch
and Elisabeth Deindl**
Depletion of γδ T Cells Leads to Reduced Angiogenesis and Increased Infiltration of
Inflammatory M1-like Macrophages in Ischemic Muscle Tissue
Reprinted from: *Metals* **2022**, *11*, 1490, doi:10.3390/cells11091490 39

Philippe Georgel
Crosstalk between Interleukin-1β and Type I Interferons Signaling in
Autoinflammatory Diseases
Reprinted from: *Metals* **2021**, *10*, 1134, doi:10.3390/cells10051134 59

Jessica M. Gullett, Rebecca E. Tweedell and Thirumala-Devi Kanneganti
It's All in the PAN: Crosstalk, Plasticity, Redundancies, Switches, and Interconnectedness
Encompassed by PANoptosis Underlying the Totality of Cell Death-Associated
Biological Effects
Reprinted from: *Metals* **2022**, *11*, 1495, doi:10.3390/cells11091495 69

Jonas Johannes Papendorf, Elke Krüger and Frédéric Ebstein
Proteostasis Perturbations and Their Roles in Causing Sterile Inflammation and
Autoinflammatory Diseases
Reprinted from: *Metals* **2022**, *11*, 1422, doi:10.3390/cells11091422 89

**Ürün Ukan, Fredy Delgado Lagos, Sebastian Kempf, Stefan Günther, Mauro Siragusa, Beate
Fisslthaler and Ingrid Fleming**
Effect of Thrombin on the Metabolism and Function of Murine Macrophages
Reprinted from: *Metals* **2022**, *11*, 1718, doi:10.3390/cells11101718 115

**Tessa Carrau, Susanne Thümecke, Liliana M. R. Silva, David Perez-Bravo, Ulrich Gärtner,
Anja Taubert, Carlos Hermosilla, Andreas Vilcinskas and Kwang-Zin Lee**
The Cellular Innate Immune Response of the Invasive Pest Insect *Drosophila suzukii* against
Pseudomonas entomophila Involves the Release of Extracellular Traps
Reprinted from: *Metals* **2021**, *10*, 3320, doi:10.3390/cells10123320 133

Natalia Landázuri, Jennifer Gorwood, Ylva Terelius, Fredrik Öberg, Koon Chu Yaiw, Afsar Rahbar and Cecilia Söderberg-Nauclér
The Endothelin Receptor Antagonist Macitentan Inhibits Human Cytomegalovirus Infection
Reprinted from: Metals **2021**, *10*, 3072, doi:10.3390/cells10113072 . . . . **147**

Hao Lin, Yuhui Fan, Andreas Wieser, Jiang Zhang, Ivonne Regel, Hanno Nieß, Julia Mayerle, Alexander L. Gerbes and Christian J. Steib
Albumin Might Attenuate Bacteria-Induced Damage on Kupffer Cells for Patients with Chronic Liver Disease
Reprinted from: Metals **2021**, *10*, 2298, doi:10.3390/cells10092298 . . . . **165**

About the Editors

Silvia Fischer

Silvia Fischer received her doctor's degree at the Institute of Biochemistry of the Justus-Liebig-University in Giessen. After her post-doc time in Los Angeles, where she studied the generation and application of liposomes, she studied regulatory mechanisms and specific properties of the endothelium, especially the regulation of the permeability of the blood-brain barrier as well as processes of angiogenesis at the Max-Planck-Institute in Bad Nauheim. Since several years she investigated the role of extracellular RNA as danger associated molecular pattern in inflammatory processes and diseases at the Institute of Biochemistry in Giessen. She could demonstrate that extracellular RNA contributes to inflammatory pathologies such as stroke, myocardial infarction, rheumatoid arthritis, or cancer growth.

Elisabeth Deindl

Elisabeth Deindl (Dr) received her doctor's degree at the ZMBH in Heidelberg, Germany, where she worked on hepatitis B viruses. Thereafter, she joined the lab of Wolfgang Schaper at the Max-Planck-Institute in Bad Nauheim, where she started to decipher the molecular mechanisms of arteriogenesis. After a short detour on stem cells, she focused again on arteriogenesis becoming a leading expert in the field. By using a peripheral model of arteriogenesis, she demonstrated that collateral artery growth is a matter of innate immunity and presents a blueprint of sterile inflammation, which is locally triggered by extracellular RNA.

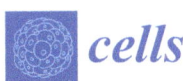

Editorial

State of the Art of Innate Immunity—An Overview

Silvia Fischer [1,*] and Elisabeth Deindl [2,3]

1. Institute of Biochemistry, Justus-Liebig-University, 35392 Giessen, Germany
2. Walter-Brendel-Centre of Experimental Medicine, University Hospital, Ludwig-Maximilians-University, 81377 Munich, Germany
3. Biomedical Center, Institute of Cardiovascular Physiology and Pathophysiology, Ludwig-Maximilians-University, Planegg-Martinsried, 82152 Munich, Germany
* Correspondence: silvia.fischer@biochemie.med.uni-giessen.de; Tel.: +49-641-9947440

Citation: Fischer, S.; Deindl, E. State of the Art of Innate Immunity—An Overview. *Cells* 2022, 11, 2705. https://doi.org/10.3390/cells11172705

Received: 24 August 2022
Accepted: 26 August 2022
Published: 30 August 2022

Publisher's Note: MDPI stays neutral with regard to jurisdictional claims in published maps and institutional affiliations.

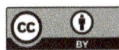

Copyright: © 2022 by the authors. Licensee MDPI, Basel, Switzerland. This article is an open access article distributed under the terms and conditions of the Creative Commons Attribution (CC BY) license (https://creativecommons.org/licenses/by/4.0/).

The innate immune system is the first line of defense against bacterial and viral infections and sterile inflammation through the recognition of pathogen-associated molecular patterns (PAMPs) as well as danger-associated molecular patterns (DAMPs) by pathogen-recognition receptors (PRRs), and produces proinflammatory and antiviral cytokines and chemokines [1].

This Special Issue of *Cells* is devoted to many aspects of innate immunity and gives an overview of different DAMPs, immune cells, special mechanisms, and therapeutic options for treating diseases related to chronic inflammation or infections.

One of the well-known DAMPs is the high-mobility group box 1 protein (HMGB1), which is either passively released by dying cells or actively secreted by immune and other cells and was described as implicated in both stimulating and inhibiting innate immunity. Andersson et al. reported that the pro- and anti-inflammatory activities of HMGB1 depend on post-translational modification of its disulfide bonds by binding to different extracellular cell surface receptors either directly or as a cofactor of PAMPs [2].

Another DAMP, extracellular ribosomal RNA, which is released under pathological conditions from damaged tissue, acts synergistically with Toll-like receptor 2 ligands, inducing the release of cytokines in a nuclear factor kappa B-dependent manner in vitro as well as in vivo. Grote et al. suggest that extracellular RNA might sensitize Toll-like receptor 2 to enhance the immune response under pathological conditions and therefore might serve as a new target for the treatment of bacterial or viral infections [3].

Arnholdt et al. demonstrate that cells related to innate immunity and influencing immunoregulatory and inflammatory processes, such as gamma delta T cells, play an important role in angiogenesis and tissue generation. By using a femoral artery ligation model in mice, depletion of this subset of T cells was demonstrated to impair angiogenesis, increase the number of leukocytes and inflammatory M1-like macrophages, and promote the formation of neutrophil extracellular traps (NETs) [4].

The topic of autoinflammation is also covered in this Special Issue. The review of P. Georgel provides some examples of autoimmune/autoinflammatory diseases caused by the deregulated expression of type I interferons and interleukin-1β. The role of interleukin-1 and type I interferons and their crosstalk in autoinflammatory diseases such as rheumatic diseases are analyzed to reveal novel therapeutic opportunities [5].

Gullet et al. discuss the key components of programmed cell death pathways and highlight the plasticity of pyroptosis, apoptosis, and necroptosis as well as significant crosstalk among these pathways. The concept of PANoptosis, an inflammatory cell death pathway that integrates components of different cell death pathways and is implicated in driving innate immune responses and inflammation, is explained [6].

A review by Papendorf et al. provides a comprehensive overview of molecular pathogenesis disorders caused by proteostasis perturbations, and current knowledge of the various mechanisms by which impaired proteostasis promotes autoinflammation is summarized [7].

To investigate the crosstalk between coagulation and innate immunity, the effect of thrombin on macrophage polarization is investigated by Ukan et al. Results demonstrate that thrombin induces an anti-inflammatory phenotype in macrophages, which shows similarities to as well as differences from the classical M2 polarization states regarding the expression of secreted modular Ca^{2+}-binding protein [8].

To investigate insect innate immunity, the in vitro cultivation of primary hemocytes from *D. Suzuki* third-instar larvae is described by Carrau et al. as a valuable tool for investigating hemocyte-derived effector mechanisms against pathogens, particularly for the formation of extracellular traps [9].

Drugs such as ganciclovir and its pro-drug valganciclovir are often used to treat viremic patients transfected with, e.g., human cytomegalovirus (HCMV). Results from Landázuri now suggest that binding and signaling through endothelin receptor B (ETBR) is crucial for viral replication and that selected ETBR blockers inhibit HCMV infections [10].

Lin et al. report that albumin attenuates chronic liver diseases (CLDs) via alleviating inflammation of Kupffer cells caused by bacterial products, which might provide a compelling rationale for albumin therapy in patients with CLDs [11].

Funding: This research received no external funding.

Conflicts of Interest: The authors declare no conflict of interest.

References

1. Brubaker, S.W.; Bonham, K.S.; Zanoi, I.; Kagan, J.C. Innate immune pattern recognition: A cell biological perspective *Annu. Rev. Immunol.* **2015**, *33*, 257. [CrossRef] [PubMed]
2. Andersson, U.; Tracey, K.J.; Yang, H. Post-translational modification of HMGB1 disulfide bonds in stimulating and inhibiting inflammation. *Cells* **2021**, *10*, 2223. [CrossRef]
3. Grote, K.; Nicolai, M.; Schubert, U.; Schieffer, B.; Troidl, C.; Preissner, K.T.; Bauer, S.; Fischer, S. Extracellular ribosomal RNA acts synergistically with toll-like receptor 2 agonists to promote inflammation. *Cells* **2022**, *11*, 1440. [CrossRef] [PubMed]
4. Arnholdt, C.; Kumaraswami, K.; Götz, P.; Kübler, M.; Lasch, M.; Deindl, E. Depletion of gdT cells leads to reduced angiogenesis and increased infiltration of inflammatory M1-like macrophages in ischemic muscle tissue. *Cells* **2022**, *11*, 1490. [CrossRef] [PubMed]
5. Georgel, P. Crosstalk between interleukin-1b and type I interferons signaling in autoinflammatory diseases. *Cells* **2021**, *10*, 1134. [CrossRef] [PubMed]
6. Gullet, J.M.; Tweedell, R.E.; Kanneganti, T.-D. It's all in the PAN: Crosstalk, plasticity, redundancies, switches, and interconnectedness encompassed by PANoptosis underlying the totality of cell death-associated biological effects. *Cells* **2022**, *11*, 1495. [CrossRef]
7. Papendorf, J.J.; Krüger, E.; Ebstein, F. Proteostasis perturbations and their roles in causing sterile inflammation and autoinflammatory diseases. *Cells* **2022**, *11*, 1422. [CrossRef] [PubMed]
8. Ukan, Ü.; Lagos, F.D.; Kempf, S.; Günther, S.; Siragusa, M.; Fisslthaler, B.; Fleming, I. Effect of thrombin on the metabolism and function of murine macrophages. *Cells* **2022**, *11*, 1718. [CrossRef]
9. Carrau, T.; Thümecke, S.; Silva, L.M.R.; Perez-Bravo, D.; Gärtner, U.; Taubert, A.; Hermosilla, C.; Vilcinskas, A.; Lee, K.-Z. The cellular innate immune response of the invasive pest insect *Drosophila suzukii* against *Pseudomas entomophila* involves the release of extracellular traps. *Cells* **2021**, *10*, 3320. [CrossRef] [PubMed]
10. Landázuri, N.; Gorwood, J.; Terellus, Y.; Öberg, F.; Yalw, K.C.; Rahbar, A.; Söderberg-Nauclér, C. The endothelin receptor antagonist macitentan inhibits human cytomegalovirus infection. *Cells* **2021**, *10*, 3072. [CrossRef] [PubMed]
11. Lin, H.; Fan, Y.; Wieser, A.; Zhang, J.; Regel, I.; Nieß, H.; Mayerle, J.; Gerbes, A.L.; Steib, C.J. Albumin might attenuate bacteria-induced damage on kupffer cells for patients with chronic liver disease. *Cells* **2021**, *10*, 2298. [CrossRef] [PubMed]

Review

Post-Translational Modification of HMGB1 Disulfide Bonds in Stimulating and Inhibiting Inflammation

Ulf Andersson [1,*], Kevin J. Tracey [2] and Huan Yang [2]

[1] Department of Women's and Children's Health, Karolinska Institute, Karolinska University Hospital, 17176 Stockholm, Sweden

[2] Institute for Bioelectronic Medicine, The Feinstein Institutes for Medical Research, 350 Community Drive, Manhasset, NY 11030, USA; kjtracey@northwell.edu (K.J.T.); hyang@northwell.edu (H.Y.)

* Correspondence: ulf.andersson@ki.se; Tel.: +46-(70)-7401740

Abstract: High mobility group box 1 protein (HMGB1), a highly conserved nuclear DNA-binding protein, is a "damage-associated molecular pattern" molecule (DAMP) implicated in both stimulating and inhibiting innate immunity. As reviewed here, HMGB1 is an oxidation-reduction sensitive DAMP bearing three cysteines, and the post-translational modification of these residues establishes its proinflammatory and anti-inflammatory activities by binding to different extracellular cell surface receptors. The redox-sensitive signaling mechanisms of HMGB1 also occupy an important niche in innate immunity because HMGB1 may carry other DAMPs and pathogen-associated molecular pattern molecules (PAMPs). HMGB1 with DAMP/PAMP cofactors bind to the receptor for advanced glycation end products (RAGE) which internalizes the HMGB1 complexes by endocytosis for incorporation in lysosomal compartments. Intra-lysosomal HMGB1 disrupts lysosomal membranes thereby releasing the HMGB1-transported molecules to stimulate cytosolic sensors that mediate inflammation. This HMGB1-DAMP/PAMP cofactor pathway slowed the development of HMGB1-binding antagonists for diagnostic or therapeutic use. However, recent discoveries that HMGB1 released from neurons mediates inflammation via the TLR4 receptor system, and that cancer cells express fully oxidized HMGB1 as an immunosuppressive mechanism, offer new paths to targeting HMGB1 for inflammation, pain, and cancer.

Keywords: HMGB1; RAGE; TLR4; DAMP; SIRT1; α7-nicotinic acetylcholine receptor; nociceptor; inflammation; cancer; COVID-19

1. Introduction

High mobility group box 1 protein (HMGB1)s a DNA-binding molecule bound to chromatin in all eukaryotic cells [1]. When passively released by dying cells or actively secreted by activated immune and other cells, it is an alarmin and damage-associated molecular pattern molecule (DAMP). In general, alarmins perform distinct intracellular tasks during homeostatic conditions but promote inflammation to initiate repair mechanisms when released extracellularly in response to danger signals [2]. However, exaggerated alarmin responses can increase tissue injury and cause organ dysfunction, a central mechanism in the pathogenesis of acute and chronic inflammatory diseases. Extracellular HMGB1 has been implicated in chemokine, cytokine, metabolic, inflammatory, neuroinflammatory, and anti-inflammatory activities, a diverse range of functions that depend on the molecular binding partners of HMGB1, its extracellular or intracellular location, and its redox state [3,4].

2. Extracellular HMGB1 Release

HMGB1 expresses 214 amino acids arranged in two consecutive DNA-binding HMG box domains (box A and box B) and an acidic C-terminal tail, containing a stretch of thirty continuous glutamic and aspartic acids (Figure 1).

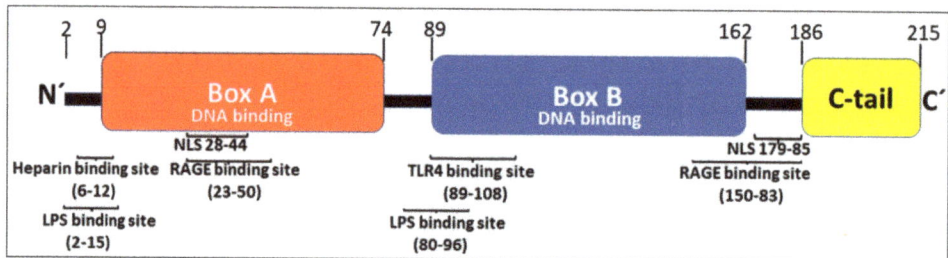

Figure 1. Position of binding sites for HMGB1-receptors, heparin, LPS, and the two nuclear localization sites (NLSs) in the HMGB1 molecule.

The two DNA-binding boxes of HMGB1 contain three cysteines and the redox state of each of these residues is critically important for the ability of the nuclear molecule to be secreted and for the extracellular receptor usage. All three cysteines reside in a fully reduced state with thiol groups (all-thiol HMGB1) in inactive cells. Mild HMGB1 oxidation generates disulfide HMGB1 characterized by a disulfide bond between Cys23 and Cys45 while keeping Cys106 in the reduced form. Further oxidation of HMGB1 will produce sulfonyl groups on any or all cysteine residues creating an isoform called sulfonyl HMGB1 [1]. Homo-dimerization of HMGB1 at Cys106 has recently but described to take place both in the nucleus and extracellularly [5]. The biological significance of this molecule needs further investigation.

Active HMGB1 release occurs in several steps. First, nuclear HMGB1 translocates to the cytoplasm, a process that requires JAK-STAT1 signaling that will generate acetylation of critical lysine residues located in the two nuclear localization sites (NLSs) [6,7] (Figure 1). Hyperacetylation of HMGB1 prevents the continuous bidirectional shuttle of HMGB1 between the cytoplasm and the nucleus present in all cells and leads to cytoplasmic accumulation of HMGB1. Nuclear hyperacetylation is also accomplished via increased histone-acetylase (HAT) activity as well as decreased histone-deacetylase (HDAC) activity [7–9]. Several agents including metformin, resveratrol, and curcumin (which all enhance sirtuin 1 (SIRT1) deacetylase activity) decrease extracellular HMGB1 release and reduce HMGB1-dependent inflammation [10–18]. Decreased activity of SIRT1, a nicotinamide adenine dinucleotide-dependent HDAC, occurs in aging and senescence, suggesting a role for HMGB1 in the inflammation associated with aging ("inflammageing") [19–21]. Additional HDACs including HDAC1 and HDAC4 have likewise been demonstrated to efficiently inhibit active HMGB1 release [8,9,22]. Ethanol reduces HDAC1/4 performance and thus enhances neuronal HMGB1 release [9]. Ischemia-reperfusion injury is another cause of reduced nuclear HDAC1 and HDAC4 activities that generate increased levels of extracellular hyperacetylated HMGB1 [8].

Intranuclear oxidation of HMGB1 to the disulfide isoform is also a prerequisite for the translocation of HMGB1 to the cytosol [23]. Nuclear peroxiredoxins I and II induce an intramolecular disulfide formation between Cys23 and Cys45 to generate disulfide HMGB1 that will be transported out of the nucleus by binding to the nuclear exportin chromosome-region maintenance 1 (CRM1) interacting with the two nuclear export signal sites present in each of the HMG boxes of HMGB1 [7].

Second, cytoplasmic HMGB1 is released extracellularly via several mechanisms. One route proceeds via exocytosis of secretory lysosomes, a pathway also used for IL-1β secretion, although HMGB1 and IL-1β are stored in separate vesicles [24] (Figure 2A). The intracellular events that control the sequestration of cytoplasmic HMGB1 in secretory lysosomes remain to be elucidated. A second route for HMGB1 to exit cells is via its expression on the surface of microparticles derived from activated platelets [25,26]. Vascular injury induces the massive extracellular release of HMGB1 from platelets displaying an important role in the pathogenesis of thrombosis formation and neutrophil activation [27–29].

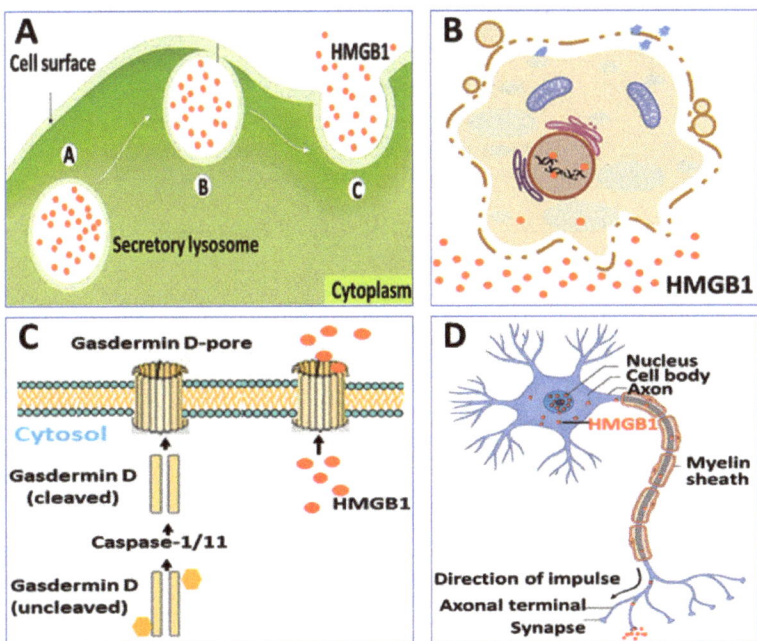

Figure 2. Selected examples of mechanisms for HMGB1 release. (**A**) HMGB1 lacks a secretory signal sequence and is instead packed into secretory lysosomes in hematopoietic cells, before being released extracellularly. (**B**) Pyroptosis and necrosis are both lytic processes that generate HMGB1 release, (**C**) Inflammasome-activated gasdermin D creates pore formation in the outer cell membrane enabling HMGB1 release even before cell lysis may occur. (**D**) Stimulated nociceptors release HMGB1 in a retrograde manner.

Programmed, proinflammatory cell death (pyroptosis) is an additional mechanism for the regulated release of HMGB1, which is hyperacetylated and expresses the disulfide redox isoform [30–32] (Figure 2B,C). This process takes place due to increased caspase-1/caspase-11 activity that generates inflammasome activation and gasdermin D cleavage inducing pore formation and eventually ruptures the outer cell membrane [33]. Gasdermin D-generated nanopore formation and pyroptosis have been implicated as the dominant pathway for HMGB1 release during gram-negative sepsis when caspase-1/caspase-11 double-deficient mice express markedly reduced systemic HMGB1 levels [34]. Recent evidence indicates that stimulated sensory neurons actively secrete HMGB1 in an antidromic fashion by molecular mechanisms that remain elusive [35] (Figure 2D). The neuronally released HMGB1 is most likely disulfide HMGB1 since it acts via TLR4 to mediate inflammation and pain [13,36–47] and disulfide HMGB1 is the single redox form of HMGB1 capable of binding to the MD-2/TLR4 receptor complex [48]. Functional consequences regarding the neuronal HMGB1-regulation of inflammation will be discussed later in this review.

Various forms of cell deaths generate passive HMGB1 release expressing different isoforms. Necrosis releases fully reduced, non-acetylated HMGB1 (the habitual nuclear HMGB1 isoform), which acts as a chemotactic factor when bound to CXCL12 generating enhanced CXCR4 signaling [49,50]. Apoptosis causes insignificant extracellular HMGB1 release since the nuclear HMGB1 strongly attached to modified DNA is retained in membrane-sealed apoptotic bodies [51]. However, if the phagocytic clearance of the apoptotic bodies fails this debris may undergo secondary-necrosis and discharge non-acetylated

HMGB1 mainly in the sulfonyl redox isoform [52]. As already described, pyroptosis generates disulfide, hyperacetylated HMGB1 [30–32].

3. HMGB1 Receptor Usage

The redox state of HMGB1 determines the ability for receptor interactions and thus the functional outcome of extracellular HMGB1 interactions. TLR4 and the receptor for advanced glycated end-products (RAGE) are the most extensively studied HMGB1 receptors. TLR4 is the HMGB1 receptor causing cytokine and type 1 interferon production [53] (Figure 3). This interaction requires disulfide HMGB1 to bind at low nanomolar avidity to the TLR4 co-receptor MD-2, in an analogous way to LPS, but attaching at another position [48].

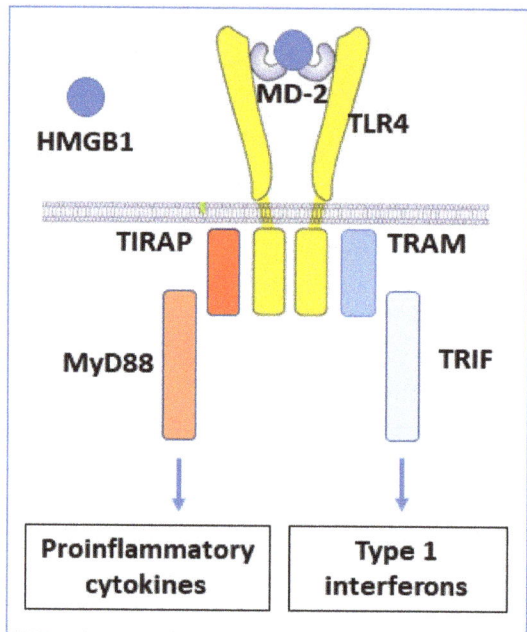

Figure 3. Disulfide HMGB1 binds to MD-2 and activates the TLR4 receptor complex via two separate intracellular signal pathways. Proinflammatory cytokines are formed when the adapter molecule TIRAP gets associated with toll-like receptor 4 and the myeloid differentiation factor 88 (MyD88) that activates the NF-κB signaling pathway. Interferon-β is produced when TRAM (TRIF-related adaptor molecule) associates with TRIF (TIR-domain-containing adapter-inducing interferon-β).

RAGE is a multi-ligand receptor expressed by many cell types, predominantly as a preformed intracellular molecule available for rapid NF-κB-controlled translocation to the cell surface [54,55]. RAGE was originally identified as an HMGB1-receptor in the context of studies of neurite outgrowth in the fetal brain without any signs of concomitant proinflammatory activity. This RAGE-binding site in HMGB1 is located in sequence 150–83 [56] (Figure 1). One additional RAGE-binding site situated in the HMGB1 box A domain (sequence 23–50) was later identified and RAGE-interaction with this site has profound proinflammatory effects [57]. Extracellular HMGB1 readily forms heterocomplexes with multiple extracellular DAMPs and PAMPs [58], which are subsequently endocytosed by HMGB1 binding to RAGE for further intracellular transport to the endolysosomal compartment [34,59–69]. Heparin, recombinant truncated HMGB1 box A protein, and acetylcholine each blocks the endocytosis of HMGB1 and its partner molecules [60,70]. HMGB1 heterocomplexes are endocytosed via RAGE expressed on macrophages and finally accumulate in the lysosomal compartment [34] (Figure 4). HMGB1, at high concentration, then accomplishes a unique function inside acidic lysosomes because HMGB1 disrupts the lysosomal membrane at low pH allowing its partner molecules to circumvent degradation and leak into the cytosol. In contrast, any molecule imported into the lysosomal system via antibodies in the absence of HMGB1 is normally degraded there. The HMGB1-imported extracellular DAMPs and PAMPs released from the ruptured lysosomes will subsequently bind and activate cognate cytosolic sensors, a mechanism that would not occur in the absence of the RAGE/HMGB1-assisted transport. Stimulation of proinflammatory cytosolic sensors generates inflammasome activation, pyroptosis, the release of proinflammatory mediators, and activation of the extrinsic coagulation cascade [34,71,72]. Inflammasomes cleave and activate inflammatory caspases such as caspase 1, 4, 5, and 11 resulting in activation of cytoplasmic gasdermin D. The truncated gasdermin D then forms oligomerized molecules producing nanopores in the plasma membrane culminating in pyroptotic cell death (Figure 2C). This process in live and dying cells mediates the release of IL-1α, IL-1β, IL-18, and HMGB1 [30,31,71] (Figure 4). Furthermore, cleaved gasdermin D also activates a membrane-located scramblase inducing phosphatidylserine externalization on the cell surface, where the molecule assembles a complex of cofactor proteases of the coagulation cascade initiating coagulation [33,73,74].

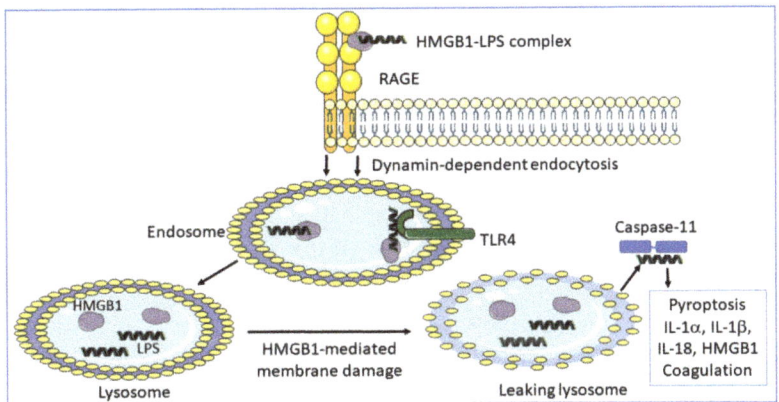

Figure 4. LPS needs HMGB1 to trigger severe inflammation. Injected LPS and type 1 interferon, (which generates HMGB1 release) in TLR4 gene-deficient mice is lethal in contrast to when administered to caspase-11 knockout mice [75,76]. The initial event in LPS toxicity is due to extracellular LPS activation of cell surface TLR4, which triggers extracellular HMGB1 release. HMGB1 has two LPS-binding sites (Figure 1) and thus forms extracellular HMGB1-LPS complexes that get endocytosed via RAGE to finally reach the cytosol culminating in caspase-11 activation (in mice; caspases 4/5 in humans) causing inflammation and coagulation.

Surprising new findings in tumor biology reveal that oxidized HMGB1 (sulfonyl HMGB1) is an anti-inflammatory molecule that signals via RAGE [77] (Table 1). Sulfonyl HMGB1 has until now been considered as a functionally inert molecule, mainly defined by an absent capacity to generate inflammation, but these new observations implicate sulfonyl HMGB1 in recruiting immunocompetent cells which inhibit cytotoxic cells, thereby impairing their ability to attack and kill the tumor cells. Immunosuppressive cells recruited by sulfonyl HMGB1 include regulatory T lymphocytes (Tregs), M2 macrophages, and myeloid-derived suppressor cells (MDSC). Sulfonyl HMGB1 also downregulates antigen-presenting cells including dendritic cells and plasmacytoid dendritic cells (summarized in Table 1).

Table 1. Extracellular HMGB1 redox forms determine functional outcomes in inflammation.

HMGB1 Redox Form	Partner Molecule	Receptor	Biological Response	Reference
All-thiol	CXCL12	CXCR4	Chemotaxis	[50]
Disulfide	None	TLR4	Cytokines	[53]
Sulfonyl	Unknown	RAGE	Accumulation of Tregs and MDSCs, enhanced M2/M1 macrophage ratio and dendritic cell tolerogenicity	[77]
Undetermined	Many PAMPs and DAMPs	RAGE	Inflammasome activation, hyperinflammation, coagulation, pyroptosis	[34]
Undetermined	None	CD24+ Siglec-10	NF-κB inhibition	[78]

Administration of HMGB1 inhibitors improved outcomes from cancer in several experimental models. Anti-HMGB1 therapy inhibited tumor growth, diminished the recruitment of immunosuppressive cells, and enhanced the antigen-presenting capacity of tumor-associated dendritic cells [77]. Furthermore, the therapeutic efficacy of checkpoint immune inhibitors was enhanced when concomitant HMGB1 blocking treatment was provided. These results suggest a very intriguing scenario where sulfonyl HMGB1 may occupy a supportive role in the resolution of inflammation, but a detrimental role in the defense against tumors. The results suggest further studies of the mechanism are warranted to determine the role of sulfonyl HMGB1/ RAGE-dependent biology in cancer because it offers an interesting experimental therapeutic strategy (Figure 5).

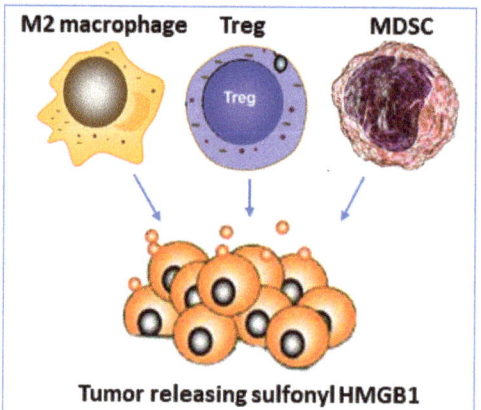

Figure 5. Fully oxidized HMGB1 inhibits cytotoxicity versus tumors. Tumor secreting sulfonyl HMGB1 which attracts M2 macrophages, regulatory T cells, and myeloid-derived suppressor cells (MDSC) which all inhibit a cytotoxic cell response against the tumor.

The immunosuppressive regulation of sulfonyl HMGB1 via RAGE is not the only HMGB1 anti-inflammatory mechanism [77]. It has previously been demonstrated that HMGB1, of undefined redox isoform, binds to CD24 (Table 1) [78]. This cell surface sialoglycoprotein is expressed by several cell types including dendritic cells, where it provides costimulatory signals to T cells but lacks a mechanism for signal transduction. HMGB1-CD24 forms a trimolecular complex on dendritic cells with the signaling receptor Siglec-10, which subsequently associates with the tyrosine phosphatase SHP-1, a negative regulator of nuclear factor-kB (NF-κB) activation [78] (Figure 6).

The consequence of these molecular events is thus downregulated inflammation. Experimental administration of CD24-Fc fusion protein inhibited inflammation in pre-clinical models of virus infection, autoimmunity, and graft-versus-host disease [79–81].

Clinical studies based on the administration of soluble CD24 and CD24Fc are in progress for patients with severe COVID-19 [82].

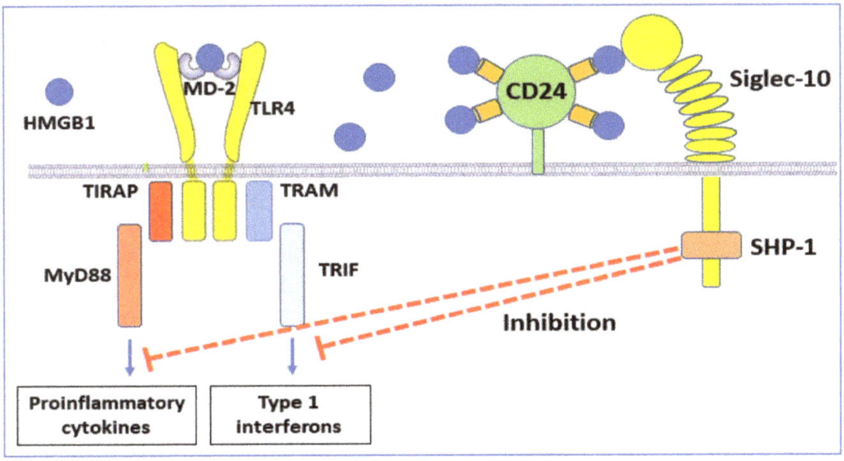

Figure 6. An anti-inflammatory HMGB1-dependent pathway. A trimolecular complex formed by HMGB1, CD24, and Siglec-10 generates intracellular cell signaling that turns off NF-κB-dependent inflammatory processes.

4. Sensory Neurons Direct Inflammation via HMGB1 Release

Sensory neurons, termed "nociceptors" mediate neuroinflammation through the retrograde or "antidromic" release of neuropeptides, neurotransmitters, and incompletely defined mediators. Recently we reported that HMGB1 is a necessary and sufficient mediator of neuroinflammation because nociceptors harvested from transgenic mice expressing channelrhodopsin-2 (ChR2) directly release HMGB1 when stimulated by light [35]. In collagen antibody-induced arthritis in mice, ablation of neuronal HMGB1 decreased hyperalgesia, delayed onset, and reduced intensity of joint inflammation and cartilage destruction compared to wild type (WT) or HMGB1 floxed ($HMGB1^{fl/fl}$) control mice (Figure 7).

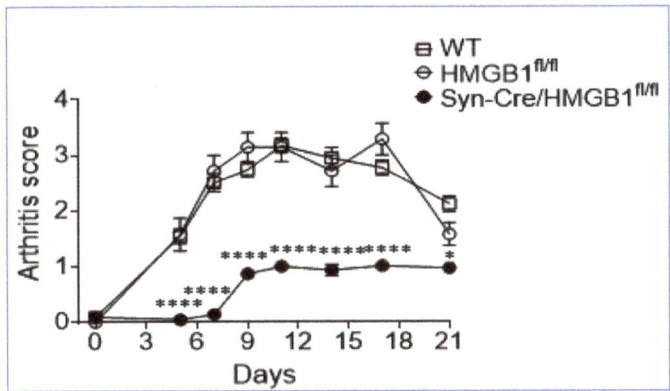

Figure 7. Ablation of neuronal HMGB1 reduces joint inflammation. Polyarthritis was induced by the administration of anti-collagen antibodies in mice. Wild type (WT) and HMGB1$^{fl/fl}$ control mice developed severe polyarthritis. Significantly delayed onset and reduced severity of polyarthritis were observed in neuronally HMGB1 gene-deficient mice (Syn-Cre/HMGB1$^{fl/fl}$). *: $p < 0.05$, ****: $p < 0.0001$ vs. HMGB1$^{fl/fl}$ control. Reproduced from Yang et al. [35].

Furthermore, sterile sciatic nerve injury produces inflammation, swelling, and hyperalgesia in the paws of wild type mice (WT) and HMGB1 floxed $HMGB1^{fl/fl}$ mice, but these responses are attenuated in neuronal-specific HMGB1 knock-out (Syn-Cre/HMGB1$^{fl/fl}$) mice (Figure 8A,B) [35]. These and other results indicate neuronal HMGB1 is required to mediate nerve injury-induced tissue inflammation and neuropathic pain.

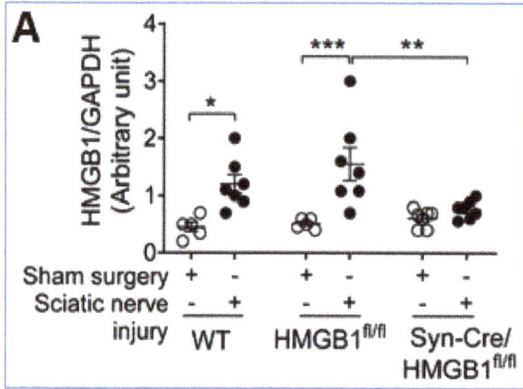
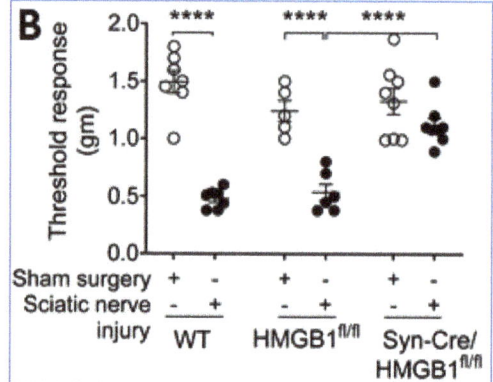

Figure 8. Ablation of neuronal HMGB1 reduces inflammation and hyperalgesia after sciatic nerve injury. Standardized sciatic nerve injury was induced via nerve ligation. (**A**) HMGB1 levels were significantly increased in paw tissue from WT and HMGB1$^{fl/fl}$ control mice in contrast to Syn-Cre/ HMGB1$^{fl/fl}$ mice (* $p < 0.05$, ** $p < 0.01$, *** $p < 0.001$). (**B**) Mechanical sensitivity assessed using von Frey filaments and the Dixon up-down method to calculate the threshold response demonstrated that hyperalgesia after sciatic nerve injury was significantly reduced in Syn-Cre/HMGB1$^{fl/fl}$ mice as compared to HMGB $^{fl/fl}$ control mice (**** $p < 0.0001$). Reproduced from Yang et al. [35].

The redox state of the neuronally released HMGB1 is yet to be defined, but it is likely the disulfide form because neuroinflammation and hyperalgesia are TLR4-dependent, and disulfide HMGB1 is a specific TLR4 ligand [83–86]. Neuronal TLR4 KO mice are also significantly protected from sciatic injury-induced allodynia and skin inflammation [87]. Other studies of global TLR4 knockout mice likewise indicate that TLR4 is required for HMGB1-mediated hyperalgesia [83,84].

Active neuronal HMGB1 release is not restricted to peripheral sensory nerves but has been demonstrated to occur in yet undefined neurons in the central nervous system too [9,46,88–90]. Cultured primary cortical neurons stimulated by TNF release HMGB1 [88]. Ethanol triggers HMGB1 release from neurons in rat hippocampal-entorhinal cortex brain slice cultures [9], as ethanol reduces HDAC activity which promotes the release of acetylated HMGB1. Targeting neuronal HMGB1 reduces the expression of TNF and IL-1β in microglia cells in the cultured brain slices. Hyperexcitatory brain neurons from Alzheimer's patients also release HMGB1, which binds to TLR4 and mediates neurite degeneration [46]. A recently developed HMGB1-specific mAb blocking the TLR4-binding epitope of HMGB1 has demonstrated beneficial therapeutic effects in mouse models of preclinical Alzheimer´s disease [46,91], and other neutralizing anti-HMGB1 mAbs exerted neuroprotection in a rat model of Parkinson´s disease [89]. In the anti-HMGB1 mAb-treated group, HMGB1 was retained in the nucleus of neurons and astrocytes, whereas in the control mAb-treated group cytoplasmic HMGB1 translocation was observed in both neurons and astrocytes.

In summary, these multiple observations suggest that HMGB1 is actively released during neuronal depolarization and plays a key etiologic role in the initiation and amplification of inflammation.

5. HMGB1 in COVID-19

There are presently almost 200,000 publications about COVID-19 listed on PubMed but only 40 of them investigated the role of HMGB1, out of which only 4 reports on elevated systemic HMGB1 levels in COVID-19 patients [92–95]. This is a remarkably small number considering that extensive necrosis and hyperinflammation in the disease should generate substantial HMGB1 release. A hyperexcited HMGB1-RAGE axis would also be expected since the respiratory tract macrophages, epithelial, and endothelial cells release large amounts of extracellular HMGB1, and its cognate receptor RAGE is constitutively abundantly expressed in the lungs only. It is therefore highly surprising that only a few papers are documenting robustly increased systemic amounts of HMGB1 during the acute stage of severe COVID-19. The HMGB1 ELISAs used in the four reports that demonstrated high HMGB1 levels included antibodies with different specificities for HMGB1 than those applied in standardized HMGB1 ELISAs used in the majority of HMGB1 studies. It is most likely that these four papers reflect COVID-19 pathophysiology. We further speculate that during the acute stage of the disease large amounts of extracellular endogenous DNA and other DAMPs are released by extensive cell death. This combined with extracellular viral RNA and other PAMPs bound to HMGB1 may interfere with HMGB1 assays. Standard HMGB1 ELISA methods commonly include buffer steps to dissociate HMGB1 and partner molecules bound to HMGB1 enabling the ELISA antibodies to recognize HMGB1. Based on our unpublished results we suspect that some standardized HMGB1 ELISAs do not perform accurately with COVID-19 plasma samples and fail to remove complex-bound molecules efficiently from HMGB1, which produces confounding results.

This view is supported by our recent analysis of plasma samples from 9 COVID-19 patients with severe hyperinflammation using ELISA methods that revealed HMGB1 levels within the normal range (Figure 9A). However, immunoblotting analysis under reducing conditions of the same samples demonstrated highly elevated HMGB1 levels as compared to normal controls indicating pathologically increased plasma concentrations (Figure 9B). Pretreatment of the plasma samples with perchloric acid [96] to dissociate molecules attached to HMGB1 shifted the ELISA results to demonstrate increased, pathological HMGB1 levels, despite that the harsh acidic handling partly damaged the samples (Figure 9A). Taken together, it seems that there are exceptional problems regarding systemic HMGB1 quantification during acute COVID-19, due to yet undefined partner molecules attaching strongly to HMGB1 and causing steric hindrance for antibody recognition.

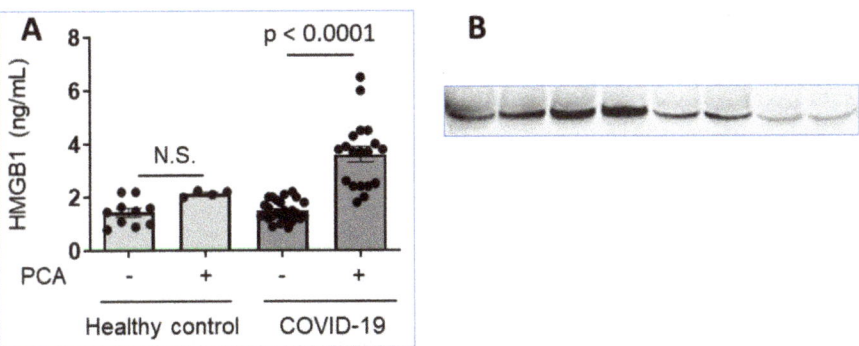

Figure 9. Plasma HMGB1 levels are increased in patients with severe COVID-19. (**A**) Multiple plasma samples from COVID-19 patients (27 samples from 9 patients) and healthy controls (14 samples from 4 healthy controls) were analyzed in HMGB1 ELISA (IBL International GmbH, Germany). The samples were either pretreated by perchloric acid (PCA) or not [96]. (**B**) Plasma samples from two COVID-19 patients and two healthy controls were subjected to SDS polyacrylamide gel electrophoresis in reducing conditions and probed with a monoclonal anti-HMGB1 antibody. Lanes 1-4 shows plasma samples from day 0, 2, 3, 4 from the admission of a patient with lethal Covid-19 infection; lanes 5–6 represent samples from a severely ill COVID-19 patient on day 0 and 1 from admission, while lanes 7–8 demonstrate results in two healthy controls.

ELISA measurement of systemic HMGB1 levels in some other clinical conditions including active systemic lupus erythematosus (SLE) or septic shock has previously been reported to underestimate results reminding of the problems that we encountered in our pilot study in COVID-19 patients. Barnay-Verdier et al. studied HMGB1 quantification using ELISA in plasma samples from patients with septic shock [96]. They compared results in plasma versus plasma subjected to perchloric acid exposure prior to ELISA. The results were straightforward, PCA-ELISA detected significantly higher amounts of HMGB1 in plasma samples compared to conventional ELISA. Another study unexpectedly found that lupus patients with active disease had HMGB1 levels measured by ELISA to be at the same or even at lower levels than in healthy controls [97]. In contrast, western blot assessment demonstrated huge differences between healthy controls and patients with active lupus, who expressed high HMGB1 levels. The plasma molecules that presumably bound and masked HMGB1 in ELISA measurements were not identified.

6. HMGB1 and Acetylcholine-Potent Antagonists Balancing Inflammation

Over the past 20 years, amazingly consistent and successful results from preclinical and in vitro studies have revealed that acetylcholine is a strong inhibitor of HMGB1-provoked inflammation and pain [60,98–110]. The two ancient molecules acetylcholine and HMGB1 have during evolution formed a functional yin-yang relationship. Homeostasis in inflammation is obtained when the functional influences mediated by HMGB1 and acetylcholine are in balance. Therapeutic results in preclinical studies using vagus nerve stimulation, choline esterase inhibitors, or $\alpha 7$-nicotinic acetylcholine receptor ($\alpha 7$nAChR) agonists are strikingly similar to those seen after HMGB1-specific blocking treatment regarding kinetics and final outcome [3,111–114]. Acetylcholine inhibits HMGB1 release [102,103,105–107,115–117], TLR4/MyD88/NF-κB signaling [118], and RAGE-mediated endocytosis of HMGB1 and HMGB1 complex-bound to DAMPs or PAMPs [60]. Each one of these inhibitory accomplishments is beneficial for controlling HMGB1-mediated inflammation. SIRT1 functions were enhanced by $\alpha 7$nAChR-specific agonist stimulation and inhibited by an $\alpha 7$nAChR- specific antagonists supporting a role for $\alpha 7$nAChR signaling to mediate increased SIRT1 activity inhibiting HMGB1 release [119]. Furthermore, electroacupuncture pretreatment using a specific acupoint termed ST36 attenuated acute lung injury through $\alpha 7$nAChR-mediated inhibition of HMGB1 release in rats after cardiopulmonary bypass [107]. It was recently demonstrated that low-intensity electroacupuncture stimulation of the ST36 acupoint excited PROKR2-expressing sensory neurons to activate the cholinergic anti-inflammatory system [116].

Enhancing nuclear HMGB1 deacetylation to inhibit the nucleocytoplasmic translocation and subsequent extracellular release may thus offer a promising treatment for HMGB1-mediated inflammation. This insight should encourage further clinical studies using non-invasive transcutaneous auricular vagus nerve stimulation or electroacupuncture stimulation at carefully selected acupoints to treat uncontrolled HMGB1-triggered inflammation and neuropathic pain [101,120]. These $\alpha 7$nAChR-mediated therapeutic means augment SIRT1 function and thus inhibit HMGB1 release and subsequent inflammation. It is thus conceivable that HMGB1 antagonists and cholinergic anti-inflammatory activation generate almost interchangeable results in preclinical treatment studies since acetylcholine inhibits extracellular HMGB1 release.

7. Key Challenges in the HMGB1 Field

Even though extracellular HMGB1 has been intensely studied for more than two decades there are basic methodological shortcomings that need urgent attention. We need improved methods to quantify extracellular levels of HMGB1 isoforms in clinical samples. The problem of steric hindrance generated by molecules complex-bound to HMGB1 in vivo has here been exemplified in the context of COVID-19, SLE, and septic shock and must be resolved via the invention of improved tools for diagnostic and therapeutic purposes. There are presently no existing methods to quantify HMGB1 redox isoforms or other posttranslational modifications. These obstacles severely delay a further exploration of the fascinating and important biology created by extracellular HMGB1.

Despite numerous successful preclinical therapeutic studies with HMGB1 antagonists in inflammation and pain conditions there is still no clinically approved treatment targeting HMGB1 specifically, which is both disappointing and inspiring. The HMGB1 protein expresses 99% identity among mammals, which should facilitate the process, while on the other hand molecules attached to the extracellular HMGB1 complicate the development of HMGB1-binding antagonists, especially when HMGB1-RAGE endocytosis needs to be targeted. One academic research group in Japan has generated an anti-HMGB1 mAb recognizing the repetitive C-terminal part of the molecule, which conceivably might be an element less engaged by partner molecules in vivo [89,121–132]. This antibody has exhibited impressive therapeutic efficacy in many animal models of neuroinflammation both in the central nervous system and in the periphery, most of which events are TLR4-dependent. Another Japanese research group recently reported a successful creation of an HMGB1-specific mAb blocking the HMGB1 sequence engaged in MD-2/TLR4 interaction. This antibody impeded HMGB1-mediated TLR4-dependent biological effects in vitro and exerted beneficial therapeutic effects in a preclinical model of Alzheimer´s disease [91]. These are indeed encouraging examples to guide and inspire further clinical development of HMGB1-targeted therapy.

Author Contributions: U.A., K.J.T. and H.Y. wrote the draft manuscript and designed the figures together. All authors have read and agreed to the published version of the manuscript.

Funding: This work was supported by grants to U.A. from the Freemason Lodge Barnhuset in Stockholm.

Institutional Review Board Statement: The study presented in Figure 9 was conducted according to the guidelines of the Declaration of Helsinki, and approved by the Swedish Ethical Review Authority (protocol code 2020-01653; approval date 8 April 2020).

Informed Consent Statement: Informed consent was obtained from all subjects involved in the study presented in Figure 9A,B.

Data Availability Statement: Raw data available upon request to corresponding author.

Conflicts of Interest: The authors declare no conflict of interest.

Abbreviations

HMGB1	high mobility group box 1 protein
RAGE	receptor for advanced glycation end-product
TLR4	toll-like receptor 4
MD-2	myeloid differentiation factor 2
TIRAP	TIR domain containing adaptor protein
TRAM	toll-receptor-associated molecule
MyD88	myeloid differentiation primary response 88
TRIF	TIR-domain-containing adapter-inducing interferon-β
CXCL12	C-X-C Motif Chemokine Ligand 12
CXCR4	C-X-C chemokine receptor type 4
NF-κB	nuclear factor kappa-light-chain-enhancer of activated B cells
LPS	lipopolysaccharide
DAMP	damage-associated molecular pattern molecule
PAMP	pathogen-associated molecular pattern molecule
HDAC	histone-deacetylase
HAT	histone-acetylase
SIRT1	sirtuin 1
CRMI	nuclear exportin chromosome-region maintenance 1
NLS	nuclear localization site

SHP-1	Src homology 2 domain-containing protein tyrosine phosphatase 1
a7nAChR	a7-nicotinic acetylcholine receptor
MDSC	myeloid-derived suppressor cells
Treg cell	regulatory T lymphocyte
M1 macrophage	proinflammatory macrophage
M2 macrophage	anti-inflammatory macrophage
Syn-Cre/HMGB1$^{fl/fl}$ mice	neuronally HMGB1 gene-deficient mice
CD24	cluster of differentiation 24
Siglec-10	Sialic acid-binding Ig-like lectin 10

References

1. Kang, R.; Chen, R.; Zhang, Q.; Hou, W.; Wu, S.; Cao, L.; Huang, J.; Yu, Y.; Fan, X.-G.; Yan, Z.; et al. HMGB1 in health and disease. *Mol. Asp. Med.* **2014**, *40*, 1–116. [CrossRef] [PubMed]
2. Oppenheim, J.J.; Yang, D. Alarmins: Chemotactic activators of immune responses. *Curr. Opin. Immunol.* **2005**, *17*, 359–365. [CrossRef] [PubMed]
3. Andersson, U.; Tracey, K.J. HMGB1 Is a Therapeutic Target for Sterile Inflammation and Infection. *Annu. Rev. Immunol.* **2011**, *29*, 139–162. [CrossRef]
4. Andersson, U.; Yang, H.; Harris, H. High-mobility group box 1 protein (HMGB1) operates as an alarmin outside as well as inside cells. *Semin. Immunol.* **2018**, *38*, 40–48. [CrossRef]
5. Kwak, M.S.; Rhee, W.J.; Lee, Y.J.; Kim, H.S.; Kim, Y.H.; Kwon, M.K.; Shin, J.-S. Reactive oxygen species induce Cys106-mediated anti-parallel HMGB1 dimerization that protects against DNA damage. *Redox Biol.* **2021**, *40*, 101858. [CrossRef]
6. Lu, B.; Nakamura, T.; Inouye, K.; Li, J.; Tang, Y.; Lundbäck, P.; Valdés-Ferrer, S.I.; Olofsson, P.S.; Kalb, T.; Roth, J.; et al. Novel role of PKR in inflammasome activation and HMGB1 release. *Nature* **2012**, *488*, 670–674. [CrossRef] [PubMed]
7. Bonaldi, T.; Talamo, F.; Scaffidi, P.; Ferrera, D.; Porto, A.; Bachi, A.; Rubartelli, A.; Agresti, A.; Bianchi, M.E. Monocytic cells hyperacetylate chromatin protein HMGB1 to redirect it towards secretion. *EMBO J.* **2003**, *22*, 5551–5560. [CrossRef]
8. Evankovich, J.; Cho, S.W.; Zhang, R.; Cardinal, J.; Dhupar, R.; Zhang, L.; Klune, J.R.; Zlotnicki, J.; Billiar, T.; Tsung, A. High Mobility Group Box 1 Release from Hepatocytes during Ischemia and Reperfusion Injury Is Mediated by Decreased Histone Deacetylase Activity. *J. Biol. Chem.* **2010**, *285*, 39888–39897. [CrossRef]
9. Zou, J.Y.; Crews, F.T. Release of Neuronal HMGB1 by Ethanol through Decreased HDAC Activity Activates Brain Neuroimmune Signaling. *PLoS ONE* **2014**, *9*, e87915. [CrossRef]
10. Hwang, J.S.; Choi, H.S.; Ham, S.A.; Yoo, T.; Lee, W.J.; Paek, K.S.; Seo, H.G. Deacetylation-mediated interaction of SIRT1-HMGB1 improves survival in a mouse model of endotoxemia. *Sci. Rep.* **2015**, *5*, 15791. [CrossRef]
11. Zhao, P.; Xu, S.; Huang, Z.; Jiang, G.; Deng, P.; Zhang, Y. Hyperbaric Oxygen via Mediating SIRT1-Induced Deacetylation of HMGB1 Improved Cerebral Ischemia/Reperfusion injury. *Eur. J. Neurosci.* **2021**, *54*, 7318–7331. [CrossRef]
12. Karkischenko, V.N.; Skvortsova, V.I.; Gasanov, M.T.; Fokin, Y.V.; Nesterov, M.S.; Petrova, N.V.; Alimkina, O.V.; Pomytkin, I.A. Inhaled [D-Ala2]-Dynorphin 1-6 Prevents Hyperacetylation and Release of High Mobility Group Box 1 in a Mouse Model of Acute Lung Injury. *J. Immunol. Res.* **2021**, *2021*, 1–10. [CrossRef] [PubMed]
13. Le, K.; Daliv, E.C.; Wu, S.; Qian, F.; Ali, A.I.; Yu, D.; Guo, Y. SIRT1-regulated HMGB1 release is partially involved in TLR4 signal transduction: A possible anti-neuroinflammatory mechanism of resveratrol in neonatal hypoxic-ischemic brain injury. *Int. Immunopharmacol.* **2019**, *75*, 105779. [CrossRef]
14. Rabadi, M.M.; Xavier, S.; Vasko, R.; Kaur, K.; Goligorksy, M.S.; Ratliff, B.B. High-mobility group box 1 is a novel deacetylation target of Sirtuin1. *Kidney Int.* **2015**, *87*, 95–108. [CrossRef] [PubMed]
15. Xu, S.; Zeng, Z.; Zhao, M.; Huang, Q.; Gao, Y.; Dai, X.; Lu, J.; Huang, W.; Zhao, K. Evidence for SIRT1 Mediated HMGB1 Release from Kidney Cells in the Early Stages of Hemorrhagic Shock. *Front. Physiol.* **2019**, *10*. [CrossRef] [PubMed]
16. Feng, X.; Chen, W.; Ni, X.; Little, P.J.; Xu, S.; Tang, L.; Weng, J. Metformin, Macrophage Dysfunction and Atherosclerosis. *Front. Immunol.* **2021**, *12*, 682853. [CrossRef] [PubMed]
17. Yu, S.; Zhou, X.; Xiang, H.; Wang, S.; Cui, Z.; Zhou, J. Resveratrol Reduced Liver Damage After Liver Resection in a Rat Model by Upregulating Sirtuin 1 (SIRT1) and Inhibiting the Acetylation of High Mobility Group Box 1 (HMGB1). *Med Sci. Monit.* **2019**, *25*, 3212–3220. [CrossRef] [PubMed]
18. Yin, Y.; Wu, X.; Peng, B.; Zou, H.; Li, S.; Wang, J.; Cao, J. Curcumin improves necrotising microscopic colitis and cell pyroptosis by activating SIRT1/NRF2 and inhibiting the TLR4 signalling pathway in newborn rats. *Innate Immun.* **2020**, *26*, 609–617. [CrossRef] [PubMed]
19. Guarente, L. Sirtuins, Aging, and Medicine. *N. Engl. J. Med.* **2011**, *364*, 2235–2244. [CrossRef] [PubMed]
20. Dobbin, M.M.; Madabhushi, R.; Pan, L.; Chen, Y.; Kim, D.; Gao, J.; Ahanonu, B.; Pao, P.-C.; Qiu, Y.; Zhao, Y.; et al. SIRT1 collaborates with ATM and HDAC1 to maintain genomic stability in neurons. *Nat. Neurosci.* **2013**, *16*, 1008–1015. [CrossRef]
21. Hubbard, B.P.; Sinclair, D.A. Small molecule SIRT1 activators for the treatment of aging and age-related diseases. *Trends Pharmacol. Sci.* **2014**, *35*, 146–154. [CrossRef] [PubMed]

22. Sixto-López, Y.; Rosales-Hernández, M.C.; De Oca, A.C.-M.; Fragoso-Morales, L.G.; Mendieta-Wejebe, J.E.; Correa-Basurto, A.M.; Abarca-Rojano, E.; Correa-Basurto, J. N-(2′-Hydroxyphenyl)-2-Propylpentanamide (HO-AAVPA) Inhibits HDAC1 and Increases the Translocation of HMGB1 Levels in Human Cervical Cancer Cells. *Int. J. Mol. Sci.* **2020**, *21*, 5873. [CrossRef]
23. Kwak, M.S.; Kim, H.S.; Lee, B.; Kim, Y.H.; Son, M.; Shin, J.-S. Immunological Significance of HMGB1 Post-Translational Modification and Redox Biology. *Front. Immunol.* **2020**, *11*. [CrossRef] [PubMed]
24. Gardella, S.; Andrei, C.; Ferrera, D.; Lotti, L.V.; Torrisi, M.R.; Bianchi, M.E.; Rubartelli, A. The nuclear protein HMGB1 is secreted by monocytes via a non-classical, vesicle-mediated secretory pathway. *EMBO Rep.* **2002**, *3*, 995–1001. [CrossRef] [PubMed]
25. Mobarrez, F.; Vikerfors, A.; Gustafsson, J.T.; Gunnarsson, I.; Zickert, A.; Larsson, A.; Pisetsky, D.S.; Wallén, H.; Svenungsson, E. Microparticles in the blood of patients with systemic lupus erythematosus (SLE): Phenotypic characterization and clinical associations. *Sci. Rep.* **2016**, *6*, 36025. [CrossRef] [PubMed]
26. Pisetsky, D.S.; Gauley, J.; Ullal, A. HMGB1 and Microparticles as Mediators of the Immune Response to Cell Death. *Antioxidants Redox Signal.* **2011**, *15*, 2209–2219. [CrossRef]
27. Vogel, S.; Bodenstein, R.; Chen, Q.; Feil, S.; Feil, R.; Rheinlaender, J.; Schäffer, T.; Bohn, E.; Frick, J.-S.; Borst, O.; et al. Platelet-derived HMGB1 is a critical mediator of thrombosis. *J. Clin. Investig.* **2015**, *125*, 4638–4654. [CrossRef]
28. Stark, K.; Philippi, V.; Stockhausen, S.; Busse, J.; Antonelli, A.; Miller, M.; Schubert, I.; Hoseinpour, P.; Chandraratne, S.; Von Brühl, M.-L.; et al. Disulfide HMGB1 derived from platelets coordinates venous thrombosis in mice. *Blood* **2016**, *128*, 2435–2449. [CrossRef]
29. Maugeri, N.; Capobianco, A.; Rovere-Querini, P.; Ramirez, G.A.; Tombetti, E.; Della Valle, P.; Monno, A.; D'Alberti, V.; Gasparri, A.M.; Franchini, S.; et al. Platelet microparticles sustain autophagy-associated activation of neutrophils in systemic sclerosis. *Sci. Transl. Med.* **2018**, *10*, eaao3089. [CrossRef]
30. Lamkanfi, M.; Sarkar, A.; Walle, L.V.; Vitari, A.C.; Amer, A.O.; Wewers, M.D.; Tracey, K.J.; Kanneganti, T.-D.; Dixit, V.M. Inflammasome-Dependent Release of the Alarmin HMGB1 in Endotoxemia. *J. Immunol.* **2010**, *185*, 4385–4392. [CrossRef] [PubMed]
31. Lu, B.; Wang, H.; Andersson, U.; Tracey, K.J. Regulation of HMGB1 release by inflammasomes. *Protein Cell* **2013**, *4*, 163–167. [CrossRef]
32. Deng, M.; Scott, M.J.; Fan, J.; Billiar, T.R. Location is the key to function: HMGB1 in sepsis and trauma-induced inflammation. *J. Leukoc. Biol.* **2019**, *106*, 161–169. [CrossRef] [PubMed]
33. Li, W.; Deng, M.; Loughran, P.A.; Yang, M.; Lin, M.; Yang, C.; Gao, W.; Jin, S.; Li, S.; Cai, J.; et al. LPS Induces Active HMGB1 Release from Hepatocytes Into Exosomes Through the Coordinated Activities of TLR4 and Caspase-11/GSDMD Signaling. *Front. Immunol.* **2020**, *11*, 229. [CrossRef] [PubMed]
34. Deng, M.; Tang, Y.; Li, W.; Wang, X.; Zhang, R.; Zhang, X.; Zhao, X.; Liu, J.; Tang, C.; Liu, Z.; et al. The Endotoxin Delivery Protein HMGB1 Mediates Caspase-11-Dependent Lethality in Sepsis. *Immunity* **2018**, *49*, 740–753.e7. [CrossRef] [PubMed]
35. Yang, H.; Zeng, Q.; Silverman, H.A.; Gunasekaran, M.; George, S.J.; Devarajan, A.; Addorisio, M.E.; Li, J.; Tsaava, T.; Shah, V.; et al. HMGB1 released from nociceptors mediates inflammation. *Proc. Natl. Acad. Sci. USA* **2021**, *118*. [CrossRef]
36. Cheng, X.; Yang, Y.-L.; Yang, H.; Wang, Y.-H.; Du, G.-H. Kaempferol alleviates LPS-induced neuroinflammation and BBB dysfunction in mice via inhibiting HMGB1 release and down-regulating TLR4/MyD88 pathway. *Int. Immunopharmacol.* **2018**, *56*, 29–35. [CrossRef] [PubMed]
37. Guo, X.; Shi, Y.; Du, P.; Wang, J.; Han, Y.; Sun, B.; Feng, J. HMGB1/TLR4 promotes apoptosis and reduces autophagy of hippocampal neurons in diabetes combined with OSA. *Life Sci.* **2019**, *239*, 117020. [CrossRef] [PubMed]
38. Laird, M.D.; Shields, J.S.; Sukumari-Ramesh, S.; Kimbler, D.E.; Fessler, R.D.; Shakir, B.; Youssef, P.; Yanasak, N.; Vender, J.R.; Dhandapani, K.M. High mobility group box protein-1 promotes cerebral edema after traumatic brain injury via activation of toll-like receptor 4. *Glia* **2013**, *62*, 26–38. [CrossRef] [PubMed]
39. Li, Y.; Zhang, L.; Tang, J.; Yang, X.; Huang, J.; Zhu, T.; Zhao, F.; Li, S.; Li, X.; Qu, Y.; et al. Role of toll-like receptor 4 in the regulation of the cell death pathway and neuroinflammation. *Brain Res. Bull.* **2019**, *148*, 79–90. [CrossRef]
40. Oladiran, O.; Shi, X.Q.; Yang, M.; Fournier, S.; Zhang, J. Inhibition of TLR4 signaling protects mice from sensory and motor dysfunction in an animal model of autoimmune peripheral neuropathy. *J. Neuroinflamm.* **2021**, *18*, 1–17. [CrossRef]
41. Paudel, Y.N.; Khan, S.U.; Othman, I.; Shaikh, M.F. Naturally Occurring HMGB1 Inhibitor, Glycyrrhizin, Modulates Chronic Seizures-Induced Memory Dysfunction in Zebrafish Model. *ACS Chem. Neurosci.* **2021**, *12*, 3288–3302. [CrossRef]
42. Paudel, Y.N.; Othman, I.; Shaikh, M.F. Anti-High Mobility Group Box-1 Monoclonal Antibody Attenuates Seizure-Induced Cognitive Decline by Suppressing Neuroinflammation in an Adult Zebrafish Model. *Front. Pharmacol.* **2021**, *11*. [CrossRef] [PubMed]
43. Paudel, Y.N.; Shaikh, M.F.; Chakraborti, A.; Kumari, Y.; Aledo-Serrano, A.; Aleksovska, K.; Alvim, M.K.M.; Othman, I. HMGB1: A Common Biomarker and Potential Target for TBI, Neuroinflammation, Epilepsy, and Cognitive Dysfunction. *Front. Neurosci.* **2018**, *12*, 628. [CrossRef]
44. Su, W.; Cui, H.; Wu, D.; Yu, J.; Ma, L.; Zhang, X.; Huang, Y.; Ma, C. Suppression of TLR4-MyD88 signaling pathway attenuated chronic mechanical pain in a rat model of endometriosis. *J. Neuroinflamm.* **2021**, *18*, 1–17. [CrossRef]
45. Sun, X.; Zeng, H.; Wang, Q.; Yu, Q.; Wu, J.; Feng, Y.; Deng, P.; Zhang, H. Glycyrrhizin ameliorates inflammatory pain by inhibiting microglial activation-mediated inflammatory response via blockage of the HMGB1-TLR4-NF-kB pathway. *Exp. Cell Res.* **2018**, *369*, 112–119. [CrossRef]

46. Fujita, K.; Motoki, K.; Tagawa, K.; Chen, X.; Hama, H.; Nakajima, K.; Homma, H.; Tamura, T.; Watanabe, H.; Katsuno, M.; et al. HMGB1, a pathogenic molecule that induces neurite degeneration via TLR4-MARCKS, is a potential therapeutic target for Alzheimer's disease. *Sci. Rep.* **2016**, *6*, 31895. [CrossRef] [PubMed]
47. Kong, Z.-H.; Chen, X.; Hua, H.-P.; Liang, L.; Liu, L.-J. The Oral Pretreatment of Glycyrrhizin Prevents Surgery-Induced Cognitive Impairment in Aged Mice by Reducing Neuroinflammation and Alzheimer's-Related Pathology via HMGB1 Inhibition. *J. Mol. Neurosci.* **2017**, *63*, 385–395. [CrossRef] [PubMed]
48. Yang, H.; Wang, H.; Ju, Z.; Ragab, A.A.; Lundbäck, P.; Long, W.; Valdés-Ferrer, S.I.; He, M.; Pribis, J.P.; Li, J.; et al. MD-2 is required for disulfide HMGB1-dependent TLR4 signaling. *J. Exp. Med.* **2015**, *212*, 5–14. [CrossRef] [PubMed]
49. Schiraldi, M.; Raucci, A.; Muñoz, L.M.; Livoti, E.; Celona, B.; Venereau, E.; Apuzzo, T.; De Marchis, F.; Pedotti, M.; Bachi, A.; et al. HMGB1 promotes recruitment of inflammatory cells to damaged tissues by forming a complex with CXCL12 and signaling via CXCR4. *J. Exp. Med.* **2012**, *209*, 551–563. [CrossRef]
50. Venereau, E.; Casalgrandi, M.; Schiraldi, M.; Antoine, D.J.; Cattaneo, A.; De Marchis, F.; Liu, J.; Antonelli, A.; Preti, A.; Raeli, L.; et al. Mutually exclusive redox forms of HMGB1 promote cell recruitment or proinflammatory cytokine release. *J. Exp. Med.* **2012**, *209*, 1519–1528. [CrossRef] [PubMed]
51. Bianchi, M.E.; Crippa, M.P.; Manfredi, A.A.; Mezzapelle, R.; Querini, P.R.; Venereau, E. High-mobility group box 1 protein orchestrates responses to tissue damage via inflammation, innate and adaptive immunity, and tissue repair. *Immunol. Rev.* **2017**, *280*, 74–82. [CrossRef]
52. Yang, H.; Wang, H.; Chavan, S.S.; Andersson, U. High Mobility Group Box Protein 1 (HMGB1): The Prototypical Endogenous Danger Molecule. *Mol. Med.* **2015**, *21*, S6–S12. [CrossRef] [PubMed]
53. Yang, H.; Hreggvidsdottir, H.S.; Palmblad, K.; Wang, H.; Ochani, M.; Li, J.; Lu, B.; Chavan, S.; Rosas-Ballina, M.; Al-Abed, Y.; et al. A critical cysteine is required for HMGB1 binding to Toll-like receptor 4 and activation of macrophage cytokine release. *Proc. Natl. Acad. Sci. USA* **2010**, *107*, 11942–11947. [CrossRef] [PubMed]
54. Bierhaus, A.; Humpert, P.M.; Morcos, M.; Wendt, T.; Chavakis, T.; Arnold, B.; Stern, D.M.; Nawroth, P.P. Understanding RAGE, the receptor for advanced glycation end products. *J. Mol. Med.* **2005**, *83*, 876–886. [CrossRef]
55. Kierdorf, K.; Fritz, G. RAGE regulation and signaling in inflammation and beyond. *J. Leukoc. Biol.* **2013**, *94*, 55–68. [CrossRef] [PubMed]
56. Merenmies, J.; Pihlaskari, R.; Laitinen, J.; Wartiovaara, J.; Rauvala, H. 30-kDa heparin-binding protein of brain (amphoterin) involved in neurite outgrowth. Amino acid sequence and localization in the filopodia of the advancing plasma membrane. *J. Biol. Chem.* **1991**, *266*, 16722–16729. [CrossRef]
57. LeBlanc, P.M.; Doggett, T.A.; Choi, J.; Hancock, M.A.; Durocher, Y.; Frank, F.; Nagar, B.; Ferguson, T.A.; Saleh, M. An Immunogenic Peptide in the A-box of HMGB1 Protein Reverses Apoptosis-induced Tolerance through RAGE Receptor. *J. Biol. Chem.* **2014**, *289*, 7777–7786. [CrossRef] [PubMed]
58. Bianchi, M.E. HMGB1 loves company. *J. Leukoc. Biol.* **2009**, *86*, 573–576. [CrossRef] [PubMed]
59. Xu, J.; Jiang, Y.; Wang, J.; Shi, X.; Liu, Q.; Liu, Z.; Li, Y.; Scott, M.J.; Xiao, G.; Li, S.; et al. Macrophage endocytosis of high-mobility group box 1 triggers pyroptosis. *Cell Death Differ.* **2014**, *21*, 1229–1239. [CrossRef] [PubMed]
60. Yang, H.; Liu, H.; Zeng, Q.; Imperato, G.H.; Addorisio, M.E.; Li, J.; He, M.; Cheng, K.F.; Al-Abed, Y.; Harris, H.E.; et al. Inhibition of HMGB1/RAGE-mediated endocytosis by HMGB1 antagonist box A, anti-HMGB1 antibodies, and cholinergic agonists suppresses inflammation. *Mol. Med.* **2019**, *25*, 1–13. [CrossRef]
61. Ling, Y.; Yang, Z.-Y.; Yin, T.; Li, L.; Yuan, W.-W.; Wu, H.-S.; Wang, C.-Y. Heparin changes the conformation of high-mobility group protein 1 and decreases its affinity toward receptor for advanced glycation endproducts in vitro. *Int. Immunopharmacol.* **2011**, *11*, 187–193. [CrossRef]
62. Porat, A.; Giat, E.; Kowal, C.; He, M.; Son, M.; Latz, E.; Ben-Zvi, I.; Al-Abed, Y.; Diamond, B. DNA-Mediated Interferon Signature Induction by SLE Serum Occurs in Monocytes Through Two Pathways: A Mechanism to Inhibit Both Pathways. *Front. Immunol.* **2018**, *9*. [CrossRef] [PubMed]
63. Lin, H.-J.; Jiang, Z.-P.; Lo, H.-R.; Feng, C.-L.; Chen, C.-J.; Yang, C.-Y.; Huang, M.-Z.; Wu, H.-Y.; Chen, Y.-A.; Chiu, C.-H.; et al. Coalescence of RAGE in Lipid Rafts in Response to Cytolethal Distending Toxin-Induced Inflammation. *Front. Immunol.* **2019**, *10*, 109. [CrossRef] [PubMed]
64. Jia, C.; Zhang, J.; Chen, H.; Zhuge, Y.; Chen, H.; Qian, F.; Zhou, K.; Niu, C.; Wang, F.; Qiu, H.; et al. Endothelial cell pyroptosis plays an important role in Kawasaki disease via HMGB1/RAGE/cathespin B signaling pathway and NLRP3 inflammasome activation. *Cell Death Dis.* **2019**, *10*, 1–16. [CrossRef] [PubMed]
65. De Mingo Pulido, Á.; Hänggi, K.; Celias, D.P.; Gardner, A.; Li, J.; Batista-Bittencourt, B.; Mohamed, E.; Trillo-Tinoco, J.; Osunmakinde, O.; Pena, R.; et al. The inhibitory receptor TIM-3 limits activation of the cGAS-STING pathway in intra-tumoral dendritic cells by suppressing extracellular DNA uptake. *Immunity* **2021**, *54*, 1154–1167.e7. [CrossRef] [PubMed]
66. Lu, J.; Yue, Y.; Xiong, S. Extracellular HMGB1 augments macrophage inflammation by facilitating the endosomal accumulation of ALD-DNA via TLR2/4-mediated endocytosis. *Biochim. Biophys. Acta Mol. Basis Dis.* **2021**, *1867*, 166184. [CrossRef] [PubMed]
67. Zhang, X.; Fernández-Hernando, C. Endothelial HMGB1 (High-Mobility Group Box 1) Regulation of LDL (Low-Density Lipoprotein) Transcytosis: A Novel Mechanism of Intracellular HMGB1 in Atherosclerosis. *Arterioscler. Thromb. Vasc. Biol.* **2020**, *41*, 217–219. [PubMed]

68. Lan, J.; Luo, H.; Wu, R.; Wang, J.; Zhou, B.; Zhang, Y.; Jiang, Y.; Xu, J. Internalization of HMGB1 (High Mobility Group Box 1) Promotes Angiogenesis in Endothelial Cells. *Arter. Thromb. Vasc. Biol.* **2020**, *40*, 2922–2940. [CrossRef]
69. Liu, L.; Yang, M.; Kang, R.; Dai, Y.; Yu, Y.; Gao, F.; Wang, H.; Sun, X.; Li, X.; Li, J.; et al. HMGB1–DNA complex-induced autophagy limits AIM2 inflammasome activation through RAGE. *Biochem. Biophys. Res. Commun.* **2014**, *450*, 851–856. [CrossRef] [PubMed]
70. Rouhiainen, A.; Nykänen, N.-P.; Kuja-Panula, J.; Vanttola, P.; Huttunen, H.J.; Rauvala, H. Inhibition of Homophilic Interactions and Ligand Binding of the Receptor for Advanced Glycation End Products by Heparin and Heparin-Related Carbohydrate Structures. *Medicines* **2018**, *5*, 79. [CrossRef] [PubMed]
71. Tan, S.-W.; Zhao, Y.; Li, P.; Ning, Y.-L.; Huang, Z.-Z.; Yang, N.; Liu, D.; Zhou, Y.-G. HMGB1 mediates cognitive impairment caused by the NLRP3 inflammasome in the late stage of traumatic brain injury. *J. Neuroinflamm.* **2021**, *18*, 1–16. [CrossRef] [PubMed]
72. Yang, X.; Cheng, X.; Tang, Y.; Qiu, X.; Wang, Z.; Fu, G.; Wu, J.; Kang, H.; Wang, J.; Wang, H.; et al. The role of type 1 interferons in coagulation induced by gram-negative bacteria. *Blood* **2020**, *135*, 1087–1100. [CrossRef] [PubMed]
73. Tang, Y.; Wang, X.; Li, Z.; He, Z.; Yang, X.; Cheng, X.; Peng, Y.; Xue, Q.; Bai, Y.; Zhang, R.; et al. Heparin prevents caspase-11-dependent septic lethality independent of anticoagulant properties. *Immunity* **2021**, *54*, 454–467.e6. [CrossRef] [PubMed]
74. Yang, X.; Cheng, X.; Tang, Y.; Qiu, X.; Wang, Y.; Kang, H.; Wu, J.; Wang, Z.; Liu, Y.; Chen, F.; et al. Bacterial Endotoxin Activates the Coagulation Cascade through Gasdermin D-Dependent Phosphatidylserine Exposure. *Immunity* **2019**, *51*, 983–996.e6. [CrossRef] [PubMed]
75. Hagar, J.A.; Powell, D.A.; Aachoui, Y.; Ernst, R.K.; Miao, E.A. Cytoplasmic LPS Activates Caspase-11: Implications in TLR4-Independent Endotoxic Shock. *Science* **2013**, *341*, 1250–1253. [CrossRef]
76. Kayagaki, N.; Wong, M.T.; Stowe, I.B.; Ramani, S.R.; Gonzalez, L.C.; Akashi-Takamura, S.; Miyake, K.; Zhang, J.; Lee, W.P.; Muszyński, A.; et al. Noncanonical Inflammasome Activation by Intracellular LPS Independent of TLR4. *Science* **2013**, *341*, 1246–1249. [CrossRef] [PubMed]
77. Hubert, P.; Roncarati, P.; Demoulin, S.; Pilard, C.; Ancion, M.; Reynders, C.; Lerho, T.; Bruyere, D.; Lebeau, A.; Radermecker, C.; et al. Extracellular HMGB1 blockade inhibits tumor growth through profoundly remodeling immune microenvironment and enhances checkpoint inhibitor-based immunotherapy. *J. Immunother. Cancer* **2021**, *9*, e001966. [CrossRef]
78. Chen, G.-Y.; Tang, J.; Zheng, P.; Liu, Y. CD24 and Siglec-10 Selectively Repress Tissue Damage–Induced Immune Responses. *Science* **2009**, *323*, 1722–1725. [CrossRef]
79. Tian, R.-R.; Zhang, M.-X.; Liu, M.; Fang, X.; Li, D.; Zhang, L.; Zheng, P.; Zheng, Y.-T.; Liu, Y. CD24Fc protects against viral pneumonia in simian immunodeficiency virus-infected Chinese rhesus monkeys. *Cell. Mol. Immunol.* **2020**, *17*, 887–888. [CrossRef]
80. Tian, R.-R.; Zhang, M.-X.; Zhang, L.-T.; Zhang, P.; Ma, J.-P.; Liu, M.; Devenport, M.; Zheng, P.; Zhang, X.-L.; Lian, X.-D.; et al. CD24 and Fc fusion protein protects SIVmac239-infected Chinese rhesus macaque against progression to AIDS. *Antivir. Res.* **2018**, *157*, 9–17. [CrossRef]
81. Toubai, T.; Rossi, C.; Oravecz-Wilson, K.; Zajac, C.; Liu, C.; Braun, T.; Fujiwara, H.; Wu, J.; Sun, Y.; Brabbs, S.; et al. Siglec-G represses DAMP-mediated effects on T cells. *JCI Insight* **2017**, *2*. [CrossRef]
82. Song, N.J.; Allen, C.; Vilgelm, A.E.; Riesenberg, B.P.; Weller, K.P.; Reynolds, K.; Chakravarthy, K.B.; Kumar, A.; Khatiwada, A.; Sun, Z.; et al. Immunological Insights into the Therapeutic Roles of CD24Fc Against Severe COVID-19. *medRxiv* **2021**, *8*, 21262258.
83. Agalave, N.M.; Larsson, M.; Abdelmoaty, S.; Su, J.; Baharpoor, A.; Lundbäck, P.; Palmblad, K.; Andersson, U.; Harris, H.; Svensson, C.I. Spinal HMGB1 induces TLR4-mediated long-lasting hypersensitivity and glial activation and regulates pain-like behavior in experimental arthritis. *Pain* **2014**, *155*, 1802–1813. [CrossRef]
84. Rudjito, R.; Agalave, N.M.; Farinotti, A.B.; Lundbäck, P.; Szabo-Pardi, T.A.; Price, T.J.; Harris, H.E.; Burton, M.D.; Svensson, C.I. Sex- and cell-dependent contribution of peripheral high mobility group box 1 and TLR4 in arthritis-induced pain. *Pain* **2020**, *162*, 459–470. [CrossRef] [PubMed]
85. Frank, M.G.; Weber, M.D.; Watkins, L.R.; Maier, S.F. Stress sounds the alarmin: The role of the danger-associated molecular pattern HMGB1 in stress-induced neuroinflammatory priming. *Brain Behav. Immun.* **2015**, *48*, 1–7. [CrossRef] [PubMed]
86. Grace, P.M.; Strand, K.A.; Galer, E.L.; Rice, K.C.; Maier, S.F.; Watkins, L.R. Protraction of neuropathic pain by morphine is mediated by spinal damage associated molecular patterns (DAMPs) in male rats. *Brain Behav. Immun.* **2017**, *72*, 45–50. [CrossRef]
87. Yang, H.; Andersson, U.; Brines, M. Neurons Are a Primary Driver of Inflammation via Release of HMGB1. *Cells* **2021**, *10*, 2791. [CrossRef] [PubMed]
88. Sun, Y.; Chen, H.; Dai, J.; Wan, Z.; Xiong, P.; Xu, Y.; Han, Z.; Chai, W.; Gong, F.; Zheng, F. Glycyrrhizin Protects Mice Against Experimental Autoimmune Encephalomyelitis by Inhibiting High-Mobility Group Box 1 (HMGB1) Expression and Neuronal HMGB1 Release. *Front. Immunol.* **2018**, *9*, 1518. [CrossRef] [PubMed]
89. Sasaki, T.; Liu, K.; Agari, T.; Yasuhara, T.; Morimoto, J.; Okazaki, M.; Takeuchi, H.; Toyoshima, A.; Sasada, S.; Shinko, A.; et al. Anti-high mobility group box 1 antibody exerts neuroprotection in a rat model of Parkinson's disease. *Exp. Neurol.* **2016**, *275*, 220–231. [CrossRef]
90. Tanaka, A.; Ito, T.; Kibata, K.; Inagaki-Katashiba, N.; Amuro, H.; Nishizawa, T.; Son, Y.; Ozaki, Y.; Nomura, S. Serum high-mobility group box 1 is correlated with interferon-α and may predict disease activity in patients with systemic lupus erythematosus. *Lupus* **2019**, *28*, 1120–1127. [CrossRef]
91. Tanaka, H.; Kondo, K.; Fujita, K.; Homma, H.; Tagawa, K.; Jin, X.; Jin, M.; Yoshioka, Y.; Takayama, S.; Masuda, H.; et al. HMGB1 signaling phosphorylates Ku70 and impairs DNA damage repair in Alzheimer's disease pathology. *Commun. Biol.* **2021**, *4*, 1–23. [CrossRef] [PubMed]

92. Bolay, H.; Karadas, O.; Öztürk, B.; Sonkaya, R.; Tasdelen, B.; Bulut, T.D.S.; Gülbahar, O.; Özge, A.; Baykan, B. HMGB1, NLRP3, IL-6 and ACE2 levels are elevated in COVID-19 with headache: A window to the infection-related headache mechanism. *J. Headache Pain* **2021**, *22*, 1–12. [CrossRef]
93. Chen, L.; Long, X.; Xu, Q.; Tan, J.; Wang, G.; Cao, Y.; Wei, J.; Luo, H.; Zhu, H.; Huang, L.; et al. Elevated serum levels of S100A8/A9 and HMGB1 at hospital admission are correlated with inferior clinical outcomes in COVID-19 patients. *Cell. Mol. Immunol.* **2020**, *17*, 992–994. [CrossRef] [PubMed]
94. Chen, R.; Huang, Y.; Quan, J.; Liu, J.; Wang, H.; Billiar, T.R.; Lotze, M.T.; Zeh, H.J.; Kang, R.; Tang, D. HMGB1 as a potential biomarker and therapeutic target for severe COVID-19. *Heliyon* **2020**, *6*, e05672. [CrossRef] [PubMed]
95. Sivakorn, C.; Dechsanga, J.; Jamjumrus, L.; Boonnak, K.; Schultz, M.J.; Dorndorp, A.M.; Phumratanaprapin, W.; Ratanarat, R.; Naorungroj, T.; Wattanawinitchai, P.; et al. High Mobility Group Box 1 and Interleukin 6 at Intensive Care Unit Admission as Biomarkers in Critically Ill COVID-19 Patients. *Am. J. Trop. Med. Hyg.* **2021**, *105*, 73–80. [CrossRef]
96. Barnay-Verdier, S.; Gaillard, C.; Messmer, M.; Borde, C.; Gibot, S.; Maréchal, V. PCA-ELISA: A sensitive method to quantify free and masked forms of HMGB1. *Cytokine* **2011**, *55*, 4–7. [CrossRef] [PubMed]
97. Abdulahad, D.A.; Westra, J.; Bijzet, J.; Limburg, P.C.; Kallenberg, C.G.; Bijl, M. High mobility group box 1 (HMGB1) and anti-HMGB1 antibodies and their relation to disease characteristics in systemic lupus erythematosus. *Arthritis Res. Ther.* **2011**, *13*, R71–R79. [CrossRef] [PubMed]
98. Cai, B.; Chen, F.; Ji, Y.; Kiss, L.; de Jonge, W.J.; Conejero-Goldberg, C.; Szabo, C.; Deitch, E.A.; Ulloa, L. Alpha7 cholinergic-agonist prevents systemic inflammation and improves survival during resuscitation. *J. Cell. Mol. Med.* **2008**, *13*, 3774–3785. [CrossRef] [PubMed]
99. Crews, F.T.; Fisher, R.; Deason, C.; Vetreno, R.P. Loss of Basal Forebrain Cholinergic Neurons Following Adolescent Binge Ethanol Exposure: Recovery with the Cholinesterase Inhibitor Galantamine. *Front. Behav. Neurosci.* **2021**, *15*, 652494. [CrossRef]
100. Hu, J.; Vacas, S.; Feng, X.; Lutrin, D.; Uchida, Y.; Lai, I.K.; Maze, M. Dexmedetomidine Prevents Cognitive Decline by Enhancing Resolution of High Mobility Group Box 1 Protein–induced Inflammation through a Vagomimetic Action in Mice. *Anesthesiology* **2018**, *128*, 921–931. [CrossRef]
101. Huston, J.M.; Gallowitsch-Puerta, M.; Ochani, M.; Ochani, K.; Yuan, R.; Rosas-Ballina, M.; Ashok, M.; Goldstein, R.S.; Chavan, S.; Pavlov, V.A.; et al. Transcutaneous vagus nerve stimulation reduces serum high mobility group box 1 levels and improves survival in murine sepsis. *Crit. Care Med.* **2007**, *35*, 2762–2768. [CrossRef] [PubMed]
102. Li, F.; Chen, Z.; Pan, Q.; Fu, S.; Lin, F.; Ren, H.; Han, H.; Billiar, T.R.; Sun, F.; Li, Q. The Protective Effect of PNU-282987, a Selective α7 Nicotinic Acetylcholine Receptor Agonist, on the Hepatic Ischemia-Reperfusion Injury Is Associated with the Inhibition of High-Mobility Group Box 1 Protein Expression and Nuclear Factor κB Activation in Mice. *Shock* **2013**, *39*, 197–203. [CrossRef]
103. Pavlov, V.A.; Ochani, M.; Yang, L.-H.; Gallowitsch-Puerta, M.; Ochani, K.; Lin, X.; Levi, J.; Parrish, W.R.; Rosas-Ballina, M.; Czura, C.J.; et al. Selective α7-nicotinic acetylcholine receptor agonist GTS-21 improves survival in murine endotoxemia and severe sepsis. *Crit. Care Med.* **2007**, *35*, 1139–1144. [CrossRef]
104. Sitapara, R.A.; Gauthier, A.G.; Valdés-Ferrer, S.I.; Lin, M.; Patel, V.; Wang, M.; Martino, A.T.; Perron, J.C.; Ashby, C.R., Jr.; Tracey, K.J.; et al. The α7 nicotinic acetylcholine receptor agonist, GTS-21, attenuates hyperoxia-induced acute inflammatory lung injury by alleviating the accumulation of HMGB1 in the airways and the circulation. *Mol. Med.* **2020**, *26*, 1–12. [CrossRef] [PubMed]
105. Wang, H.; Liao, H.; Ochani, M.; Justiniani, M.; Lin, X.; Yang, L.; Al-Abed, Y.; Wang, H.; Metz, C.; Miller, E.J.; et al. Cholinergic agonists inhibit HMGB1 release and improve survival in experimental sepsis. *Nat. Med.* **2004**, *10*, 1216–1221. [CrossRef]
106. Wang, Q.; Wang, F.; Li, X.; Yang, Q.; Li, X.; Xu, N.; Huang, Y.; Zhang, Q.; Gou, X.; Chen, S.; et al. Electroacupuncture pretreatment attenuates cerebral ischemic injury through α7 nicotinic acetylcholine receptor-mediated inhibition of high-mobility group box 1 release in rats. *J. Neuroinflamm.* **2012**, *9*, 24. [CrossRef] [PubMed]
107. Wang, Z.; Hou, L.; Yang, H.; Ge, J.; Wang, S.; Tian, W.; Wang, X.; Yang, Z. Electroacupuncture Pretreatment Attenuates Acute Lung Injury Through α7 Nicotinic Acetylcholine Receptor-Mediated Inhibition of HMGB1 Release in Rats After Cardiopulmonary Bypass. *Shock* **2018**, *50*, 351–359. [CrossRef] [PubMed]
108. Wazea, S.A.; Wadie, W.; Bahgat, A.K.; El-Abhar, H.S. Galantamine anti-colitic effect: Role of alpha-7 nicotinic acetylcholine receptor in modulating Jak/STAT3, NF-κB/HMGB1/RAGE and p-AKT/Bcl-2 pathways. *Sci. Rep.* **2018**, *8*, 5110. [CrossRef] [PubMed]
109. Zhang, J.; Xia, F.; Zhao, H.; Peng, K.; Liu, H.; Meng, X.; Chen, C.; Ji, F. Dexmedetomidine-induced cardioprotection is mediated by inhibition of high mobility group box-1 and the cholinergic anti-inflammatory pathway in myocardial ischemia-reperfusion injury. *PLoS ONE* **2019**, *14*, e0218726. [CrossRef] [PubMed]
110. Zhang, J.; Yong, Y.; Li, X.; Hu, Y.; Wang, J.; Wang, Y.-Q.; Song, W.; Chen, W.-T.; Xie, J.; Chen, X.-M.; et al. Vagal modulation of high mobility group box-1 protein mediates electroacupuncture-induced cardioprotection in ischemia-reperfusion injury. *Sci. Rep.* **2015**, *5*, 15503. [CrossRef]
111. Andersson, U.; Tracey, K.J. Neural reflexes in inflammation and immunity. *J. Exp. Med.* **2012**, *209*, 1057–1068. [CrossRef]
112. Andersson, U.; Tracey, K.J. Reflex Principles of Immunological Homeostasis. *Annu. Rev. Immunol.* **2012**, *30*, 313–335. [CrossRef]
113. Pavlov, V.A.; Chavan, S.S.; Tracey, K.J. Molecular and Functional Neuroscience in Immunity. *Annu. Rev. Immunol.* **2018**, *36*, 783–812. [CrossRef] [PubMed]
114. Pavlov, V.; Chavan, S.S.; Tracey, K.J. Bioelectronic Medicine: From Preclinical Studies on the Inflammatory Reflex to New Approaches in Disease Diagnosis and Treatment. *Cold Spring Harb. Perspect. Med.* **2019**, *10*, a034140. [CrossRef] [PubMed]

115. Xia, Y.-Y.; Xue, M.; Wang, Y.; Huang, Z.-H.; Huang, C. Electroacupuncture Alleviates Spared Nerve Injury-Induced Neuropathic Pain and Modulates HMGB1/NF-κB Signaling Pathway In The Spinal Cord. *J. Pain Res.* **2019**, *12*, 2851–2863. [CrossRef]
116. Liu, S.; Wang, Z.; Su, Y.; Qi, L.; Yang, W.; Fu, M.; Jing, X.; Wang, Y.; Ma, Q. A neuroanatomical basis for electroacupuncture to drive the vagal–adrenal axis. *Nature* **2021**, *598*, 641–645. [CrossRef] [PubMed]
117. Wang, Z.; Liu, T.; Yin, C.; Li, Y.; Gao, F.; Yu, L.; Wang, Q. Electroacupuncture Pretreatment Ameliorates Anesthesia and Surgery-Induced Cognitive Dysfunction via Activation of an α7-nAChR Signal in Aged Rats. *Neuropsychiatr. Dis. Treat.* **2021**, *17*, 2599–2611. [CrossRef] [PubMed]
118. Zi, S.-F.; Li, J.-H.; Liu, L.; Deng, C.; Ao, X.; Chen, D.-D.; Wu, S.-Z. Dexmedetomidine-mediated protection against septic liver injury depends on TLR4/MyD88/NF-κB signaling downregulation partly via cholinergic anti-inflammatory mechanisms. *Int. Immunopharmacol.* **2019**, *76*, 105898. [CrossRef]
119. Li, D.-J.; Huang, F.; Ni, M.; Fu, H.; Zhang, L.-S.; Shen, F.-M. α7 Nicotinic Acetylcholine Receptor Relieves Angiotensin II–Induced Senescence in Vascular Smooth Muscle Cells by Raising Nicotinamide Adenine Dinucleotide–Dependent SIRT1 Activity. *Arter. Thromb. Vasc. Biol.* **2016**, *36*, 1566–1576. [CrossRef] [PubMed]
120. Aranow, C.; Atish-Fregoso, Y.; Lesser, M.; Mackay, M.; Anderson, E.; Chavan, S.; Zanos, T.P.; Datta-Chaudhuri, T.; Bouton, C.; Tracey, K.J.; et al. Transcutaneous auricular vagus nerve stimulation reduces pain and fatigue in patients with systemic lupus erythematosus: A randomised, double-blind, sham-controlled pilot trial. *Ann. Rheum. Dis.* **2020**, *80*, 203–208. [CrossRef] [PubMed]
121. Nishibori, M.; Mori, S.; Takahashi, H.K. Anti-HMGB1 monoclonal antibody therapy for a wide range of CNS and PNS diseases. *J. Pharmacol. Sci.* **2019**, *140*, 94–101. [CrossRef] [PubMed]
122. Fu, L.; Liu, K.; Wake, H.; Teshigawara, K.; Yoshino, T.; Takahashi, H.; Mori, S.; Nishibori, M. Therapeutic effects of anti-HMGB1 monoclonal antibody on pilocarpine-induced status epilepticus in mice. *Sci. Rep.* **2017**, *7*, 1–13. [CrossRef] [PubMed]
123. Haruma, J.; Teshigawara, K.; Hishikawa, T.; Wang, D.; Liu, K.; Wake, H.; Mori, S.; Takahashi, H.; Sugiu, K.; Date, I.; et al. Anti-high mobility group box-1 (HMGB1) antibody attenuates delayed cerebral vasospasm and brain injury after subarachnoid hemorrhage in rats. *Sci. Rep.* **2016**, *6*, 37755. [CrossRef] [PubMed]
124. Masai, K.; Kuroda, K.; Isooka, N.; Kikuoka, R.; Murakami, S.; Kamimai, S.; Wang, D.; Liu, K.; Miyazaki, I.; Nishibori, M.; et al. Neuroprotective Effects of Anti-high Mobility Group Box-1 Monoclonal Antibody Against Methamphetamine-Induced Dopaminergic Neurotoxicity. *Neurotox. Res.* **2021**, *39*, 1511–1523. [CrossRef]
125. Nakajo, M.; Uezono, N.; Nakashima, H.; Wake, H.; Komiya, S.; Nishibori, M.; Nakashima, K. Therapeutic time window of anti-high mobility group box-1 antibody administration in mouse model of spinal cord injury. *Neurosci. Res.* **2018**, *141*, 63–70. [CrossRef] [PubMed]
126. Nakamura, Y.; Morioka, N.; Abe, H.; Zhang, F.F.; Hisaoka-Nakashima, K.; Liu, K.; Nishibori, M.; Nakata, Y. Neuropathic Pain in Rats with a Partial Sciatic Nerve Ligation Is Alleviated by Intravenous Injection of Monoclonal Antibody to High Mobility Group Box-1. *PLoS ONE* **2013**, *8*, e73640. [CrossRef]
127. Nosaka, N.; Hatayama, K.; Yamada, M.; Fujii, Y.; Yashiro, M.; Wake, H.; Tsukahara, H.; Nishibori, M.; Morishima, T. Anti-high mobility group box-1 monoclonal antibody treatment of brain edema induced by influenza infection and lipopolysaccharide. *J. Med Virol.* **2018**, *90*, 1192–1198. [CrossRef] [PubMed]
128. Okuma, Y.; Liu, K.; Wake, H.; Zhang, J.; Maruo, T.; Date, I.; Yoshino, T.; Ohtsuka, A.; Otani, N.; Tomura, S.; et al. Anti-high mobility group box-1 antibody therapy for traumatic brain injury. *Ann. Neurol.* **2012**, *72*, 373–384. [CrossRef]
129. Okuma, Y.; Wake, H.; Teshigawara, K.; Takahashi, Y.; Hishikawa, T.; Yasuhara, T.; Mori, S.; Takahashi, H.K.; Date, I.; Nishibori, M. Anti–High Mobility Group Box 1 Antibody Therapy May Prevent Cognitive Dysfunction After Traumatic Brain Injury. *World Neurosurg.* **2019**, *122*, e864–e871. [CrossRef]
130. Uezono, N.; Zhu, Y.; Fujimoto, Y.; Yasui, T.; Matsuda, T.; Nakajo, M.; Abematsu, M.; Setoguchi, T.; Mori, S.; Takahashi, H.K.; et al. Prior Treatment with Anti-High Mobility Group Box-1 Antibody Boosts Human Neural Stem Cell Transplantation-Mediated Functional Recovery After Spinal Cord Injury. *Stem Cells* **2018**, *36*, 737–750. [CrossRef]
131. Wang, D.; Liu, K.; Wake, H.; Teshigawara, K.; Mori, S.; Nishibori, M. Anti-high mobility group box-1 (HMGB1) antibody inhibits hemorrhage-induced brain injury and improved neurological deficits in rats. *Sci. Rep.* **2017**, *7*, 46243. [CrossRef] [PubMed]
132. Zhu, Y.; Uezono, N.; Yasui, T.; Nakajo, M.; Nagai, T.; Wang, D.; Nishibori, M.; Nakashima, K. Combinatrial treatment of anti-High Mobility Group Box-1 monoclonal antibody and epothilone B improves functional recovery after spinal cord contusion injury. *Neurosci. Res.* **2021**, *172*, 13–25. [CrossRef] [PubMed]

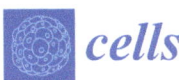

Article

Extracellular Ribosomal RNA Acts Synergistically with Toll-like Receptor 2 Agonists to Promote Inflammation

Karsten Grote [1], Marina Nicolai [2], Uwe Schubert [3], Bernhard Schieffer [1], Christian Troidl [4,5], Klaus T. Preissner [5], Stefan Bauer [2,†] and Silvia Fischer [3,5,*,†]

1. Cardiology & Angiology, Medical School, Philipps-University, 35043 Marburg, Germany; grotek@staff.uni-marburg.de (K.G.); schieferb@staff.uni-marburg.de (B.S.)
2. Institute of Immunology, Medical School, Philipps-University, 35043 Marburg, Germany; nicolai5@staff.uni-marburg.de (M.N.); bauerst@staff.uni-marburg.de (S.B.)
3. Institute of Biochemistry, Medical School, Justus-Liebig-University, 35392 Giessen, Germany; uwe.schubert@biochemie.med.uni-giessen.de
4. Medical Clinic I, Cardiology/Angiology, Campus Kerckhoff, Justus-Liebig-University, 61231 Bad Nauheim, Germany; christian.troidl@innere.med.uni-giessen.de
5. Department Cardiology, Kerckhoff-Heart Research Institute, Medical School, Justus-Liebig-University, 35392 Giessen, Germany; klaus.t.preissner@biochemie.med.uni-giessen.de
* Correspondence: silvia.fischer@biochemie.med.uni-giessen.de
† These authors contributed equally to this work.

Abstract: Self-extracellular RNA (eRNA), which is released under pathological conditions from damaged tissue, has recently been identified as a new alarmin and synergistic agent together with toll-like receptor (TLR)2 ligands to induce proinflammatory activities of immune cells. In this study, a detailed investigation of these interactions is reported. The macrophage cell line J774 A.1 or C57 BL/6 J wild-type mice were treated with 18S rRNA and different TLR2 agonists. Gene and protein expression of tumor necrosis factor *(Tnf)-α*; interleukin *(Il)-1β*, *Il-6*; or monocyte chemoattractant protein *(Mcp)-1* were analyzed and furthermore *in vitro* binding studies to TLR2 were performed. The TLR2/TLR6-agonist Pam$_2$ CSK$_4$ (Pam2) together with 18S rRNA significantly increased the mRNA expression of inflammatory genes and the release of TNF-α from macrophages in a TLR2- and nuclear factor kappa B (NF-κB)-dependent manner. The injection of 18S rRNA/Pam2 into mice increased the cytokine levels of TNF-α, IL-6, and MCP-1 in the peritoneal lavage. Mechanistically, 18S rRNA built complexes with Pam2 and thus enhanced the affinity of Pam2 to TLR2. These results indicate that the alarmin eRNA, mainly consisting of rRNA, sensitizes TLR2 to enhance the innate immune response under pathological conditions. Thus, rRNA might serve as a new target for the treatments of bacterial and viral infections.

Keywords: extracellular RNA; inflammation; cytokines; macrophages; endothelial cells; toll-like receptors

Citation: Grote, K.; Nicolai, M.; Schubert, U.; Schieffer, B.; Troidl, C.; Preissner, K.T.; Bauer, S.; Fischer, S. Extracellular Ribosomal RNA Acts Synergistically with Toll-like Receptor 2 Agonists to Promote Inflammation. *Cells* **2022**, *11*, 1440. https://doi.org/10.3390/cells11091440

Academic Editors: Pascal Colosetti and Alessandro Poggi

Received: 28 January 2022
Accepted: 22 April 2022
Published: 24 April 2022

Publisher's Note: MDPI stays neutral with regard to jurisdictional claims in published maps and institutional affiliations.

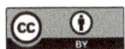

Copyright: © 2022 by the authors. Licensee MDPI, Basel, Switzerland. This article is an open access article distributed under the terms and conditions of the Creative Commons Attribution (CC BY) license (https://creativecommons.org/licenses/by/4.0/).

1. Introduction

Toll-like receptors (TLRs) are the best-characterized members of the family of pattern recognition receptors (PRRs) on host cells in innate immunity and trigger inflammation, induced by pathogen-associated molecular patterns (PAMPs) of infectious microbes as well as damage-associated molecular patterns (DAMPs) as endogenous alarmins. On a structural basis, each TLR contains a variable number of extracellular leucine-rich-repeats (LRR), which are involved in ligand recognition [1], a transmembrane domain, and an intracellular tail containing the Toll/IL-1 receptor (TIR) domain [2]. In immune cells, TLR1, TLR2, TLR4, TLR5, and TLR6 are expressed on the cell surface and recognize mainly bacterial products such as lipopeptides, peptidoglycans, lipopolysaccharide (LPS), or flagellin, whereas endosomal TLRs, such as TLR3, TLR7, and TLR9 respond to nucleic acid structures, which are only accessible after uptake of these microbial products by host cells [3].

The recognition of DAMPs, released by dying or damaged cells under stress conditions such as ischemia/reperfusion or mechanical trauma, promotes sterile inflammation, which is important for restoring tissue homeostasis, tissue repair, and regeneration. On the other hand, DAMPs can also lead to the development of numerous inflammatory diseases or cancer [4]. DAMPs or alarmins include cytosolic, mitochondrial, or nuclear components such as heat shock proteins, high mobility group box 1 (HMGB1), histones, and self-nucleic acids (including nuclear DNA and several types of RNA, especially rRNA).

Self-extracellular RNA (eRNA) released from damaged tissue or cells was identified by our group as a new alarmin by contributing to disease progression in ischemic stroke, thrombosis, myocardial infarction, atherosclerosis, rheumatoid arthritis, and cancer [5–12].

eRNA is not only released by passive but also by active processes, which are dependent on an increase in the intracellular Ca^{2+} concentration leading to the release of microvesicle-associated eRNA [13,14]. Analysis of eRNA in cell supernatants or plasma samples by gel-electrophoresis revealed that rRNA is the main component of eRNA [13,15]. Accordingly, the amount of rRNA present in all eukaryotic cells was determined to be about 80–90% of the total cellular RNA [16]. In previous studies, eRNA was shown to induce prothrombotic, permeability-increasing, and inflammatory responses in immune and vascular cells [5–8,17]. Additionally, lower concentrations of eRNA can serve as a potent adjuvant, particularly for TLR2 ligands on macrophages, to increase their proinflammatory potential in a synergistic manner [14,18]. Moreover, eRNA can sensitize astrocytes, active players in cerebral innate immunity, towards exogenous and endogenous activators of inflammation (such as HMGB1) in a synergistic manner via TLR2-NF-κB-dependent signaling pathways [14].

The present study aimed to gain further insight into the mechanism of the synergistic action of eRNA and TLR2 agonists by using different TLR ligands, rRNA fragments, and by performing *in vitro* TLR2-binding studies.

2. Materials and Methods

2.1. Cell Culture

The monocyte/macrophage cell line J774 A.1 was grown in Dulbecco's modified Eagle medium (DMEM) and Glutamax medium (Gibco, Darmstadt, Germany) containing 10% fetal calf serum (FCS, Gibco) and 1% penicillin/streptomycin (Sigma-Aldrich, Munich, Germany). The endothelial cell line MyEND, showing typical endothelial properties, was grown in DMEM with 10% FCS and 1% penicillin/streptomycin, as recently described [19].

The following agents were used for cell treatments: $Pam_2 CSK_4$, $Pam_3 CSK_4$ (Pam3), MAb-mTLR2, and mouse IgG from invivoGen (Toulouse, France); PD98059, SB203580, and SP600125 from Calbiochem (Merk, Darmstadt, Germany); and Bay 11–7082 from Enzo Life Sciences (Lörrach, Germany). The macrophage-activating lipopeptide of 2 kDa (MALP-2) was synthesized and purified as described before [20]. Before stimulation, cells were washed once with phosphate-buffered saline (PBS, Sigma-Aldrich) and incubated for the indicated periods in FCS-free cell culture medium containing the different agents at the indicated concentrations. The stimulation of cells with eRNA/$Pam_2 CSK_4$, 18S rRNA/$Pam_2 CSK_4$, 18S rRNA/$Pam_3 CSK_4$, and 18S rRNA/MALP-2 mixtures was performed after preincubating both agents in double-distilled water for 30 min at 37 °C.

2.2. Mice

Mice were housed in individually ventilated cages (IVC) under specific pathogen-free (SPF) conditions in the local animal facility. Eight to ten-weeks-old male and female C57 BL/6 J wild-type mice were intraperitoneally injected with 10 ng $Pam_2 CSK_4$, 1 μg 18S rRNA, or a combination of both in 250 μL PBS. The mixture was prepared as for the cell culture experiments. After 4 h, peritoneal lavage with 3 mL of PBS was performed and the blood was collected. All experiments were approved by the governmental animal ethics committee (G13/2018) and conformed to the guidelines from directive 2010/63/EU of the European Parliament.

2.3. Isolation and Quantification of RNA

eRNA, which was used to stimulate cells, was isolated from confluent cultures of mouse fibroblasts using a commercially available kit (Peqlab, Erlangen, Germany) and extracted additionally two times with Trizol according to the manufacturer's instructions (kit from Thermo Fisher Scientific, Waltham, MA, USA). eRNA from cell supernatants was isolated as previously described [18]. Briefly, cell supernatants were first centrifuged for 5 min at 200× g to remove cells and cell debris. To prevent degradation of RNA, RNase inhibitor (4 U/mL, RNasin, Invitrogen) was added and samples were concentrated using centricon tubes (cut off 10 kDa; Millipore, Burlington, MA, USA) that were centrifuged at 3400× g for 12 min at 4 °C and subsequently washed with autoclaved sterile water. The same amounts of lysis buffer (peqGOLD total RNA kit from Peqlab) were added to the concentrated cell supernatants and RNA was isolated in accordance with the instructions of the manufacturer. RNA from lysates or cell supernatants was quantified using the NanoDrop 2000 (Thermo Fisher Scientific) and the quality of RNA was confirmed by electrophoresis on 1% agarose gels followed by ethidium bromide staining or by using the Agilent 2100 bioanalyzer and the Agilent RNA 6000 Nano Kit (Agilent Technologies, Konstanz, Germany), which demonstrated that the major components of isolated RNAs were 28S and 18S rRNA. Furthermore, the purity of RNA was confirmed by performing the endotoxin test using the Pierce™ LAL chromogenic endotoxin quantification kit (Thermo Fisher Scientific).

2.4. In Vitro Transcription of Human 18S rRNA

Human 18S rRNA (NR_145820.1) was amplified from genomic HEK293 DNA using the primer pair 5′-TAC CTG GTT GAT CCT GCC AGT AGC-3′ and 5′-TAA TGA TCC TTC CGC AGG TTC ACC TAC-3′ and cloned into pGEM®-T Easy Vector (Promega, Mannheim, Germany). Fragments of 18S rRNA (18S-1, 18S-2 and 18S-3) were amplified from full-length human 18S rRNA plasmid using the following primers: 18S-1: 5′-TAC CTG GTT GAT CCT GCC AG-3′ and 5′-GCC GTC CCT CTT AAT CAT GG-3′, 18S-2: 5′-CGG GGG CAT TCG TAT TGC GC-3′ and 5′-TAA TGA TCC TTC CGC AGG TTC-3′, 18S-3: 5′-GAC CCG CCG GGC AGC TTC CG-3′, and 5′-CTG CCG GCG TAG GGT AGG CAC-3′. For in-vitro transcription, a pGEM plasmid containing human 18S rRNA was linearized with Pvu II and purified with GeneJet PCR purification kit (ThermoFisher, Germany) according to the manufacturer's recommendation or alternatively extracted with phenol/chloroform, precipitated, and solubilized in reaction buffer. RNA was produced *in vitro* using T7-ScribeTM Standard RNA IVT Kit, CELLSCRIPTTM according to the manufacturer's recommendation. After synthesis and removal of DNA by DNase I digestion, the RNA mixture was desalted with Micro Bio-Spin™ Chromatography Columns (BIO RAD).

2.5. Electrophoretic Mobility Shift Assay (EMSA)

18S rRNA alone or preincubated with different concentrations of Pam2 for 30 min at 37 °C in the absence or presence of 1% SDS were separated on 0.7% agarose gels.

2.6. TLR2 Fusion Protein

The extracellular domain of murine toll-like receptor 2 (aa 1–587) was fused to the human IgG1-Fc protein and expressed in HEK293 cells [21]. Following the concentration of the 5-L cell supernatant with a Vivaflow 200 (Sartorius) ultrafiltration cassette (50 kDa molecular weight cut-off), the TLR2 fusion protein was purified by protein A affinity chromatography, and the purity was verified by SDS-polyacrylamide gel electrophoresis (PAGE) and Coomassie staining.

2.7. TLR2 Binding Assay

Maxisorp NUNC-immuno plates were coated with streptavidin (from Streptomyces avdinii, Sigma) at 1 µg/well in PBS and incubated at 4 °C overnight. All incubations were performed in a humid chamber. To avoid unspecific binding, the plates were blocked with PBS containing 1% BSA (Sigma-Aldrich) for 1 h at 37 °C. After the blocking procedure, the plates were washed three times with pre-warmed PBS.

To investigate the interactions of Pam2 with human 18S rRNA and TLR2 fusion protein, Pam2-Biotin (Pam2-Biotin-Aca-Aca-NH2, Genaxxon bioscience) was preincubated with human 18S rRNA in ultra-pure water (10 µL) for 30 min at 37 °C. Subsequently, TLR2 fusion protein and medium were added (pure Opti-MEM™ medium, Gibco) for an additional 30 min at 37 °C. This mixture was added to the streptavidin-coated plates (50 µL/well) and incubated for 15 min at 37 °C, followed by three washing steps with PBS.

For the detection of TLR2, each well was incubated with an anti-human IgG-peroxidase conjugated antibody (1:1000, Dako) for 1 h at 37 °C. After the last washing step, a substrate buffer with 20 mg o-phenylenediamine dihydrochloride (OPD, Sigma) and 30% of H_2O_2 was applied to the wells (50 µL) and incubated for approximately 20 min at room temperature in the dark. The reaction was stopped by adding 25 µL/well 2 M H_2SO_4, and absorption was measured with a photometer at 450–650 nm

2.8. Quantitative Real-Time PCR

Following the treatment of J774 A.1 or MyEND cells with various agonists as indicated in the legends of the corresponding figures, cells were washed twice with PBS, lysed, and RNA was isolated with the GenElute Mammalian Total RNA Miniprep Kit (Sigma). For real-time PCR analysis, 1 µg of RNA was reverse-transcribed using the High-Capacity cDNA Reverse Transcription Kit (Applied Biosystems, Carlsbad, CA, USA), and DNA amplification was performed with a StepOne Plus cycler (Applied Biosystems) and analyzed with the StepOne™ software (v2.3) in a reaction volume of 10 µL using the SensiMix Sybr Kit (Bioline, Luckenwalde, Germany) with 50 pmol of each primer. To avoid amplification of the genomic DNA, primers were designed to span exon–exon junctions. The real-time PCR was performed under the following conditions: an initial denaturation step at 95 °C for 8.5 min followed by 45 cycles, consisting of denaturation (95 °C, 30 s), annealing (60 °C, 30 s) and elongation (72 °C, 30 s). Melt curve analysis was performed to control the specific amplification. Results were normalized to the expression levels (E) of actin and expressed as the ratio of E(target)/E(Actin). The following mouse primers were used: *Tnf-α* forward 5′-ACT GAA CTT CGG GGT GAT CG-3′, *Tnf-α* reverse 5′-TGG TTT GTG AGT GTG AGG GTC-3′, *Il-1β* forward 5′-GGA TGA GGA CAT GAG CAC CT-3′, *Il-1β* reverse 5′-GGA GCC TGT AGT GCA GTT GT-3′, *Il-6* forward 5′-CTC TGC AAG AGA CTT CCA TCC A-3′, *Il-6* reverse 5′-TTG TGA AGT AGG GAA GGCCG-3′, *Mcp-1* forward 5′-AAG CTG TAGTTT TTG TCA CCA AGC-3′, *Mcp-1* reverse 5′-GAC CTT AGG GCA GAT GCA GTT-3′, *Tlr2* forward 5′-TCT TGT TTC TGA GTG TAG GGG C-3′, *Tlr2* reverse 5′-CAT CCT CTG AGA TTT GAC GCT TTG-3′, *Tlr6* forward 5′-TGA ATG ATG AAA ACT GTC AAA GGT TAA-3′, *Tlr6* reverse 5′-GGG TCA CAT TCA ATA AGG TTG GA-3′, *actin* forward 5′-CGC GAG CAC AGC TTC TTT G-3′, and *actin* reverse 5′-CGT CAT CCA TGG CGA ACT GG-3′.

2.9. Enzyme-Linked Immunosorbent Assay (ELISA)

Supernatants from J774 A.1 cells, MyEND cells, as well as samples from peritoneal lavage were analyzed by ELISA. ELISAs for TNF-α (detection limit = 8 pg/mL), Il-1β (detection limit = 8 pg/mL), IL-6 (detection limit = 4 pg/mL), and MCP-1 (detection limit = 15 pg/m) were performed using the commercially available kit from eBioscience (Frankfurt, Germany).

2.10. Statistical Analysis

All data were represented as means ± SEM. Two-tailed unpaired Student t-test was used to compare two independent groups; one-way ANOVA followed by Fisher´s LSD post hoc test was used when more than two groups with one independent variable were compared and two-way ANOVA followed by Fisher´s LSD post hoc or Tukey's multiple comparison tests were used when more than two groups with two independent variables were compared (GraphPad Prism, version 7.0; GraphPad Software, La Jolla, CA). A value of $P < 0.05$ was considered statistically significant. The numbers of independent experiments were indicated in the respective figure legends.

3. Results

3.1. Synergistic Activity of 18S rRNA and $Pam_2 CSK_4$

In previous studies, we demonstrated that eRNA synergistically enhanced TLR2 ligand-induced expression of cytokines and their secretion from murine macrophages (differentiated from bone marrow-derived stem cells) by shifting the dose-response curve (and the IC50 value) for the TLR2 ligand Pam2 to much lower concentrations [18]. As eRNA appears to be heterogeneous with regard to the composition of RNA and mainly consists of rRNA, we wanted to study whether purified full-length 18S rRNA, synthesized by *in vitro* transcription, could duplicate the observed results using the macrophage cell line J774 A.1. The observed data were initially compared with those of eRNA isolated from mouse fibroblasts. The preincubated mixtures consisting of low concentrations of Pam2 (0.1 ng/mL) and either eRNA or 18S rRNA significantly increased the mRNA expression of inflammatory cytokines such as *Tnf-α*, *Il-1β*, *Il-6*, or *Mcp-1* (Figure 1A–D), as well as the protein release of TNF-α from macrophages as compared to each of the RNA-forms alone as agonists (Figure 1E). In all experiments, early time points were used to avoid secondary effects such as autocrine effects of TNF-α [18]. Furthermore, 18S rRNA/Pam2 had a slightly higher (although not significant) potency compared to eRNA/Pam2 in mediating cytokine expression. 18S rRNA, eRNA, and Pam2 at low concentrations alone showed no or only minor effects on the cytokine expression without any significant differences between them (Figure 1A–E).

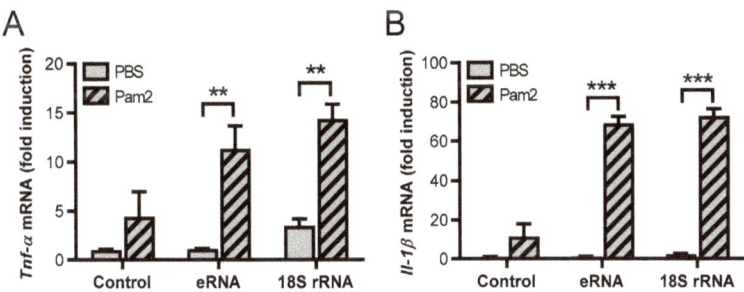

Figure 1. *Cont.*

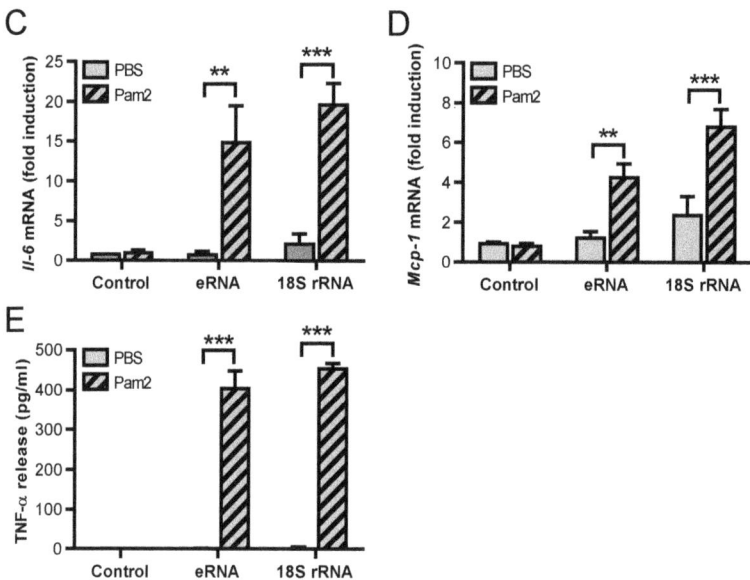

Figure 1. Synergistic activity of 18S rRNA and $Pam_2 CSK_4$. Macrophages (J774 A.1 cells) were treated for 2 h with $Pam_2 CSK_4$ (Pam2, 0.1 ng/mL) and either self-extracellular RNA (eRNA, 1 µg/mL) or 18S rRNA (1 µg/mL) alone or with the preincubated mixture of Pam2 with either eRNA or 18S rRNA. PBS-treated cells without any additives served as control. Real-time PCR was used to determine transcript levels of *Tnf-α* (**A**), *Il-1β* (**B**), *Il-6* (**C**), or *Mcp-1* (**D**). TNF-α protein levels in cellular supernatants were quantified by ELISA (**E**). Values are expressed as mean ± SEM; $N = 3$; ** $p < 0.01$, *** $p < 0.001$ between indicated groups.

3.2. Signaling Pathways Involved in 18S rRNA/$Pam_2 CSK_4$-Induced Activities

While primary macrophages were previously used to study the activities of Pam2/eRNA, the involvement of TLR2 in the induction of gene expression by Pam2 and 18S rRNA could now be confirmed with the macrophage cell line J774 A.1. 18S rRNA/Pam2-induced cytokine induction was inhibited by a neutralizing antibody against TLR2, whereas the corresponding control IgG did not show any effect (Figure S1A–D). In accordance with the eRNA/Pam2-induced signaling pathways identified in primary macrophages, the blockade of the NF-κB pathway by Bay completely abolished the mRNA expression of *Tnf-α*, *Il-1β*, and *Il-6*, as well as the release of TNF-α in J774 A.1 cells. Also, the activation of the mitogen-activated protein (MAP)-kinase p38 was involved in 18S rRNA/Pam2-mediated mRNA expression of *Il-1β*, as shown in experiments using the p38 MAP-kinase inhibitor SB203580 (Figure S1A–D). Likewise, the release of TNF-α—but not the mRNA expression of *Tnf-α*—was dependent on MAP-kinase p38-signaling (Figure S1A,D). The activation of MAP-kinase 42/44 as well as of c-Jun N-terminal kinase (JNK) was not involved in inflammatory activities of 18S rRNA/Pam2, as cytokine induction was not blocked by MAP-kinase 42/44 pathway inhibitor PD98059 or the JNK inhibitor SP600125, respectively (Figure S1A–D). These results indicate that J774 A.1 cells proved to be a suitable cell line for further studies since the inflammatory potential of 18S rRNA/Pam2 in the J774 A.1 macrophage cell line appeared to be transmitted by the same mechanisms as in primary macrophages. Therefore, all the following experiments were performed using the macrophage cell line.

Previous investigations of our group with endothelial cells demonstrated that eRNA acts via the activation of vascular endothelial growth factor (VEGF) receptor 2 (VEGF-R2) by increasing the binding of VEGF to its receptor [22]. Likewise, in J774 A.1 cells, the potent and selective VEGF-R2 tyrosine kinase inhibitor SU5416 [23] significantly decreased 18S rRNA/Pam2-induced expression of *Tnf-α*, *Il-1β*, and *Il-6*, as well as the release of TNF-α (Figure 2A–D). In contrast, the cytokine expression induced by higher concentrations of Pam2 was not decreased by SU5416. These data indicate that VEGF-R2 is involved in the synergistic activities of 18S rRNA/Pam2 but not in TLR2 activation induced by higher concentrations of active Pam2 alone.

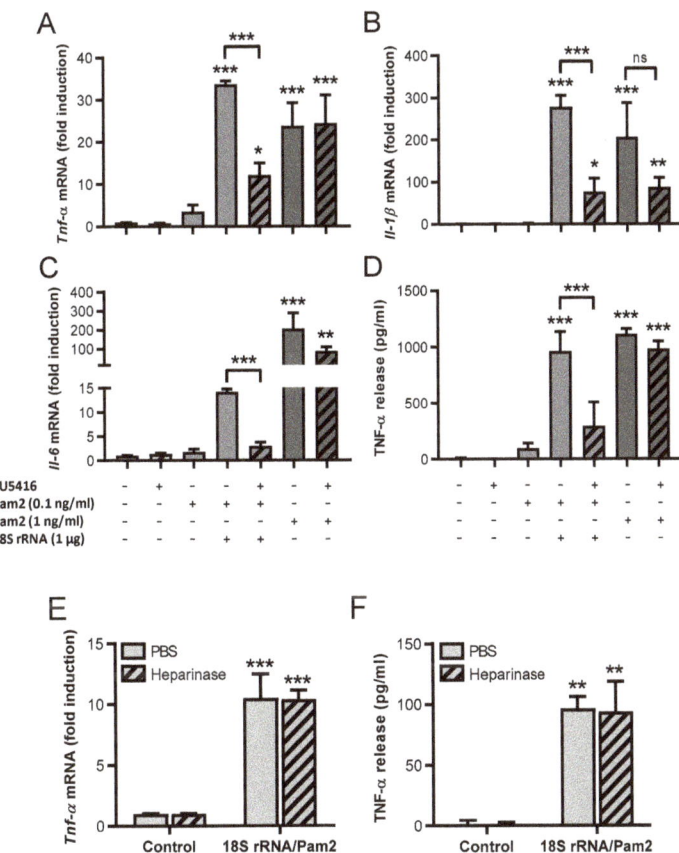

Figure 2. Synergistic activity of 18S rRNA and Pam$_2$ CSK$_4$ after blocking VEGF-R2 activation and heparinase treatment. (**A–D**): Macrophages (J774 A.1 cells) were treated for 2 h with a preincubated mixture of Pam$_2$ CSK$_4$ (Pam2, 0.1 ng/mL) and 18S rRNA or Pam2 alone (1 ng/mL), both without or after pretreatment of cells with SU5416 (10 mM) and additionally with Pam2 alone (0.1 ng/mL). Real-time PCR was used to determine transcript levels of *Tnf-α* (**A**), *Il-1β* (**B**), or *Il-6* (**C**). TNF-α protein levels in cellular supernatants were quantified by ELISA (**D**). (**E,F**) Macrophages (J774 A.1) were pretreated for 1 h with heparinase (50 mU/mL), stimulated with a preincubated mixture of Pam$_2$ CSK$_4$ (Pam2, 0.1 ng/mL) and 18S rRNA (1 µg/mL) for 2 h, and *Tnf-α* expression was analyzed by real-time PCR, (**E**) and the release of TNF-α protein levels was quantified by ELISA (**F**). PBS-treated cells without any additives served as control. Values are expressed as mean ± SEM; N = 3–6; * $p < 0.05$, ** $p < 0.01$, *** $p < 0.001$ versus control value or between indicated groups.

To investigate if regulatory proteins such as growth factors, which are known to bind to cell membrane-bound heparan sulfate proteoglycans, are involved in the 18S rRNA/Pam2-induced effects, cells were pretreated with heparinase to remove the glycosaminoglycans. Yet, pretreated macrophages did not change the expression and release of TNF-α in response to the 18S rRNA/Pam2 agonist (Figure 2E,F), indicating that heparan sulfate proteoglycans are not involved in cellular activation.

3.3. Synergistic Effects of 18S rRNA with Other TLR Ligands

To further analyze the availability and specificity of 18S rRNA for other TLR ligands, MALP-2 (another TLR2/TLR6 agonist) and the TLR2/TLR1 ligand Pam3 were used. Alone, both agonists induced *Tnf-α* mRNA expression in a concentration-dependent manner in J774 A.1 cells (Figure S2). To investigate potential synergistic effects with 18S rRNA, MALP-2 and Pam3 were used at low concentrations from 0.1–10 ng/mL, which per se had no or only a moderate influence on *Tnf-α* mRNA expression. The presence of 18S rRNA (1 μg/mL) synergistically increased MALP-2- and Pam3-induced *Tnf-α* mRNA expression as well as TNF-α release (Figure 3A,B). Of note, compared to Pam2 and 18S rRNA, higher concentrations of each respective TLR2 ligand were required (1 ng/mL for MALP-2 and Pam3 vs. 0.1 ng/mL for Pam2) to observe the described cell activation. The same results were obtained for *Il-6*, whereby *Il-1β* gene expression was only significantly increased by 18S rRNA/MALP-2 (Figure 3C,D). Also, the *Mcp-1* transcript level was not further elevated (Figure 3E). 18S rRNA alone (left pair of bars without MALP-2 or Pam3) was unable to induce cytokine expression.

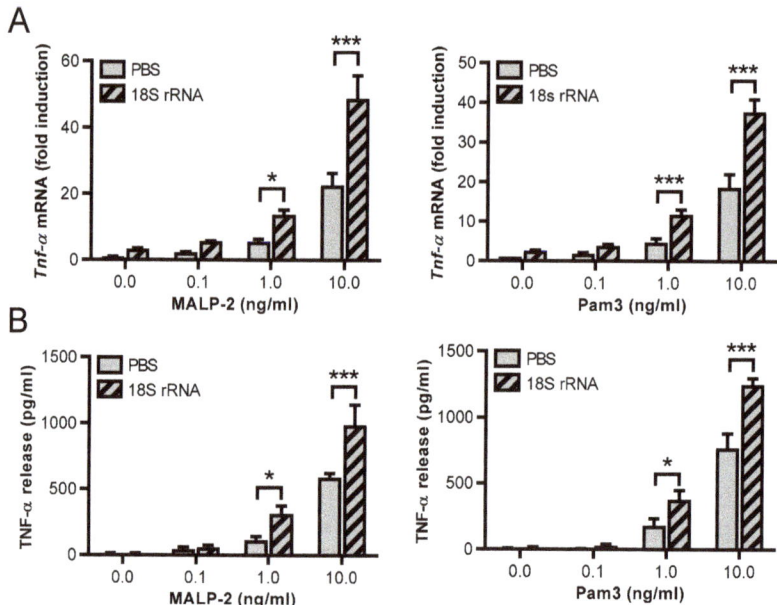

Figure 3. Cont.

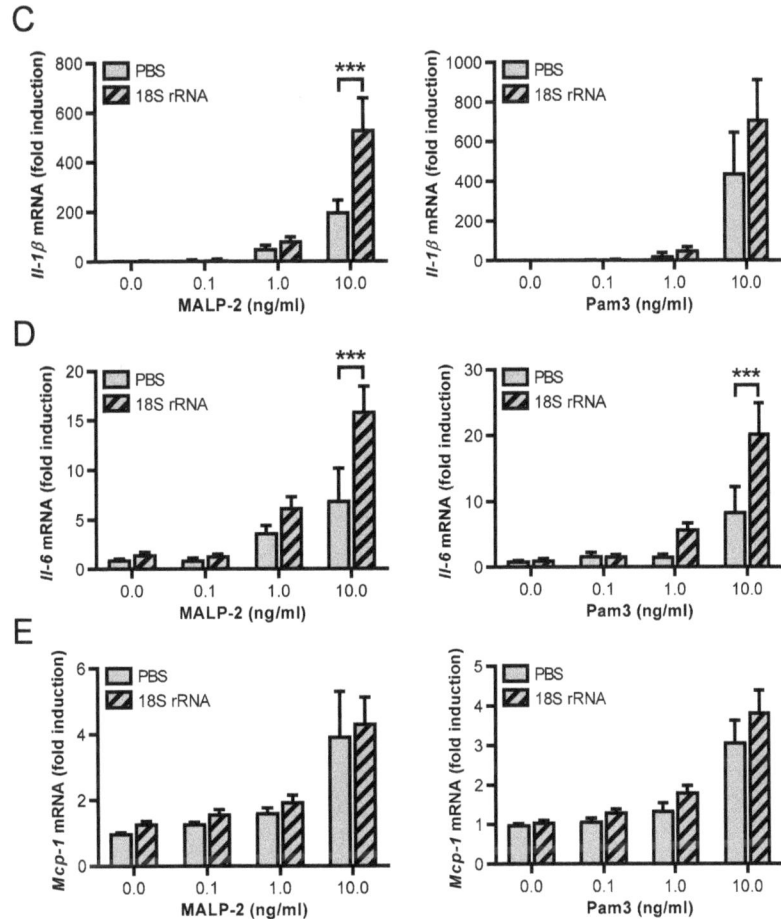

Figure 3. Synergistic activity of 18S rRNA together with the TLR ligands MALP-2 and Pam$_3$ CSK$_4$. Macrophages (J774 A.1 cells) were treated for 2 h with different concentrations of MALP-2, Pam3, or 18S rRNA (1 µg/mL) alone or with a preincubated mixture of different concentrations of MALP-2 or Pam3 together with 18S rRNA. PBS-treated cells without any additives served as control. Real-time PCR was used to determine transcript levels of *Tnf-α* (**A**), *Il-1β* (**C**), *Il-6* (**D**), or *Mcp-1* (**E**). TNF-α protein levels in cellular supernatants were quantified by ELISA (**B**). Values are expressed as mean ± SEM; N = 3–10; * $p < 0.05$, *** $p < 0.001$ between indicated groups.

3.4. Detection of 18S rRNA/Pam2 Complexes and Influence of 18S rRNA on Pam2 Binding to TLR2

To investigate a possible interaction of 18S rRNA with Pam2, we performed electrophoretic mobility shift assays. Preincubation of 18S rRNA with increasing concentrations of Pam2 for 30 min at 37 °C resulted in a dose-dependent shift of a higher molecular band in the gel, indicating the formation of 18S rRNA/Pam2 complexes. The formation of this complex was prevented by the addition of detergent (1% SDS) during preincubation (Figure 4A).

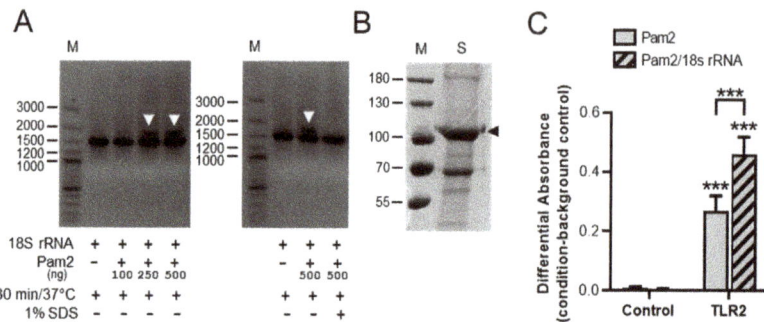

Figure 4. Detection of 18S rRNA/Pam2 complexes and binding assay of Pam2 to TLR2. 18S rRNA alone or preincubated with different concentrations of Pam2 for 30 min at 37 °C in the absence or presence of 1% SDS were separated on 0.7% agarose gels. Arrowheads indicate 18S rRNA/Pam2 complex, M = DNA marker (size in bp) (**A**). SDS-PAGE and Coomassie staining of the extracellular domain of TLR2 fused to IgG1-Fc protein, expressed in HEK293 and purified from cell supernatants, was performed. Arrowhead indicates TLR2-Fc, M = protein marker (size in kDa), S = purified and concentrated supernatant from HEK293 cells (**B**). Pam2-Biotin (7.5 ng/mL) was preincubated for 30 min in the absence or presence of 18S rRNA (0.1 µg/mL) and subsequently with the TLR2 fusion protein (10 µg/mL) (**C**). The binding of Pam2-Biotin to TLR2 was measured after binding to streptavidin and detection of bound TLR2 by IgG-peroxidase-conjugated antibody. After adding the peroxidase substrate, the absorbance of the product was measured at 450–650 nm. The mean values are presented as mean ± SEM; N = 3–4; *** $p < 0.001$ versus corresponding control values or between indicated groups.

To investigate whether the binding affinity of Pam2 to TLR2 is influenced by the presence of 18S rRNA, *in vitro* binding assays were performed. For these studies, the extracellular domain of murine TLR2 was fused to the IgG1-Fc protein and expressed in HEK293 cells. Following purification of the fusion protein from cell supernatants, the purity of the construct was verified by SDS-gel electrophoresis and used for interaction studies (Figure 4B). The binding of Pam2 to TLR2 fusion protein was significantly increased in the presence of 18S rRNA, which corresponds with the high inflammatory potency of the 18S rRNA/Pam2 complex in the previous cell assays (Figure 4C).

3.5. Synergistic Activities of Different 18S rRNA Fragments Together with Pam$_2$ CSK$_4$

In order to investigate specific regions of 18S rRNA that might be responsible for the observed synergistic effects with the indicated PAMPs, different parts of the 18S rRNA were cloned. Afterwards, the respective RNA fragments of different sizes were *in vitro* transcribed (18S-1 = 5′-fragment, 18S-2 = 3′-fragment, 18S-3 = partial 3′-fragment, 18S = full-length) (Figure 5A). Following the stimulation of J774 A.1 cells with Pam2 in the presence of such fragments in comparison to the full-length 18S rRNA revealed that the different fragments were quite similar in their synergistic potential. However, the 18S rRNA fragment 18S-1 transcribed from the initial 5′-region of 18S rRNA (1–930 bp) increased *Tnf-α*, *Il-1β*, or *Il-6* mRNA expression, as well as TNF-α released the most, even though these differences were not significant compared to the other fragments and the full-length 18S rRNA (Figure 5B–E).

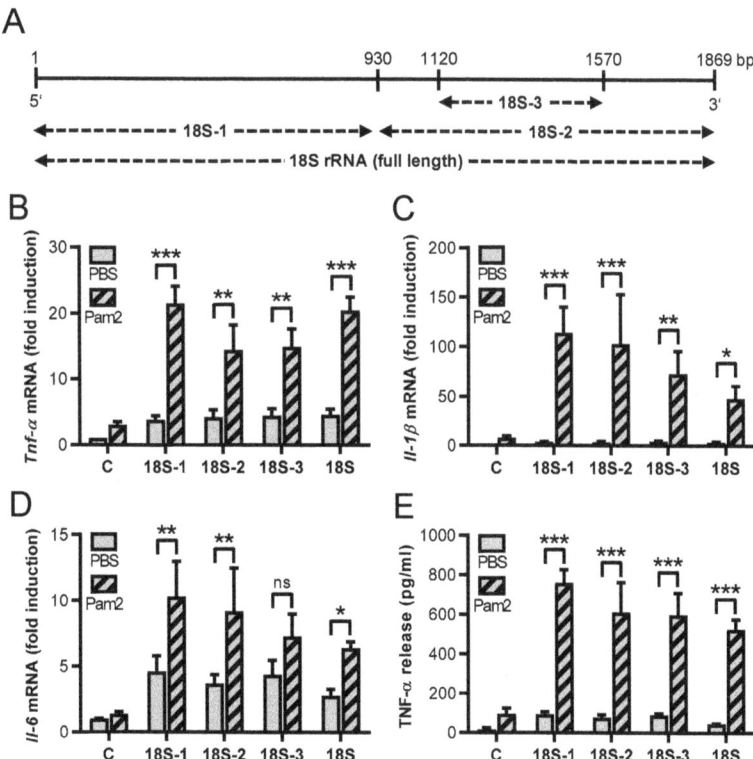

Figure 5. Synergistic activities of 18S rRNA fragments with Pam$_2$ CSK$_4$. The 18S rRNA fragments of different sizes were generated by *in vitro* transcription (**A**). Macrophages (J774 A.1 cells) were treated for 2 h with Pam$_2$ CSK$_4$ (Pam2, 0.1 ng/mL), 18S rRNA (1 μg/mL), or 18S rRNA fragments (18S-1, 18S-2, 18S-3; each 1 μg/mL) alone or with preformed complexes together with Pam2 each. PBS-treated cells without any additives served as control. Real-time PCR was used to determine transcript levels of *Tnf-α* (**B**), *Il-1β* (**C**), or *Il-6* (**D**). TNF-α protein levels in cellular supernatants were quantified by ELISA (**E**). Values are expressed as mean ± SEM; N = 6–12; * $p < 0.05$, ** $p < 0.01$, *** $p < 0.001$ between indicated groups.

3.6. Synergistic Effects of 18S rRNA and Pam$_2$ CSK$_4$ In Vivo

To evaluate the possible synergistic effects of 18S rRNA and Pam2 *in vivo*, the 18S rRNA fragment 18S-1 (1 μg) preincubated with Pam2 (10 ng) was intraperitoneally injected into C57 BL/6 J mice. 18S-1/Pam2 was found to significantly increase the protein levels of TNF-α, IL-6, and MCP-1, but not of IL-1β (at the detection limit of the ELISA) in the peritoneal lavage, whereas 18S-1 or Pam2 alone had no effect at these concentrations (Figure 6A–D).

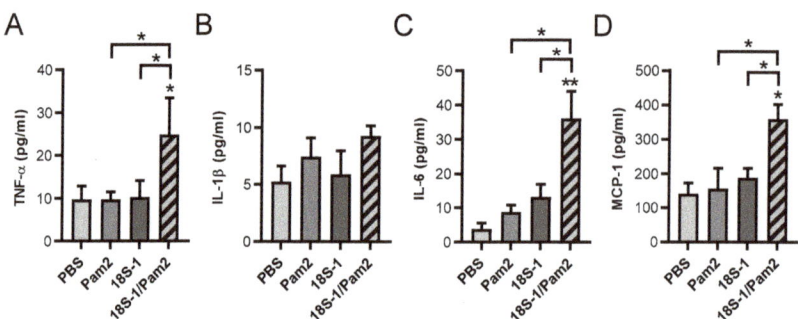

Figure 6. Synergistic activity of 18S rRNA and Pam$_2$ CSK$_4$ *in vivo*. C57 BL/6 J mice were intraperitoneally injected with either 10 ng Pam$_2$ CSK$_4$ (Pam2) or 1 µg 18S-1 rRNA alone or with preformed complexes of both in 250 µL PBS. PBS injection alone was used as sham control (PBS). After 4 h, peritoneal lavage was collected and TNF-α (**A**), IL-1β (**B**), IL-6 (**C**), and MCP-1 (**D**) protein levels were quantified by ELISA. Values are expressed as mean ± SEM; N = 4–9; * $p < 0.05$, ** $p < 0.01$ versus control value (PBS) or between indicated groups.

3.7. Lack of Synergism between 18S rRNA and Pam$_2$ CSK$_4$ on Cytokine Induction in Endothelial Cells

In addition to the macrophage-like J774 A.1 cell line, the potential synergistic effects of 18S rRNA and Pam2 were tested on endothelial cells, which likewise express TLRs for pathogen recognition and immune defense. To this end, the endothelial MyEND cell line was used, which was recently characterized with regard to its endothelial-specific properties and the expression of *Tlr2* and *Tlr6* [19]. Following 3 h of stimulation, Pam2 alone increased the mRNA levels of *Tnf-α* and *Il-6*, as well as the protein secretion of IL-6 in a dose-dependent manner, being significant at ≥10 ng/mL Pam2. Contrary to J774 A.1 cells, TNF-α protein was not detectable in MyEND cells (Figure S3A–D), indicating a different posttranscriptional regulation of the mRNA or a different proteolytic activation of the protein in these cell types. As opposed to J774 A.1 cells, inactive low concentrations of Pam2 (up to 1 ng/mL) in the presence of 18S rRNA (1 µg/mL) were ineffective to exhibit any synergistic effects on the mRNA expression levels of *Tnf-α* or *Il-6* as well as on IL-6 protein secretion in MyEND cells (Figure 7A–C). As in J774 A.1 cells, 18S rRNA alone (left pair of bars without Pam2) was unable to induce cytokine expression in MyEND cells as well.

These differences between macrophages and endothelial cells with regard to the synergistic activities of 18S rRNA/Pam2 on cytokine expression could be due to different expression levels or a different regulation pattern of the Pam2 receptors, TLR2 and TLR6, in these cell types. In fact, *Tlr2* and *Tlr6* expression was significantly lower expressed in MyEND cells compared to J774 A.1 cells (Figure 8A,B). Furthermore, Pam2-increased *Tlr2* expression in macrophages was considerably more effective than in endothelial cells. However, the presence of 18S rRNA did not show any significant increase of Pam2-induced *Tlr2* mRNA expression in both cell types (Figure 8C,D). The expression of *Tlr6* mRNA was not changed by Pam2 alone or in the presence of 18S rRNA in macrophages or endothelial cells (Figure 8E,F).

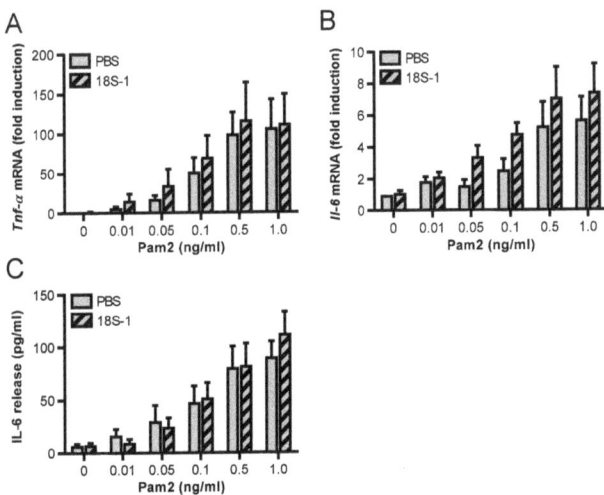

Figure 7. Lack of synergistic activity of 18S rRNA and Pam$_2$ CSK$_4$ in endothelial cells. Endothelial cells (MyEND cells) were treated for 3 h with different concentrations of Pam$_2$ CSK$_4$ (Pam2) and 18S rRNA (1 µg/mL) alone or with preformed complexes of different concentrations of Pam2 together with 18S rRNA. PBS-treated cells without any additives served as control. Tnf-α (**A**) and Il-6 (**B**) mRNA levels were quantified by real-time PCR. Release of IL-6 (**C**) protein in cellular supernatants was quantified by ELISA. Values are expressed as mean ± SEM; N = 3–8.

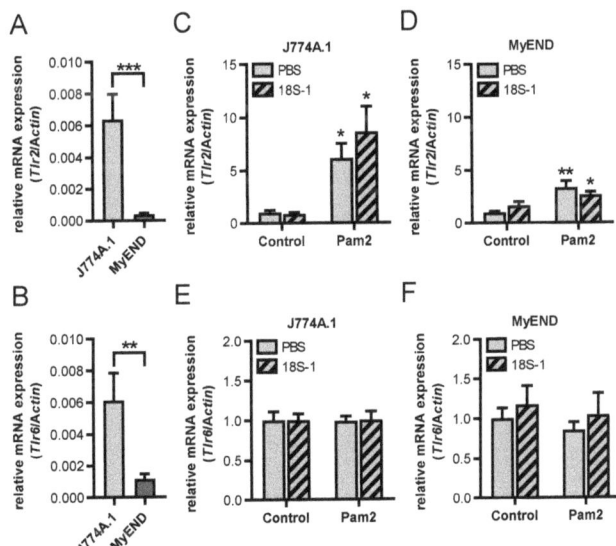

Figure 8. Influence of 18S rRNA on Pam$_2$ CSK$_4$-dependent $Tlr2$ and $Tlr6$ expression. $Tlr2$ (**A**) and $Tlr6$ (**B**) mRNA levels under basal conditions were quantified by real-time PCR in macrophages (J774 A.1 cells) and endothelial cells (MyEND cells). MyEND and J774 A.1 cells were treated for 3 h with 18S rRNA (1 µg/mL) alone or with preformed complexes of Pam$_2$ CSK$_4$ (Pam2, 100 pg/mL). PBS-treated cells without any additives served as control. $Tlr2$ (**C**,**D**) and $Tlr6$ (**E**,**F**) mRNA levels were quantified by real-time PCR. Values are expressed as mean ± SEM; N = 4–8; * $p < 0.05$, ** $p < 0.01$, *** $p < 0.001$ versus control value or between indicated groups.

4. Discussion

To study the established synergistic activities of eRNA with TLR2 ligands in more detail, in-vitro-transcribed 18S rRNA was used, which increased the expression of inflammatory genes such as *Tnf-α*, *Il-1β*, *Il-6*, and *Mcp-1*, as well as the release of TNF-α from the macrophage cell line J774 A.1 in a TLR2-dependent manner. Thus, we confirmed our previous results obtained with eRNA and primary bone marrow-derived macrophages and could further document that mainly rRNA is responsible for the described activities of eRNA [18].

Except for TLR3, most TLRs (including TLR1, TLR2, TLR4, TLR5, TLR7, TLR8, and TLR9) use the intracellular adaptor proteins myeloid differentiation primary response 88 (MyD88) and IL-1 receptor-associated kinases (IRAK-4 and -1) via their death domain interactions to activate the canonical NF-κB and MAP-kinase pathways, leading to the generation of proinflammatory cytokines such as TNF-α, IL-1β, or IL-6 [24–26]. According to our previous results, the signaling pathways induced by 18S rRNA/Pam2 also involved the activation of the NF-κB- and of MAP-kinase 38-dependent pathways [18,27].

Unlike other TLRs, which are functionally active as homodimers, TLR2 is known to exist as a heterodimer together with TLR1 or TLR6, respectively [28], to attain specificity for different lipopeptide ligands. The dimers utilize two TIR domain-containing adaptor proteins, MyD88 and TIR domain-containing adaptor protein (TIRAP), and subsequently activate NF-κB- and MAP-kinase-dependent signaling pathways [28]. In this regard, Pam2 is known to bind and activate TLR2/TLR6 dimers [29]. However, Pam2 is also active as an agonist in TLR6-deficient cells [30,31], indicating that TLR2 alone may also function as a Pam2 receptor. The synergistic activity of 18S rRNA on Pam2-induced, TLR2-dependent cytokine upregulation seems to involve the activation of VEGF-R2 as well because the overall cell activation was significantly decreased by SU5416 as a specific inhibitor of the tyrosine phosphorylation of VEGF-R2 [23]. Since the induced cytokine expression after stimulation of TLR2 by higher concentrations of Pam2 was unaffected by SU5416, a new coreceptor function of VEGF-R2 in the presence of low, by itself ineffective concentrations of Pam2 together with 18S rRNA is proposed.

It is already known that the TLRs require coreceptors. For example, the TLR2 heterodimer TLR2/TLR1 needs the coreceptor CD14, and the heterodimer TLR2/TLR6 additionally requires CD36, which both were supposed to act as an intermediate complex facilitating the loading of ligands to both TLR2 heterodimers [32]. Additionally, integrins can function as coreceptors for TLR2. Although membrane integrin α3β1 does not directly bind the lipopeptide ligand Pam3, blocking of the α3-subunit decreased TLR2-mediated IL-6 release from macrophages [33]. Furthermore, the functional association of other receptors such as C-X-C motif chemokine receptor 4 (CXCR4), a seven-transmembrane G-protein-coupled chemokine receptor, with TLR2 inside lipid rafts, led to a downregulation of the TLR2 response [34,35]. Moreover, proteins such as mannan-binding lectin (MBL), which modify TLR3 activation by interacting with poly(I:C), suppressed the poly(I:C)-induced activation of the TLR3 pathway and the subsequent cytokine production [36]. Additionally, several studies demonstrated that certain TLR ligand combinations induced a synergistic production of proinflammatory cytokines, which likely occur at the transcriptional level and involve the activation of multiple signaling pathways and transcription factor families [37–41]. Based on our present data, VEGF-R2 can be designated as an additional coreceptor for TLR2.

Many cytokines such as VEGF (or other basic proteins) can bind to membrane-bound heparan sulfate proteoglycans to become presented to their cognate signaling receptors such as VEGF-R2. However, this type of interaction appears not to be involved in the synergistic action of 18S rRNA/Pam2, since the pretreatment of macrophages with heparinase to remove cell membrane-localized heparan sulfate glycosaminoglycans and any associated proteins did not influence the 18S rRNA/Pam2-mediated cytokine induction. Although the mechanism for the coreceptor role of VEGF-R2 in 18S rRNA/Pam2-induced cytokine expression needs to be investigated in more detail, our results demonstrate that rRNA appears to induce interactions between VEGF-R2 and TLR2, which are necessary for the increased inflammatory response towards Pam2. These data are reminiscent of the previously characterized interaction between VEGF-R2 and its coreceptor neuropilin-1, which was reinforced by eRNA as well [6,22]. Accordingly, the expression of specific cofactors (e.g., CD36, CD14) can vary between different organs and cell types, which might explain the cell-type specificity of 18S rRNA/Pam2-mediated synergistic effects (https://www.proteinatlas.org/ENSG00000135218-CD36/tissue accessed on 27 January 2022). Ongoing studies are currently in progress to clarify these differences.

The synergistic influence of 18S rRNA on TLR2 activation also depends on the type of TLR2 ligand. While the release of cytokines induced by MALP-2, another TLR2/TLR6 activator, was also increased in the presence of 18S rRNA, the ligand concentration needed for this activation was much higher compared to Pam2 and comparable to the extent of activation for the TLR2/TLR1 ligand Pam3. These results indicate that rRNA might increase the binding of Pam2 to its receptor to a much higher degree in comparison to the other investigated agonists. This was confirmed by in-vitro binding assays, demonstrating that the binding affinity of the TLR2 ligand Pam2 to TLR2 was increased in the presence of 18S rRNA, which might be the reason for the observed higher inflammatory response in the cellular studies.

In accordance with our findings, it has been suggested that both the acyl groups as well as the N-terminal peptide moieties of the lipopeptide ligands are critical for their TLR2-dependent activating efficiency [30,42,43]. In this study, we were able to prove for the first time our hypothesis on the existence of a complex between 18S rRNA and Pam2 that is most likely based on the ionic interaction of positively charged amino acids in Pam2 and the negatively charged rRNA backbone. Therefore, the above-cited data could likewise depend on these structural features of rRNA. Yet, whether differences in fatty acid composition or other structural features of lipopeptides may influence the interactions between rRNA and TLR2 to promote the observed strong synergistic inflammatory response is currently under investigation.

The 18S rRNA secondary structure contains a high number of double-stranded regions and loops. To investigate whether the synergistic effect of 18S rRNA/Pam2 depends on sequence specificity and/or length, different fragments of 18S rRNA were generated. However, these 18S rRNA fragments did not show any significant differences in the expression of cytokines in the presence of Pam2. Consequently, the size, as well as the sequence of rRNA motifs, are likely not responsible for its synergistic influence, but it cannot be ruled out that secondary structural features of rRNA such as double-/single-stranded regions or stem-loops regions play a particular role. Therefore, the generation of 18S rRNA fragments with different secondary structures (hairpins, loops, etc.) will be investigated in future experiments.

We previously demonstrated, by blocking the TNF-α receptor, that longer periods of treatment of macrophages with eRNA/Pam2 included autocrine effects of TNF-α, resulting in an increased inflammatory potential [18]. It is well known that cellular interactions of TNF-α lead to the activation of NF-κB, and thereby increase not only its own expression and release at longer stimulation times but also that of other cytokines such as IL-6 [44,45]. Thus, to study only direct effects to elucidate the mechanism of activation of macrophages by 18S rRNA/Pam2 in vitro, only early time points were assessed. However, the release of cytokines, except for TNF-α, is too low after 2h of stimulation and, therefore, only the release of TNF-α was measured.

For in vivo experiments, we studied peritoneal cytokine production as an innate immune response towards the administration of the 18S rRNA/Pam2 complex. The model provides the opportunity to explore the effects of resident and recruited cells in the defined compartment of the peritoneum. In addition, for practical analytical reasons, a much larger lavage volume and higher cytokine concentrations in the peritoneum are an advantage compared to the respective analysis in blood. In fact, the preformed 18S rRNA/Pam2 complex was found to induce peritoneal cytokine production of TNF-α, IL-6, and MCP1, but not IL-1β *in vivo* in the peritoneum of mice, thereby corroborating the indicated cellular experiments. These data confirmed our previous *in vitro* findings, which demonstrated that IL-1β was not detectable in supernatants of macrophages even after 24 h of stimulation with eRNA/Pam2. Subsequently, activation of the inflammasome, which leads to the caspase-1-dependent release of Il-1β, seems not to be involved in synergistic activities of eRNA/Pam2 with the TLR2 activation [18,46]. However, it needs to be verified whether these complexes between eRNA and DAMPs/PAMPs can be formed *in vivo* as well, such as upon tissue damage or during infections. Several endogenous DAMPs such as HMGB1 were already shown to increase the sensitivity of PRRs and thereby promote the inflammatory response of viral or bacterial components [47,48]. Accordingly, it has been suggested that DAMPs, which accumulate during cell damage and aging, may play a role in the elevated severity and susceptibility of virus infections in the elderly [49]. Thus, the presence of small amounts of self eRNA released by processes of cell damage or during processes of sterile inflammation appears to sensitize the immune response by activating TLRs, induced by either a body's DAMPs such as HMGB1 or by PAMPs during viral or bacterial load [9,14].

5. Conclusions

Taken together, our results indicate that the DAMP rRNA, released from damaged tissue under situations of sterile inflammations, serves as a strong cofactor in facilitating TLR2 ligand-induced proinflammatory activities. This sensitization reaction might favor the development of specific endogenous antagonists such as RNase1 to prevent hyperinflammatory reactions during processes of sterile inflammation or infectious diseases.

Supplementary Materials: The following are available online at https://www.mdpi.com/article/10.3390/cells11091440/s1, Figure S1: Signaling pathways involved in 18S rRNA and $Pam_2\ CSK_4$-induced cytokine expression; Figure S2: MALP-2-and $Pam_3\ CSK_4$-induced *Tnf-α* mRNA expression; Figure S3: $Pam_2\ CSK_4$-induced TNF-α and IL-6 expression in endothelial cells.

Author Contributions: K.G., U.S., M.N. and S.F. performed experiments; K.G., S.B., M.N. and S.F. performed the analysis and interpretation of data; S.F., K.G., S.B., K.T.P., C.T. and B.S. designed the research; and S.F., K.G., K.T.P. and S.B. wrote the paper. All authors have read and agreed to the published version of the manuscript.

Funding: Studies were generously supported in part by a grant from the von-Behring-Röntgen Foundation (Marburg, Germany, grant number. 65–0021) to S. Fischer, K. Grote, and S. Bauer.

Institutional Review Board Statement: The animal study protocol was approved by the governmental animal ethics committee (G13/2018).

Data Availability Statement: The data presented in the current study are available on request from the corresponding author.

Acknowledgments: We thank Silke Brauschke and Michael Malysa for excellent technical assistance.

Conflicts of Interest: The authors declare no conflict of interest.

References

1. Kawai, T.; Akira, S. Toll-like receptors and their crosstalk with other innate receptors in infection and immunity. *Immunity* **2011**, *34*, 637–650. [CrossRef] [PubMed]
2. Takeda, K.; Kaisho, T.; Akira, S. Toll-like receptors. *Annu. Rev. Immunol.* **2003**, *21*, 335–376. [CrossRef] [PubMed]
3. Akira, S.; Uematsu, S.; Takeuchi, O. Pathogen recognition and innate immunity. *Cell* **2006**, *124*, 783–801. [CrossRef] [PubMed]
4. Chen, N.; Zhou, M.; Dong, X.; Qu, J.; Gong, F.; Han, Y.; Qiu, Y.; Wang, J.; Liu, Y.; Wei, Y.; et al. Epidemiological and clinical characteristics of 99 cases of 2019 novel coronavirus pneumonia in Wuhan, China: A descriptive study. *Lancet* **2020**, *395*, 507–513. [CrossRef]
5. Fischer, S.; Cabrera-Fuentes, H.A.; Noll, T.; Preissner, K.T. Impact of extracellular RNA on endothelial barrier function. *Cell Tissue Res.* **2014**, *355*, 635–645. [CrossRef]

6. Fischer, S.; Gerriets, T.; Wessels, C.; Walberer, M.; Kostin, S.; Stolz, E.; Zheleva, K.; Hocke, A.; Hippenstiel, S.; Preissner, K.T. Extracellular RNA mediates endothelial-cell permeability via vascular endothelial growth factor. *Blood* **2007**, *110*, 2457–2465. [CrossRef]
7. Fischer, S.; Gesierich, S.; Griemert, B.; Schänzer, A.; Acker, T.; Augustin, H.G.; Olsson, A.-K.; Preissner, K.T. Extracellular RNA liberates Tumor-Necrosis-Factor-α to promote tumor cell trafficking and progression. *Cancer Res.* **2013**, *73*, 5080–5089. [CrossRef]
8. Fischer, S.; Grantzow, T.; Pagel, J.-I.; Tschernatsch, M.; Sperandio, M.; Preissner, K.T.; Deindl, E. Extracellular RNA promotes leukocyte recruitment in the vascular system by mobilizing proinflammatory cytokines. *Thromb. Haemost.* **2012**, *108*, 730–741.
9. Fischer, S.; Preissner, K.T. Extracellular nucleic acids as novel alarm signals in the vascular system: Mediators of defence and disease. *Hämostaseologie* **2013**, *33*, 37–42. [CrossRef]
10. Preissner, K.T.; Fischer, S.; Deindl, E. Extracellular RNA as a Versatile DAMP and Alarm Signal That Influences Leukocyte Recruitment in Inflammation and Infection. *Front. Cell. Dev. Biol.* **2020**, *8*, 619221. [CrossRef]
11. Preissner, K.T.; Herwald, H. Extracellular nucleic acids in immunity and cardiovascular responses: Between alert and disease. *Thromb. Haemost.* **2017**, *117*, 1272–1282. [CrossRef] [PubMed]
12. Zernecke, A.; Preissner, K.T. Extracellular ribonucleic acids (RNA) enter the stage in cardiovascular disease. *Circ. Res.* **2016**, *118*, 469–479. [CrossRef] [PubMed]
13. Elsemüller, A.K.; Tomalla, V.; Gärtner, U.; Troidl, K.; Jeratsch, S.; Graumann, J.; Baal, N.; Hackstein, H.; Lasch, M.; Deindl, E.; et al. Characterization of mast cell-derived rRNA-containing microvesicles and their inflammatory impact on endothelial cells. *FASEB J.* **2019**, *33*, 5457–5467. [CrossRef] [PubMed]
14. Fischer, S.; Nasyrov, E.; Brosien, M.; Preissner, K.T.; Marti, H.H.; Kunze, R. Self-extracellular RNA promotes pro-inflammatory response of astrocytes to exogenous and endogenous danger signals. *J. Neuroinflamm.* **2021**, *18*, 252. [CrossRef] [PubMed]
15. Cabrera-Fuentes, H.A.; Ruiz-Meana, M.; Simsekyilmaz, S.; Kostin, S.; Inserte, J.; Saffarzadeh, M.; Galuska, S.P.; Vijayan, V.; Barba, I.; Barreto, G.; et al. RNase1 prevents the damaging interplay between extracellular RNA and tumour necrosis factor-alpha in cardiac ischaemia/reperfusion injury. *Thromb. Haemost.* **2014**, *112*, 1110–1119. [CrossRef] [PubMed]
16. Palazzo, A.F.; Lee, E.S. Non-coding RNA: What is functional and what is junk? *Front. Genet.* **2015**, *6*, 2. [CrossRef] [PubMed]
17. Cabrera-Fuentes, H.A.; Lopez, M.L.; McCurdy, S.; Fischer, S.; Meiler, S.; Baumer, Y.; Galuska, S.P.; Preissner, K.T.; Boisvert, W.A. Regulation of monocyte/macrophage polarisation by extracellular RNA. *Thromb. Haemost.* **2015**, *113*, 473–481. [CrossRef] [PubMed]
18. Noll, F.; Behnke, J.; Leiting, S.; Troidl, K.; Alves, G.T.; Muller-Redetzky, H.; Preissner, K.T.; Fischer, S. Self-extracellular RNA acts in synergy with exogenous danger signals to promote inflammation. *PLoS ONE* **2017**, *12*, e0190002. [CrossRef]
19. Troidl, K.; Schubert, C.; Vlacil, A.K.; Chennupati, R.; Koch, S.; Schütt, J.; Oberoi, R.; Schaper, W.; Schmitz-Rixen, T.; Schieffer, B.; et al. The Lipopeptide MALP-2 Promotes Collateral Growth. *Cells* **2020**, *9*, 997. [CrossRef]
20. Mühlradt, P.F.; Kiess, M.; Meyer, H.; Süssmuth, R.; Jung, G. Isolation, structure elucidation, and synthesis of a macrophage stimulatory lipopeptide from Mycoplasma fermentans acting at picomolar concentration. *J. Exp. Med.* **1997**, *185*, 1951–1958. [CrossRef]
21. Rutz, M.; Metzger, J.; Gellert, T.; Luppa, P.; Lipford, G.B.; Wagner, H.; Bauer, S. Toll-like receptor 9 binds single-stranded CpG-DNA in a sequence- and pH-dependent manner. *Eur. J. Immunol.* **2004**, *34*, 2541–2550. [CrossRef] [PubMed]
22. Fischer, S.; Nishio, M.; Peters, S.C.; Tschernatsch, M.; Walberer, M.; Weidemann, S.; Heidenreich, R.; Couraud, P.O.; Weksler, B.B.; Romero, I.A.; et al. Signaling mechanism of extracellular RNA in endothelial cells. *FASEB J.* **2009**, *23*, 2100–2109. [CrossRef] [PubMed]
23. Fong, T.A.; Shawver, L.K.; Sun, L.; Tang, C.; App, H.; Powell, T.J.; Kim, Y.H.; Schreck, R.; Wang, X.; Risau, W.; et al. SU5416 is a potent and selective inhibitor of the vascular endothelial growth factor receptor (Flk-1/KDR) that inhibits tyrosine kinase catalysis, tumor vascularization, and growth of multiple tumor types. *Cancer Res.* **1999**, *59*, 99–106. [PubMed]
24. Hayden, M.S.; Ghosh, S. Shared principles in NF-kappaB signaling. *Cell* **2008**, *132*, 344–362. [CrossRef]
25. Uematsu, S.; Akira, S. Toll-like receptors and innate immunity. *J. Mol. Med.* **2006**, *84*, 712–725. [CrossRef]
26. West, A.P.; Koblansky, A.A.; Ghosh, S. Recognition and signaling by toll-like receptors. *Annu. Rev. Cell Dev. Biol.* **2006**, *22*, 409–437. [CrossRef] [PubMed]
27. Black, R.A.; Rauch, C.T.; Kozlosky, C.J.; Peschon, J.J.; Slack, J.L.; Wolfson, M.F.; Castner, B.J.; Stocking, K.L.; Reddy, P.; Srinivasan, S.; et al. A metalloproteinase disintegrin that releases tumor-necrosis factor-alpha from cells. *Nature* **1997**, *385*, 729–733. [CrossRef]
28. Ozinsky, A.; Underhill, D.M.; Fontenot, J.D.; Hajjar, A.M.; Smith, K.D.; Wilson, C.B.; Schroeder, L.; Aderem, A. The repertoire for pattern recognition of pathogens by the innate immune system is defined by cooperation between toll-like receptors. *Proc. Natl. Acad. Sci. USA* **2000**, *97*, 13766–13771. [CrossRef]
29. Kang, J.Y.; Nan, X.; Jin, M.S.; Youn, S.J.; Ryu, Y.H.; Mah, S.; Han, S.H.; Lee, H.; Paik, S.G.; Lee, J.O. Recognition of lipopeptide patterns by Toll-like receptor 2-Toll-like receptor 6 heterodimer. *Immunity* **2009**, *31*, 873–884. [CrossRef]
30. Buwitt-Beckmann, U.; Heine, H.; Wiesmüller, K.H.; Jung, G.; Brock, R.; Akira, S.; Ulmer, A.J. Toll-like receptor 6-independent signaling by diacylated lipopeptides. *Europ. J. Immunol.* **2005**, *35*, 282–289. [CrossRef]
31. Buwitt-Beckmann, U.; Heine, H.; Wiesmüller, K.H.; Jung, G.; Brock, R.; Akira, S.; Ulmer, A.J. TLR1- and TLR6-independent recognition of bacterial lipopeptides. *J. Biol. Chem.* **2006**, *281*, 9049–9057. [CrossRef] [PubMed]

32. Jimenez-Dalmaroni, M.J.; Xiao, N.; Corper, A.L.; Verdino, P.; Ainge, G.D.; Larsen, D.S.; Painter, G.F.; Rudd, P.M.; Dwek, R.A.; Hoebe, K.; et al. Soluble CD36 ectodomain binds negatively charged diacylglycerol ligands and acts as a co-receptor for TLR2. *PLoS ONE* **2009**, *4*, e7411. [CrossRef] [PubMed]
33. Marre, M.L.; Petnicki-Ocwieja, T.; DeFrancesco, A.S.; Darcy, C.T.; Hu, L.T. Human integrin α(3)β(1) regulates TLR2 recognition of lipopeptides from endosomal compartments. *PLoS ONE* **2010**, *5*, e12871. [CrossRef] [PubMed]
34. Hajishengallis, G.; Wang, M.; Liang, S.; Triantafilou, M.; Triantafilou, K. Pathogen induction of CXCR4/TLR2 cross-talk impairs host defense function. *Proc. Natl. Acad. Sci. USA* **2008**, *105*, 13532–13537. [CrossRef] [PubMed]
35. Van Bergenhenegouwen, J.; Plantinga, T.S.; Joosten, L.A.; Netea, M.G.; Folkerts, G.; Kraneveld, A.D.; Garssen, J.; Vos, A.P. TLR2 & Co: A critical analysis of the complex interactions between TLR2 and coreceptors. *J. Leukoc. Biol.* **2013**, *94*, 885–902. [PubMed]
36. Liu, H.; Zhou, J.; Ma, D.; Lu, X.; Ming, S.; Shan, G.; Zhang, X.; Hou, J.; Chen, Z.; Zuo, D. Mannan binding lectin attenuates double-stranded RNA-mediated TLR3 activation and innate immunity. *FEBS Lett.* **2014**, *588*, 866–872. [CrossRef]
37. Bagchi, A.; Herrup, E.A.; Warren, H.S.; Trigilio, J.; Shin, H.S.; Valentine, C.; Hellman, J. MyD88-dependent and MyD88-independent pathways in synergy, priming, and tolerance between TLR agonists. *J. Immunol.* **2007**, *178*, 1164–1171. [CrossRef]
38. Bohnenkamp, H.R.; Papazisis, K.T.; Burchell, J.M.; Taylor-Papadimitriou, J. Synergism of Toll-like receptor-induced interleukin-12p70 secretion by monocyte-derived dendritic cells is mediated through p38 MAPK and lowers the threshold of T-helper cell type 1 responses. *Cell Immunol.* **2007**, *247*, 72–84. [CrossRef]
39. Jin, M.S.; Lee, J.O. Structures of TLR-ligand complexes. *Curr. Opin. Immunol.* **2008**, *20*, 414–419. [CrossRef]
40. Mäkelä, S.M.; Strengell, M.; Pietilä, T.E.; Osterlund, P.; Julkunen, I. Multiple signaling pathways contribute to synergistic TLR ligand-dependent cytokine gene expression in human monocyte-derived macrophages and dendritic cells. *J. Leukoc. Biol.* **2009**, *85*, 664–672. [CrossRef]
41. Napolitani, G.; Rinaldi, A.; Bertoni, F.; Sallusto, F.; Lanzavecchia, A. Selected Toll-like receptor agonist combinations synergistically trigger a T helper type 1-polarizing program in dendritic cells. *Nat. Immunol.* **2005**, *6*, 769–776. [CrossRef] [PubMed]
42. Lien, E.; Sellati, T.J.; Yoshimura, A.; Flo, T.H.; Rawadi, G.; Finberg, R.W.; Carroll, J.D.; Espevik, T.; Ingalls, R.R.; Radolf, J.D.; et al. Toll-like receptor 2 functions as a pattern recognition receptor for diverse bacterial products. *J. Biol. Chem.* **1999**, *274*, 33419–33425. [CrossRef] [PubMed]
43. Nishiguchi, M.; Matsumoto, M.; Takao, T.; Hoshino, M.; Shimonishi, Y.; Tsuji, S.; Begum, N.A.; Takeuchi, O.; Akira, S.; Toyoshima, K.; et al. Mycoplasma fermentans lipoprotein M161Ag-induced cell activation is mediated by Toll-like receptor 2: Role of N-terminal hydrophobic portion in its multiple functions. *J. Immunol.* **2001**, *166*, 2610–2616. [CrossRef] [PubMed]
44. Georgieva, E.; Leber, S.L.; Wex, C.; Garbers, C. Perturbation of the actin cytoskeleton in human hepatoma cells influences Interleukin-6 (IL-6) signaling, but not soluble IL-6 receptor generation or NF-κB activation. *Int. J. Mol. Sci.* **2021**, *22*, 7171. [CrossRef]
45. Hayden, M.S.; Ghosh, S. Regulation of NF-κB by TNF family cytokines. *Sem. Immunol.* **2014**, *26*, 253–266. [CrossRef]
46. Schroder, K.; Tschopp, J. The inflammasomes. *Cell* **2010**, *140*, 821–832. [CrossRef]
47. Yanai, H.; Ban, T.; Wang, Z.; Choi, M.K.; Kawamura, T.; Negishi, H.; Nakasato, M.; Lu, Y.; Hangai, S.; Koshiba, R.; et al. HMGB proteins function as universal sentinels for nucleic-acid-mediated innate immune responses. *Nature* **2009**, *462*, 99–103. [CrossRef]
48. Youn, J.H.; Oh, Y.J.; Kim, E.S.; Choi, J.Y.; Shin, J.-S. High mobility group box 1 protein binding to lipopolysaccharide facilitates transfer of lipopolysaccharide to CD14 and enhances lipopolysaccharide-mediated TNF-alpha production in monocytes. *J. Immunol.* **2008**, *180*, 5067–5074. [CrossRef]
49. Samy, R.P.; Lim, L.H. DAMPs and influenza virus infection in ageing. *Ageing Res. Rev.* **2015**, *24*, 83–97. [CrossRef]

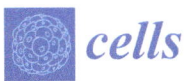

Article

Depletion of γδ T Cells Leads to Reduced Angiogenesis and Increased Infiltration of Inflammatory M1-like Macrophages in Ischemic Muscle Tissue

Christoph Arnholdt [1,2], Konda Kumaraswami [1,2], Philipp Götz [1,2], Matthias Kübler [1,2], Manuel Lasch [1,2,3] and Elisabeth Deindl [1,2,*]

1 Walter-Brendel-Centre of Experimental Medicine, University Hospital, Ludwig-Maximilians-Universität München, 81377 Munich, Germany; christoph.arnholdt@med.uni-muenchen.de (C.A.); kumaraswami.konda@med.uni-muenchen.de (K.K.); p.goetz@med.uni-muenchen.de (P.G.); matthias.kuebler@med.uni-muenchen.de (M.K.); manuel_lasch@gmx.de (M.L.)
2 Biomedical Center, Institute of Cardiovascular Physiology and Pathophysiology, Faculty of Medicine, Ludwig-Maximilians-Universität München, 82152 Planegg-Martinsried, Germany
3 Department of Otorhinolaryngology, Head and Neck Surgery, University Hospital, Ludwig-Maximilians-Universität München, 81377 Munich, Germany
* Correspondence: elisabeth.deindl@med.uni-muenchen.de; Tel.: +49-(0)-89-2180-76504

Citation: Arnholdt, C.; Kumaraswami, K.; Götz, P.; Kübler, M.; Lasch, M.; Deindl, E. Depletion of γδ T Cells Leads to Reduced Angiogenesis and Increased Infiltration of Inflammatory M1-like Macrophages in Ischemic Muscle Tissue. *Cells* 2022, *11*, 1490. https://doi.org/10.3390/cells11091490

Academic Editor: Alessandro Poggi

Received: 25 March 2022
Accepted: 27 April 2022
Published: 29 April 2022

Publisher's Note: MDPI stays neutral with regard to jurisdictional claims in published maps and institutional affiliations.

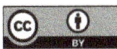

Copyright: © 2022 by the authors. Licensee MDPI, Basel, Switzerland. This article is an open access article distributed under the terms and conditions of the Creative Commons Attribution (CC BY) license (https://creativecommons.org/licenses/by/4.0/).

Abstract: γδ T cells, a small subset of T cells in blood, play a substantial role in influencing immunoregulatory and inflammatory processes. The functional impact of γδ T cells on angiogenesis in ischemic muscle tissue has never been reported and is the topic of the present work. Femoral artery ligation (FAL) was used to induce angiogenesis in the lower leg of γδ T cell depleted mice and wildtype and isotype antibody-treated control groups. Gastrocnemius muscle tissue was harvested 3 and 7 days after FAL and assessed using (immuno-)histological analyses. Hematoxylin and Eosin staining showed an increased area of tissue damage in γδ T cell depleted mice 7 days after FAL. Impaired angiogenesis was demonstrated by lower capillary to muscle fiber ratio and decreased number of proliferating endothelial cells (CD31$^+$/BrdU$^+$). γδ T cell depleted mice showed an increased number of total leukocytes (CD45$^+$), neutrophils (MPO$^+$) and neutrophil extracellular traps (NETs) (MPO$^+$/CitH3$^+$), without changes in the neutrophils to NETs ratio. Moreover, the depletion resulted in a higher macrophage count (DAPI/CD68$^+$) caused by an increase in inflammatory M1-like macrophages (CD68$^+$/MRC1$^-$). Altogether, we show that depletion of γδ T cells leads to increased accumulation of leukocytes and M1-like macrophages, along with impaired angiogenesis.

Keywords: angiogenesis; γδ T cells; gamma delta T cells; proliferation; macrophages; macrophage polarization; neutrophils; neutrophil extracellular traps; NETs; ischemia

1. Introduction

The occlusion of arterial vessels, being the main cause of the most prevalent forms of cardiovascular diseases (CVD), namely coronary heart disease (CHD), cerebrovascular accidents (CVA) and peripheral artery diseases (PAD), can often only be treated by invasive medical methods, which always present a certain risk for the patient. CVD in general have been the leading cause of death for years [1] and belong to the severe pathologies identified in SARS-CoV-2 patients [2,3]. Despite some improvements in the prevention and treatment of CHD and PAD, these diseases still represent a substantial medical burden worldwide [4]. The reduced perfusion in the affected tissue caused by the narrowing or complete occlusion of a vessel leads—without immediate treatment—to insufficient supply of oxygen and nutrients in the peripheral tissue, and after some time to ischemic tissue damage [5]. Ischemia in turn works as a stimulus to increase capillarity. This process is called angiogenesis [6,7] and can be explained by the development of new capillaries from the pre-existing vasculature, either by sprouting or by splitting; the most studied variant of angiogenesis is sprouting angiogenesis. Here, hypoxia leads to an increased release of vascular endothelial growth factor (VEGF-A), followed by a cascade which ultimately causes endothelial cells (ECs) to proliferate into the surrounding matrix and form solid sprouts [6]. Splitting angiogenesis, on the other hand, also known as intussusceptive angiogenesis, represents a process of reorganization and a strong increase in the capillary network by splitting existing vessels into two [6–8]. Unregulated angiogenesis, however, can represent the onset of cancer and various ischemic and inflammatory diseases [9]. The balance of various pro- and anti-angiogenic cytokines and enzymes, the influence of different cell types (such as ECs and pericytes and their interaction) and the components of the extracellular matrix regulate the growth and remodeling of capillary networks. Hereby, the supply of oxygen and nutrients can be ensured [10].

Under stimulation of various influencing factors, such as fMet-Leu-Phe (fMLP) or tumor necrosis factor α (TNF-α), neutrophils can release a large amount of VEGF-A and thus make a crucial contribution to angiogenic growth by enhancing endothelial cell (EC) proliferation [11–13]. In addition, several studies have shown a positive angiogenic effect through neutrophil extracellular traps (NETs) [14,15]. However, the enhancement of angiogenesis depends on a sensitive balance of NET formation, since excessive accumulation of NETs may in turn lead to cytotoxic damage to ECs and impaired tissue repair [16,17]. Macrophages also play a fundamental role in the angiogenic cascade by secreting growth factors, cytokines and enzymes, and facilitating neovascularization by modifying the extracellular matrix [18–21]. In addition, the polarization of macrophages was detected to have a crucial impact on angiogenesis: tissue containing predominantly anti-inflammatory and regenerative macrophages of the M2 phenotype showed enhanced angiogenesis, whereas an accumulation of pro-inflammatory M1-like macrophages led to a deteriorating angiogenic process [22,23].

B and T lymphocytes represent, among many other cell types, the cellular components of the immune system, which are also particularly essential elements of the adaptive immune system. In addition to their role as actors in the immune defense, it has been shown that different subgroups of B and T lymphocytes have a critical role in regulating angiogenesis as well [24–27]. With only 3–5% of all $CD3^+$ cells and compared to $\alpha\beta$ T cells, $\gamma\delta$ T cells present only a small fraction of all T lymphocytes in peripheral blood [28]. The difference between these two subgroups lies in the different structure of the T cell receptor, which consists in the $\alpha\beta$ T cells of an alpha and a beta chain, whereas a gamma and a delta chain form the receptor of $TCR\gamma\delta^+$ T cells. In contrast to $\alpha\beta$ T cells, $\gamma\delta$ T cells do not contain CD4 or CD8 co-receptors; thus, antigen recognition is not restricted to MHC molecules [29]. However, $\gamma\delta$ T cells interact with a broad range of different antigens, such as small peptides, proteins, phospholipids or sulfatides. $\gamma\delta$ T cells, natural killer (NK) cells and other cell types express the receptor natural killer group 2 member D (NKG2D). This receptor can bind MHC class 1-related ligands, such as MHC class I chain-related protein A and B (MICA and MICB) and UL16-binding protein (ULBP) [30], whose expression can be induced by stress, transformation of cells and DNA damage, and thus activate $\gamma\delta$ T cells [31–35].

These data indicate that the depletion of $\gamma\delta$ T cells might have an influencing effect on the recruitment of leukocytes, polarization of macrophages and angiogenesis in ischemic muscle tissue. Interestingly, the direct impact of $\gamma\delta$ T cells on sterile, ischemia-induced angiogenesis has never been investigated and is the subject of the present study.

2. Materials and Methods

2.1. Animal Protocol and Treatments

The following procedures were all performed after approval from the Bavarian Animal Care and Use Committee (ethical approval code: ROB-55.2Vet-2532.Vet_02-17-99) in strict accordance with German and NIH animal welfare and legislation guidelines. To investigate the role of $\gamma\delta$ T cells, 8–10 week old C57BL/6J (Charles River Laboratories, Sulzfeld, Germany) mice with $\gamma\delta$ T cell depletion were compared to wildtype C57BL/6J mice without any treatment and—as negative control to exclude unrecognized side effects caused by the depleting antibody—to C57BL/6J mice treated with an isotype control antibody (ISO). For γδ T cell depletion, a single dose of 200–250 µg of anti-γδ TCR mAb clone UC7-13D5 (cat. no. 107517, BioLegend, San Diego, CA, USA) was injected intravenously (i.v.) one day before the surgical intervention. The control group was treated with the same concentration of Ultra-LEAF™ Purified Armenian Hamster IgG isotype control antibody clone HTK888 (cat. no. 400959, BioLegend). All mice were administered 1.25 mg bromodeoxyuridine (BrdU, dissolved in phosphate-buffered saline (PBS)) (Sigma-Aldrich, St. Louis, MO, USA) i.p. daily, beginning directly after surgery.

2.2. Experimental Procedures and Tissue Harvesting

Before the surgery, a combination of anesthetics consisting of midazolam (5.0 mg/kg, Ratiopharm GmbH, Ulm, Germany), fentanyl (0.05 mg/kg, CuraMED Pharma, Karlsruhe, Germany) and medetomidine (0.5 mg/kg, Pfister Pharma, Berlin, Germany) were injected subcutaneously. After anesthetizing, unilateral ligation of the right femoral artery was performed, while the same operation was done on the left side without closing the surgical thread to obtain an internal sham control [5]. The operation led to unilateral initiation of angiogenesis in the gastrocnemius muscle, which could be investigated by further tissue processing. Tissue collection was performed on day 3 or day 7 after ligation of the femoral artery. For this purpose, after another anesthesia, the hindlimb was perfused first with adenosine buffer (5% bovine serum albumin (BSA, Sigma-Aldrich) and 1% adenosine (Sigma-Aldrich, dissolved in PBS)) and for fixation of the muscle tissue with 3% paraformaldehyde (PFA, Merck, Darmstadt, Germany; dissolved in PBS, pH 7.4). Finally, gastrocnemius muscle from both legs was harvested and stored at $-80\ °C$ after being embedded in Tissue-Tek compound (Sakura Finetek Germany GmbH, Staufen, Germany).

2.3. Histology and Immunohistology

The cryopreserved tissue blocks of the gastrocnemius muscle were cut into 8–10 µm thick slices. Gastrocnemius muscle sections of day 3 aFAL were used for neutrophil and NETs staining, whereas ECs, leukocytes, macrophages, activated VEGF receptor 2 (Tyr1175) and the extent of ischemic tissue damage were analyzed in tissue samples isolated 7 days aFAL.

To investigate the area of ischemic muscle tissue out of the total gastrocnemius muscle on day 7 aFAL, Hematoxylin and Eosin (H&E) staining was conducted.

Endothelial cells were stained along with BrdU and leukocytes (CD45). Therefore, cryo-sections were incubated with pre-warmed 1N HCL at 37 °C for 30 min in a humid chamber. The tissue was then permeabilized using 0.2% Triton X-100 solution (AppliChem GmbH, Darmstadt, Germany; 10 min at room temperature (RT)) in $1 \times$ PBS/0.5% BSA/0.1% Tween-20 (AppliChem GmbH) and blocked with 10% goat serum (Abcam, cat. ab7481, Cambridge, UK; dissolved in $1 \times$ PBS/0.5% BSA/0.1% Tween-20) for 1 h at RT. BrdU staining was now performed using the primary antibody mRat BrdU (Abcam, ab6326; diluted 1:50 in blocking solution; incubated at 4 °C overnight) and the secondary antibody GantiRat Alexa Fluor 546 (Thermo Fisher Scientific, A11081, Waltham, MA, USA; diluted 1:100 in PBST; incubated at RT for 1 h). After secondary blocking with $1 \times$ PBS/4% BSA/0.1% Tween-20 (for 30 min at RT), endothelial cells were stained using the antibody Ranti-mouse CD31-Alexa Fluor® 647 (BioLegend, 102516, diluted 1:50 in $1 \times$ PBS/0.1% Tween-20 (PBS-T); for 2 h at RT), and leukocytes were stained using anti-CD45-Alexa Fluor® 488 antibody (BioLegend, 11-0451-85, diluted 1:100 in PBS-T for 2 h at RT).

To characterize angiogenesis by VEGF receptor 2 activation at tyrosine 1175 in addition to quantification of capillaries in relation to the number of muscle fibers and Brdu$^+$ ECs per muscle fiber, co-staining of CD31 and phospho-VEGF receptor 2 at tyrosine 1175 (19A10) rabbit mAb (Cell Signaling Technology, 2478, Danvers, MA, USA; dilution 1:100 in PBS) was performed. Donkey anti-rabbit IgG Alexa Fluor® 488 antibody (Thermo Fisher Scientific, A-21206, dilution 1:200 in PBS) served as a secondary antibody for the phospho-VEGFR-2 (Tyr1175) antibody. All remaining staining steps were analogous to the CD31/CD45/BrdU staining.

To study neutrophils and NETs on muscle tissue collected 3 days aFAL, fixation was performed with 4% PFA (for 10 min at RT), permeabilization with 0.2% Triton X-100 (dissolved in 1 × PBS/0.5% BSA/0.1% Tween-20 for 2 min at RT) and blocking with 10% donkey serum (Abcam, ab7475; dissolved in 1 × PBS/0.5% BSA/0.1% Tween-20 for 1 h at RT). Subsequently, incubation with primary antibodies anti-citrullinated histone H3 (Cit-H3; polyclonal rabbit anti-Histone H3 (citrulline R2 + R8 + R17), Abcam, ab5103, diluted 1:100 in blocking solution) and anti-myeloperoxidase (MPO; R&D Systems, AF3667, Minneapolis, MN, USA; diluted 1:20 in blocking solution) at 4 °C overnight and incubation with secondary antibodies donkey anti-goat Alexa Fluor 594 (Thermo Fisher Scientific, A-11058, diluted 1:100 in PBS-T) and donkey anti-rabbit Alexa Fluor 488 antibody (Thermo Fisher Scientific, A-21206, diluted 1:200 in PBS-T) for 1 h at RT was performed.

To investigate macrophages and their polarization, sections were fixed (4% PFA, 5 min at RT), blocked (4% BSA, 1 h at RT) and incubated with the primary antibody anti-MRC1 (mannose receptor C-type 1; Abcam, ab64693, diluted 1:200 in PBS; incubation overnight at 4 °C) and secondary antibody donkey anti-rabbit IgG Alexa Fluor 546 (Thermo Fisher Scientific, A-10040, dilution 1:200 in PBS-T; incubation for 1 h at RT). Additionally, incubation with anti-CD68 Alexa Fluor 488 antibody (Abcam, ab201844, diluted 1:200 in PBS-T) overnight at 4 °C was performed.

For more detailed classification of macrophage populations into pro- and anti-inflammatory macrophages, sections were permeabilized (0.2% Triton X-100 in PBS; 10 min at RT) and incubated with either purified anti-mouse IL-10 antibody (BioLegend, 5050001, dilution 1:50 in PBS) or TNF-α monoclonal antibody (MP6-XT22, Thermo Fisher Scientific, 14-7321-81, diluted 1:100 in PBS) overnight at 4 °C. For IL-10, as well as TNF-α, secondary antibody donkey anti-rat IgG Alexa Fluor Plus 647 (Thermo Fisher Scientific, A48272, diluted 1:200 in PBS; incubation for 1 h at RT) was used.

Additionally, to label nucleic DNA, all sections were counter-stained with DAPI (Thermo Fisher Scientific, 62248, diluted 1:1000 in PBS; incubation for 10 min at RT) and mounted with Dako mounting medium (Agilent, Santa Clara, CA, USA).

Using the 20× objective (415 µm × 415 µm) of a confocal LSM 880 (Carl-Zeiss Jena GmbH, Jena, Germany) and the 20× objective (630 µm × 475 µm) of an epifluorescence microscope (Leica DM6 B, Leica microsystems, Wetzlar, Germany), stained gastrocnemius muscle tissue was analyzed. To comparatively analyze the CD31/CD45/BrdU/DAPI, CD31/Phospho-VEGF receptor 2 (Tyr1175) and CD68/MRC1/TNF-α or IL-10/DAPI stains of the 3 groups (wildtype, isotype control, and TCR γ/δ depletion), epifluorescence microscope was used. For this purpose, we selected 5 defined areas of ischemic muscle tissue to count cells. To evaluate angiogenesis, we first counted all $CD45^+/DAPI^+$ cells (leukocytes) and then inferred $CD31^+/CD45^-$ cells as ECs. To analyze proliferating ECs, we also checked for colocalization with an intranuclear positive BrdU signal. Macrophages ($CD68^+$ cells) were first counted and then differentiated by their polarization using the anti-MRC1 antibody. H&E stainings were also imaged using the epifluorescence microscope. For neutrophils and NETs quantification, 5 confocal pictures were analyzed.

To obtain a negative control of our immunohistochemical staining and to guarantee a valid assessment of the immunofluorescence images, the primary antibody was omitted for unconjugated antibodies (BrdU, MRC1, MPO, CitH3, phospho-VEGF receptor 2 (Tyr1175), IL-10, TNF-α), whereas the sham-operated muscles were comparatively assessed for conjugated antibodies (CD31, CD45, CD68, DAPI).

For all immunohistochemical studies, gastrocnemius muscles of 5 mice per group were evaluated. In addition, for all quantitative studies, we evaluated 5 images from ischemic regions of the gastrocnemius muscle per mouse per group.

The open-source program ImageJ (Wayne Rasband, retired from National Institutes of Health) and ZEN 3.2 software (blue edition, Carl Zeiss AG, Wetzlar, Germany) were used for cell counting and measurements of the percentage of tissue.

2.4. Statistical Analyses

Statistical analyses and graph plottings were performed using GraphPad Prism 8 (GraphPad Software, La Jolla, CA, USA). All data are stated as means ± standard error of the mean (SEM). Statistically significant results were considered at $p \leq 0.05$.

2.5. Graphical Abstract

The graphical abstract was created with Biorender.com (accessed on 24 April 2022).

3. Results

To investigate the influence of γδ T lymphocytes on angiogenesis in ischemic muscle tissue, we used the well-established murine hindlimb model of ischemia [5]. For that purpose, the right femoral artery was ligated in a surgical procedure, while the left leg was sham operated. This led to unilateral reduced perfusion of the lower leg, resulting in ischemia in the gastrocnemius muscle. All investigations were performed comparatively between wildtype (WT), isotype antibody-treated (ISO), and γδ T cell depleted (TCRγδ depl.) mice.

3.1. γδ T Cell Depleted Mice Show Increased Ischemic Tissue Damage

To evaluate and compare the tissue damage of WT, ISO and γδ T cell depleted mice, H&E stains were performed on gastrocnemius muscles collected on day 7 after femoral artery ligation. As expected, no ischemic damage was found in samples of sham-operated legs in any group of mice (data not shown). In the gastrocnemius muscles of the occluded side, ischemic damage was found in all muscles (Figure 1a,b), with a significantly increased area of ischemic tissue damage in the γδ T cell depleted group (Figure 1c), while gastrocnemius muscles of the ISO and the WT group showed an almost similar extent of tissue damage.

3.2. γδ T Cell Depletion Leads to Reduced Capillarity

To investigate the specific influence of γδ T cells on angiogenesis, the capillary to muscle fiber ratio of ischemic muscle tissue collected 7 days aFAL was analyzed using CD31/CD45/BrdU/DAPI staining. CD31 antibody was used as an endothelial cell marker, CD45 as a panleukocyte marker, BrdU in combination with CD31 as a marker for proliferating ECs, and DAPI to stain nuclei. To exclude CD31$^+$ leukocytes, only CD31$^+$/CD45$^-$/DAPI$^+$ cells were counted as ECs. γδ T cell depleted mice showed a decreased capillary to muscle fiber ratio compared to WT and ISO mice (Figure 2a,c). In addition, a decreased ratio of proliferating ECs per muscle fiber was observed in γδ T cell depleted mice (Figure 2b,c). WT and ISO mice showed both a similar capillary to muscle fiber ratio and a similar ratio of proliferating ECs per muscle fiber (2 a,b,c). The non-ischemic muscles isolated from sham-operated mice in all three groups showed no significant differences in capillarity or in the ratio of proliferating ECs per muscle fiber (data not shown).

3.3. γδ T Cell Depletion Leads to Reduced Activation of VEGF Receptor 2 (Tyr1175)

To examine the influence of γδ T cells on the phosphorylation of VEGF receptor 2 at tyrosine 1175, and thus its activation, muscle tissue collected on day 3 aFAL was triple stained for phospho-VEGF receptor 2 (Tyr1175), CD31 and DAPI. γδ T cell depleted mice showed significantly decreased activated VEGF receptor 2 (Tyr1175) compared to WT and ISO mice (Figure 3a,b). In nonischemic muscle tissue of sham-operated mice, no significant difference in the number of activated VEGF receptor 2 (Tyr1175) was found in all three groups (data not shown).

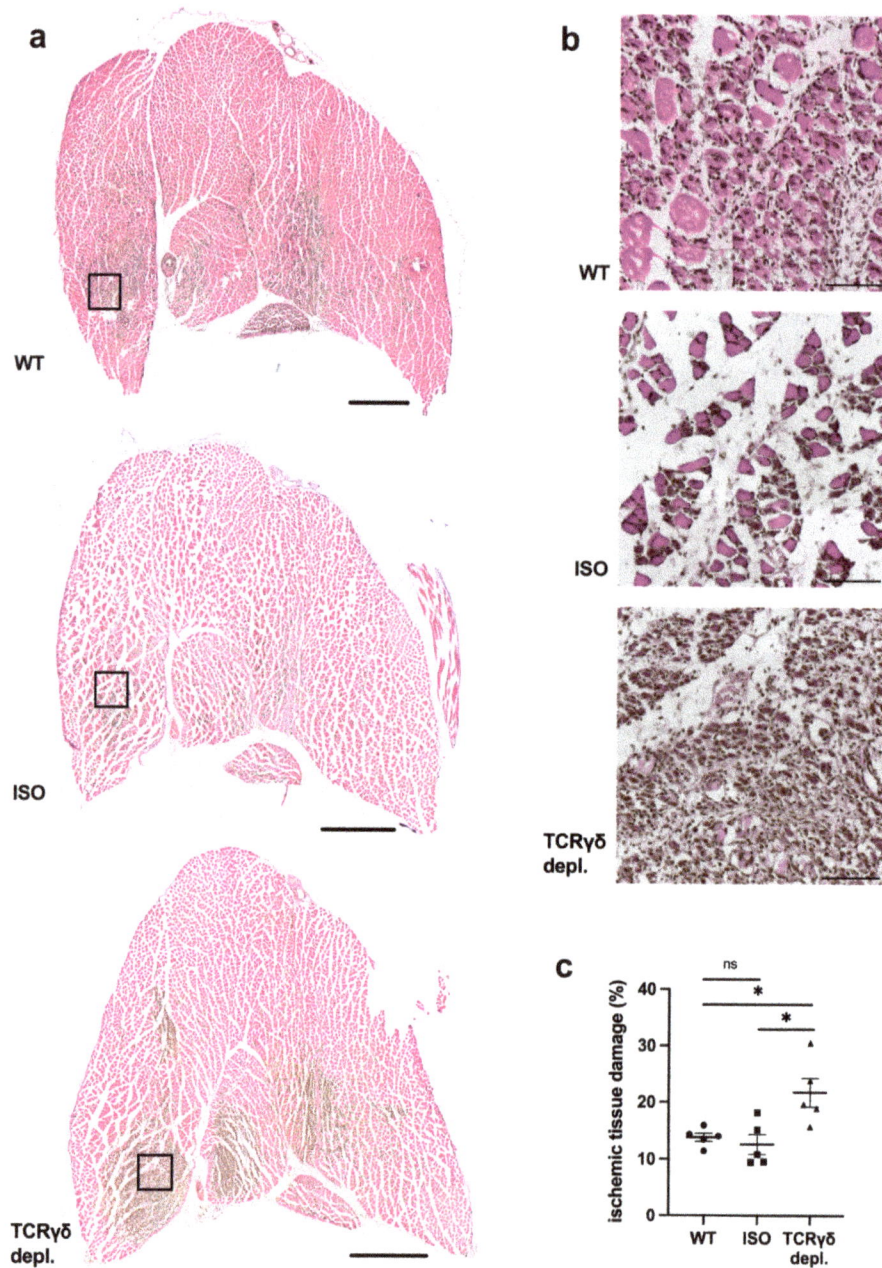

Figure 1. γδ T cell depleted mice show increased ischemic tissue damage. (**a**) Representative H&E pictures of gastrocnemius muscles of wildtype (WT) (top), isotype antibody-treated (ISO) (middle) and γδ T cell depleted mice (bottom) 7 days after femoral artery ligation (aFAL). Scale bars: 1000 μm. (**b**) Detailed images of the black boxes shown in (**a**). Scale bars: 100 μm. (**c**) The scatter plot shows the area of ischemic tissue damage (%) of WT, ISO and TCRγδ T cell depleted mice 7 days aFAL. Data are means ± SEM, n = 5 per group. * p < 0.05, ns ≥ 0.05 (WT vs. ISO vs. TCRγδ depletion) by one-way ANOVA with the Tukey's multiple comparisons test.

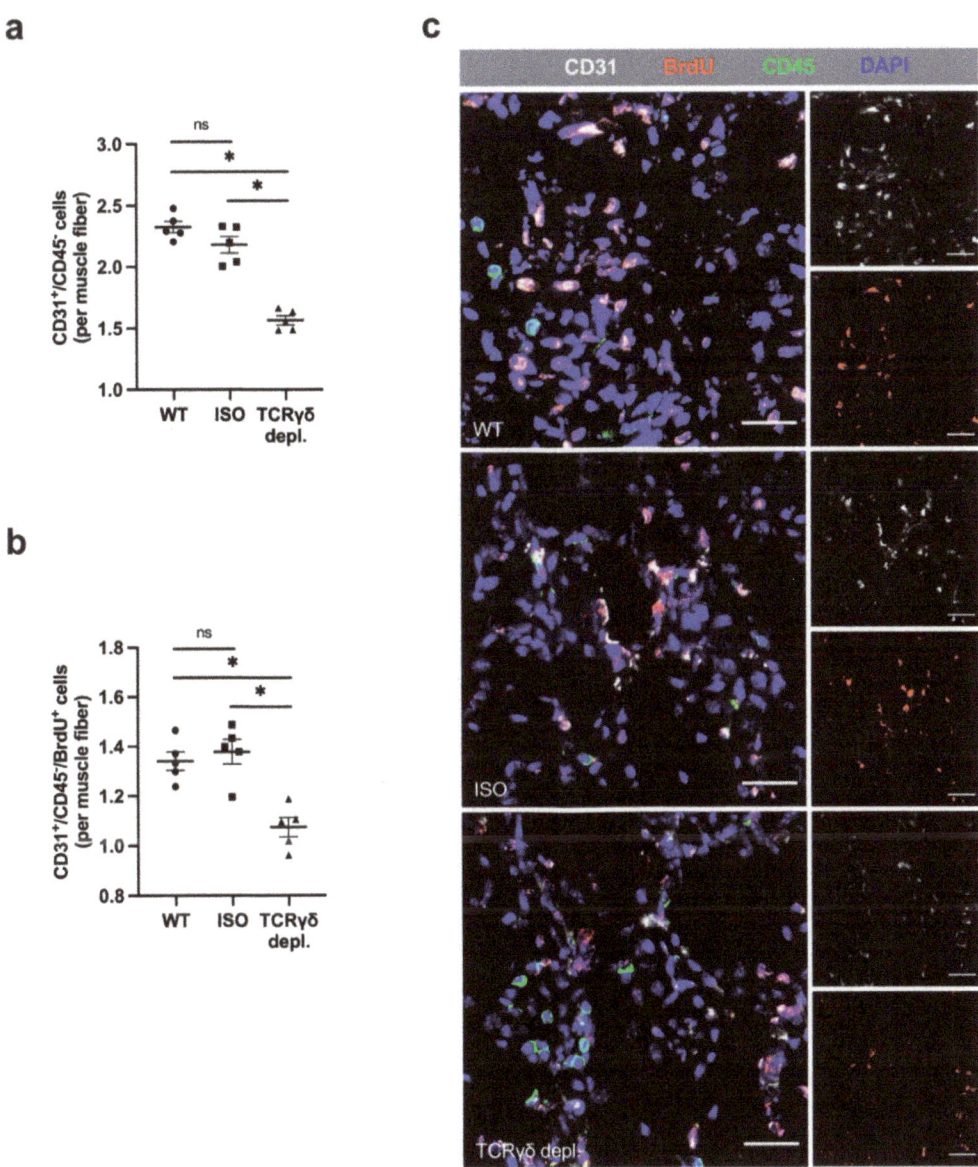

Figure 2. Absence of γδ T cells decreases angiogenesis. Scatter plots show the number of (**a**) endothelial cells (CD31$^+$/CD45$^-$) and (**b**) proliferating endothelial cells (CD31$^+$/CD45$^-$/BrdU$^+$) per muscle fiber of ischemic gastrocnemius muscles of WT, ISO and γδ T cell depleted mice 7 days after femoral artery ligation (aFAL). Data are means ± SEM, n = 5 per group. * p < 0.05, ns ≥ 0.05 (WT vs. ISO vs. TCRγδ T cell depletion) by one-way ANOVA with the Tukey's multiple comparisons test. (**c**) Representative images of ischemic gastrocnemius muscles of WT (top), isotype antibody-treated (middle) and TCRγδ T cell depleted mice (bottom) 7 days aFAL. Single channel pictures (small images) show endothelial cells (CD31, gray) and proliferating cells (BrdU, red). Merged images also show leukocytes (CD45, green) and nuclei (DAPI, blue). Scale bars: 30 μm.

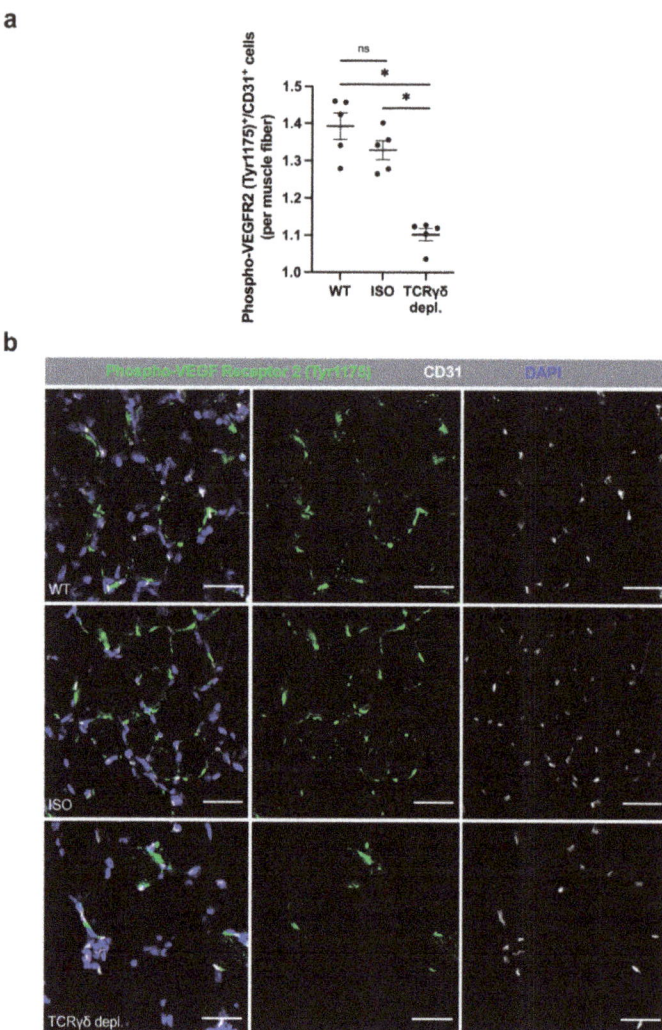

Figure 3. γδ T cell depletion leads to reduced activation of VEGF receptor 2 (Tyr1175). (**a**) The scatter plot shows the number of VEGF receptor 2 (Tyr1175)/CD31 double-positive endothelial cells (Phospho-VEGF receptor 2 (Tyr1175)$^+$/CD31$^+$) per muscle fiber in ischemic gastrocnemius muscles of WT, ISO and TCRγδ T cell depleted mice 3 days after femoral artery ligation (aFAL). Data are means ± SEM, n = 5 per group. * $p < 0.05$, ns ≥ 0.05 (WT vs. ISO vs. TCRγδ depletion) by one-way ANOVA with the Tukey's multiple comparisons test. (**b**) Representative images of ischemic gastrocnemius muscles of wildtype (WT, top), isotype antibody-treated (ISO, middle) and TCRγδ T cell depleted mice (TCRγδ depl., bottom) 3 days aFAL. The VEGF receptor 2 was stained with an antibody recognizing the activated phospho-VEGF receptor 2 (Tyr1175) form (green). Endothelial cells were stained with an antibody against CD31 (white), while nuclei were labeled using DAPI (blue). Scale bars: 30 μm.

3.4. γδ T Cell Depleted Mice Show Enhanced Leukocyte Infiltration

To investigate the infiltration of leukocytes in ischemic tissue, we analyzed the tissue obtained on day 7 aFAL using the pan-leukocyte marker CD45. The ischemic area of the γδ T cell depleted group showed a significantly increased number of CD45$^+$ leukocytes per mm² and accordingly total number of leukocytes compared to the wildtype and isotype control groups (Figure 4a,b). Without initiation of ischemia (sham operation), there was no detectable difference in the number of CD45⁺ cells in the tissue among all three different treatment groups (Supplementary Materials, Figure S1).

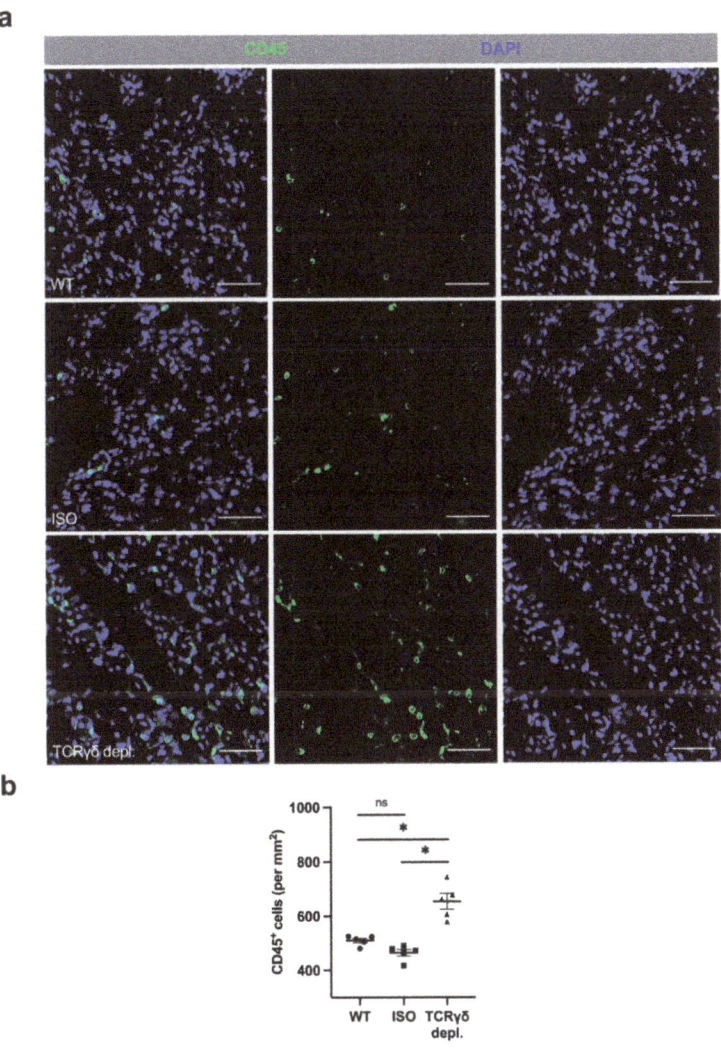

Figure 4. Mice lacking γδ T cells showed increased accumulation of leukocytes in ischemic muscle tissue. (**a**) Representative immunofluorescence images of analyzed gastrocnemius muscles of WT (top), isotype antibody-treated (middle) and TCR γδ T cell depleted mice (bottom) 7 days after femoral artery ligation (aFAL). Leukocytes were stained with an antibody against CD45 (green), while nuclei were labeled using DAPI (blue). Scale bars: 50 μm. (**b**) The scatter plot shows the absolute number of leukocytes (CD45⁺) per mm² in ischemic gastrocnemius muscle tissue from WT, ISO and TCR γδ T cell depleted mice 7 days aFAL. Data shown are means ± SEM, n = 5 per group, a defined area of 1.5 mm² of ischemic muscle was analyzed per mouse. * $p < 0.05$, ns ≥ 0.05 (WT vs. ISO vs. TCR γδ depletion) by one-way ANOVA with the Tukey's multiple comparisons test.

3.5. γδ T Cell Depleted Mice Show Higher Amount of Neutrophils

In order to assess the total number of neutrophils and the formation of NETs, muscle tissue collected on day 3 aFAL was triple stained for myeloperoxidase (MPO), for citrullinated histone H3 (CitH3) as well as for DAPI. MPO$^+$/DAPI$^+$ cells were counted as neutrophils and MPO$^+$/CitH3$^+$/DAPI$^+$ cells were classified as NETs. The evaluation showed a significantly increased number of neutrophils in muscle tissue of γδ T cell depleted mice compared to WT and isotype control antibody-treated mice (Figure 5a,d). In addition, the amount of NETs per mm^2 was significantly increased in comparison to the control groups (Figure 5b,d). However, the percentage of NETs related to the total number of neutrophils showed no significant differences in all three groups (Figure 5c,d). In nonischemic muscles of sham-operated mice, almost no neutrophils or NETs could be found in all three groups (Supplementary Materials, Figure S2). Moreover, there was no difference in the NETs to neutrophil ratio (data not shown).

3.6. γδ T Cell Depletion Leads to Increased Number of Macrophages with Inflammatory M1-like Polarization

To analyze the number and polarization of recruited macrophages in the gastrocnemius muscle, tissue collected 7 days aFAL was stained for CD68 and the mannose receptor C-type 1 (MRC1) to differentiate between M1-like polarized macrophages and M2-like polarized macrophages. CD68$^+$/MRC1$^+$/DAPI$^+$ signals were interpreted as M2-like polarized macrophages, whereas M1-like polarized macrophages were defined as MRC1-negative cells (CD68$^+$/MRC1$^-$/DAPI$^+$).

A significantly increased total number of macrophages was found in γδ T cell depleted mice in comparison to wildtype and isotype control antibody-treated mice (Figure 6a,d). Examination of macrophage polarization showed a significant increase in the absolute count of MRC1-negative macrophages (M1-like macrophages) in γδ T cell depleted mice compared to the two control groups, whereas no difference in the number of M2-like macrophages was found in all three groups (Figure 6b,c,d). To further investigate whether MRC1-negative macrophages (CD68$^+$/MRC1$^-$) show inflammatory features, co-staining of CD68 and MRC1, together with TNF-α as a pro-inflammatory marker, was performed (see Supplementary Materials, Figure S3). Indeed, our results evidenced that virtually all CD68$^+$/MRC1$^-$ macrophages expressed TNF-α and identified them as inflammatory macrophages. In contrast, all CD68$^+$/MRC1$^+$ macrophages expressed IL-10, identifying them as anti-inflammatory macrophages (see Supplementary Materials, Figure S4).

In non-ischemic muscles of sham-operated mice, no difference was found between all three groups either regarding the number of macrophages or their polarization (Supplementary Materials, Figure S5).

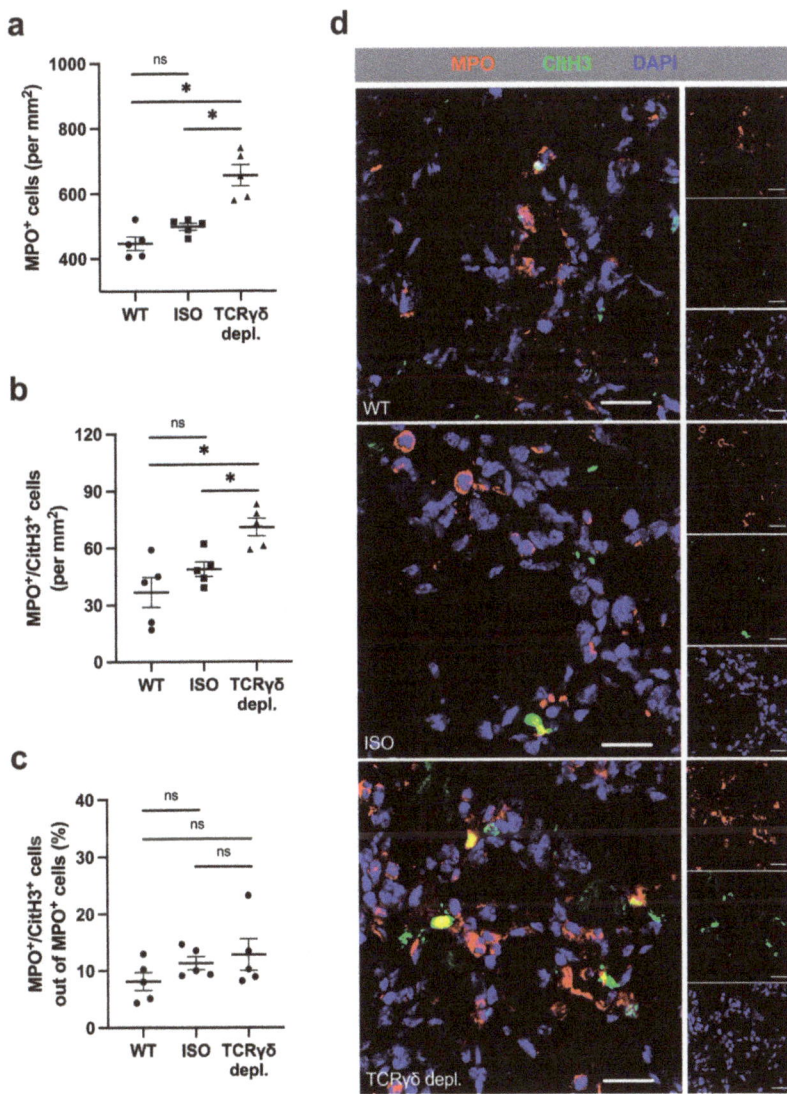

Figure 5. Absence of γδ T cells results in increased accumulation of neutrophils without affecting the formation of neutrophil extracellular traps. The scatter plots show (**a**) the total number of neutrophils (myeloperoxidase; MPO$^+$ cells) per mm^2 (upper plot), (**b**) the occurrence of NETs (MPO$^+$/CitH3$^+$ (citrullinated histone 3)) per mm^2 (middle plot), and (**c**) the relative proportion of NETs positive MPO$^+$ cells of all MPO$^+$ cells (lower plot) in the ischemic gastrocnemius muscle tissue of mice of the WT, isotype antibody-treated and γδ T cell depleted group 3 days after femoral artery ligation (aFAL). Data are means ± SEM, n = 5 per group. * p < 0.05, ns ≥ 0.05 (WT vs. ISO vs. TCR γδ depletion) by one-way ANOVA with the Tukey's multiple comparisons test. A defined area of 1.5 mm^2 of ischemic gastrocnemius muscle tissue was analyzed per mouse. (**d**) Representative immunofluorescence images of ischemic gastrocnemius muscles from WT (top), ISO (middle) and TCR γδ T cell depleted mice (bottom) 3 days aFAL. Images show neutrophils (MPO$^+$/DAPI$^+$), NETs (MPO$^+$/CitH3$^+$/DAPI$^+$) and nuclei (DAPI$^+$) labeled with anti-MPO (red), anti-CitH3 (green) and DAPI (blue). Scale bars: 20 μm.

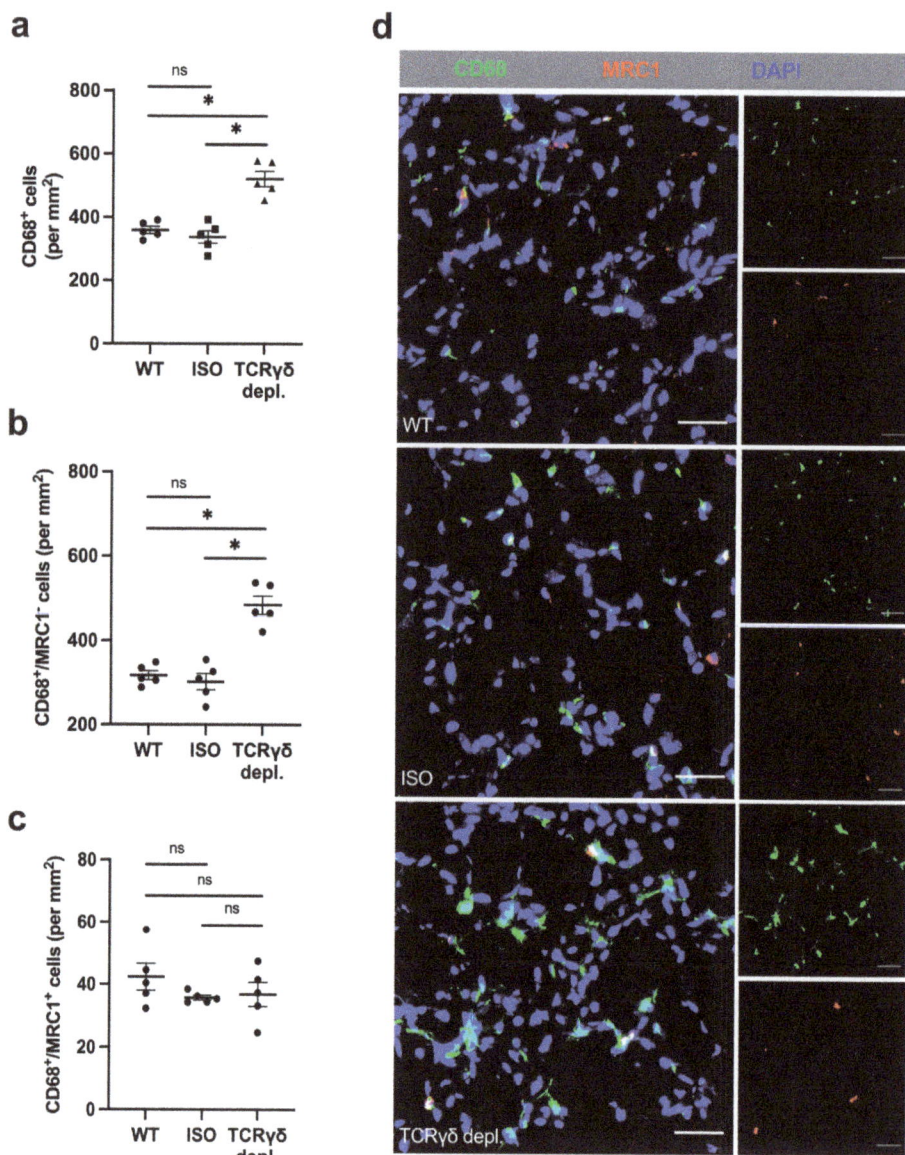

Figure 6. Depletion of γδ T cells leads to an increased number of M1-like polarized macrophages. Scatter plots show the absolute number of (**a**) all macrophages (CD68$^+$) per mm^2 (top plot), (**b**) MRC1-negative macrophages (CD68$^+$/MRC1$^-$ (mannose receptor C-type 1)) (middle plot) and (**c**) MRC1-positive macrophages (CD68$^+$/MRC1$^+$) (bottom plot) in ischemic gastrocnemius muscle tissue of wildtype (WT), isotype (ISO) and TCR γδ T cell depleted mice 7 days aFAL. Data are means ± SEM, n = 5 per group. * p < 0.05, ns ≥ 0.05 (WT vs. ISO vs. TCR γδ depletion) by one-way ANOVA with the Tukey's multiple comparisons test. (**d**) Representative immunofluorescence images of analyzed ischemic muscle tissue of WT, ISO and TCR γδ T cell depleted mice. Macrophages (CD68$^+$/DAPI$^+$) were stained with antibodies targeting CD68 (green), MRC1 (red) and DAPI (blue). CD68$^+$/MRC1$^-$/DAPI$^+$ cells were defined as M1-like polarized macrophages and CD68$^+$/MRC1$^+$/DAPI$^+$ cells as M2-like polarized macrophages. Scale bars: 30 μm.

4. Discussion

In the present study, the influence of γδ T lymphocytes on the process of angiogenesis was studied. Our data demonstrated that the depletion of γδ T cells results in increased ischemic tissue damage and impaired angiogenesis. Increased infiltration of immune cells (CD45+ cells) was based on an increased number of neutrophils and macrophages. In addition, we found that the higher number of macrophages in γδ T cell depleted mice was due to a strong increase in inflammatory TNF-α$^+$ M1-like polarized macrophages.

Neutrophils represent the first recruited cells of the innate immune system in our murine ischemic hindlimb model leading to inflammation and angiogenesis [36]. Their influence on angiogenesis is characterized by phagocytosis, removal of cell debris, participation in tissue repair and delivery of various growth factors [36]. Under hypoxic conditions, neutrophils play an important role in the initiation of angiogenesis by secreting VEGF-A and providing MMPs [37–39]. MMPs released by neutrophils, especially MMP-9, are responsible for the degradation of extracellular matrix components and through this mechanism are able to release further growth factors, including VEGF-A, which are bound to the extracellular matrix. The singularity of neutrophils among immune cells is their ability to release MMP-9 without the tissue inhibitor of metalloproteinases (TIMP), an endogenous inhibitor of MMP-9, and thus can positively influence angiogenesis [38]. However, our data, showing increased numbers of neutrophils with decreased angiogenesis in the γδ T cell depleted group, suggest that neutrophils may have had a negative effect on the angiogenic process. In addition to the pro-angiogenic properties of neutrophils, many reports have uncovered limiting effects on angiogenesis as well: In vitro studies have shown that upon proinflammatory stimulation, neutrophils can release proteolytically active elastase, which can cleave plasminogen to angiostatin fragments [40]. The resulting angiostatin fragments, comprising kringle domains 1–3, show an inhibitory effect on endothelial cell proliferation by degrading basic-fibroblast growth factor (bFGF) and VEGF [40,41]. Furthermore, the release of α-defensins by neutrophils can inhibit angiogenesis by preventing endothelial cell adhesion and blocking VEGF-induced endothelial cell proliferation [42]. In an ischemia-reperfusion injury (IRI) model in the lung, liver, kidney and intestine, Funken et al. showed that the absence of γδ T cells led to increased neutrophil recruitment, which is in line with our results [43]. The simultaneously higher tissue damage could also be a result of the release of reactive oxygen species (ROS) as neutrophils are known to release ROS, which may entail endothelial dysfunction and increased tissue damage [44].

Moreover, neutrophils have multiple strategies in the context of immune regulation, pathogen clearance and disease pathology. Phagocytosis, secretion of specialized granules and release of NETs are the three most important mechanisms to exert these tasks [45]. In particular, the formation of NETs and their impact on inflammatory processes has received increasing attention in recent years. Here, we evaluated by immunohistological analysis the neutrophil-derived formation of neutrophil extracellular traps (NETs) using MPO/CitH3 co-staining. We found an increased number of NETs, but no difference in the ratio of NETs to neutrophils. Hence, the depletion of γδ T cells does not influence the formation of NETs in our experimental setup. NETs are described as extracellular, web-like structures consisting of globular protein domains and DNA from neutrophils [46]. Regarding angiogenesis, different evidence was obtained: Aldabbous et al. demonstrated a positive angiogenic effect of NETs in studies of patients with pulmonary hypertension in vivo and in vitro [14]. However, a highly increased incidence of NETs did not seem to have any further beneficial effect on angiogenesis. Rather, a balance of NETs seems to be important for a positive angiogenic microenvironment [16]. Especially in wound healing, NET formation was not associated with improved angiogenesis, but with increased tissue damage [17,47]. Based on our data showing an increased occurrence of NETs caused by an increased number of neutrophils, we suggest that γδ T-cell depletion led to a pro-inflammatory NET formation that contributed to increased tissue damage and decreased angiogenesis.

Leukocytes with their manifold properties play a crucial role in the context of angiogenesis. The ischemic stimulus of damaged tissue resulting in inflammation leads to infiltration of leukocytes, whose transmigration to the tissue is facilitated by increased permeability of the endothelium [48]. Infiltrated leukocytes begin to remove cell debris, enhance local inflammation, and recruit additional immune cells, including neutrophils and macrophages. The release of pro-angiogenic factors, including VEGF-A [49], and proteins such as matrix metalloproteinase 9 (MMP9), responsible for remodeling of the extracellular matrix, contribute to further alteration of the microenvironment [23,36,50]. Rani et al. showed in a mouse model, studying the inflammatory process of acute lung injury (ALI) after trauma-hemorrhage (TH), that an absence of γδ T cells leads to an increase in inflammatory cells, such as monocytes or granulocytes [51]. These findings correspond to our results of increased infiltration of leukocytes, i.e., neutrophils and macrophages, and indicate that γδ T cells have a regulatory effect on the recruitment of different leukocyte subtypes. Another aspect that is in line with our findings of increased tissue damage is the fact that prolonged infiltration of leukocytes in ischemic tissue damage may also result in anti-angiogenic effects [50,52]. Several studies have shown that mice lacking γδ T cells displayed a prolonged inflammatory phase, whereas WT mice recovered faster from ischemia [53,54]. Furthermore, a rescue experiment showed that external administration of wildtype γδ T cells to the aforementioned mice led to resolution of inflammation and recovery [53].

Macrophages are well known as fundamental modulators of inflammation and angiogenesis. They represent an extremely plastic cell population due to their different phenotypes, which can affect angiogenesis, for example, through the release of paracrine-acting substances or directly as cellular chaperones that promote the fusion of vascular sprouts [48,55]. Depending on the prevailing stimuli, macrophages can polarize to pro-inflammatory M1 macrophages or to anti-inflammatory, regenerative M2 macrophages. However, the M1/M2 nomenclature is only valid for in vitro conditions and reflects the extreme edges of possible polarizations [56,57]. Accordingly, for in vivo situations, very often the terms M1-like and M2-like macrophages are used to indicate that these macrophages show pro-inflammatory features as M1 macrophages do, or anti-inflammatory, regenerative properties like M2 macrophages [58–60]. Accordingly, we denoted in our study $CD68^+/MRC1^-/TNF-\alpha^+$ macrophages as pro-inflammatory M1-like polarized macrophages and $CD68^+/MRC1^+/IL-10^+$ macrophages as anti-inflammatory regenerative M2-like polarized macrophages.

By release of cytokines such as TNF-α or IL-10 and other paracrine signals, macrophages are considered to play an important role as enhancers of angiogenesis at the side of ischemic tissue [10,61–63]. At the onset of inflammation, M0-like monocytes mature into the pro-inflammatory M1-like macrophages with the function of phagocytosis, leukocyte recruitment and delivery of both pro-angiogenic factors (VEGF-A) and pro-inflammatory cytokines, such as TNF-α or IL-1β [23,61]. The pro-angiogenic influence of macrophages of the M1 phenotype is limited due to several reasons. One important reason is the matrix metalloproteinase-9 zymogen (proMMP-9) secreted by M1-like macrophages, which loses its pro-angiogenic effect through complexation with the tissue inhibitors of metalloproteinases metallopeptidase inhibitor 1 (TIMP-1) [64]. Polarization of macrophages to the M2 phenotype leads to downregulation of TIMP-1 expression, resulting in the release of TIMP-1 deficient, pro-angiogenic proMMP-9 [64]. Thus, the higher absolute number of M1-like macrophages in the tissue of γδ T cell depleted mice only leads to an increased level of TIMP-1 complexed pro-MMP-9, which cannot contribute to angiogenic processes. The pro-inflammatory phase is followed by the regenerative phase with the polarization of the initially classically activated macrophages (M1-like macrophages) to the alternatively activated M2-like macrophages [65,66]. M2-like macrophages can resolve the inflammatory conditions, provide tissue repair, and facilitate growth, tissue remodeling and thus angiogenesis [67,68]. Compared to WT and ISO mice, γδ T cell depleted mice showed in our experimental setup a strong predominance of pro-inflammatory M1-like macrophages along with an increased extent of tissue damage and reduced angiogenesis. Thus, the increased infiltration of macrophages ($CD68^+$ cells) in γδ T cell depleted mice, which predominantly displayed M1-like polarization, may indicate an impaired switch to M2-like macrophages, which could be responsible for the reduced angiogenesis and the increased tissue damage. However, this is only an assumption, since mechanistic correlations are difficult to provide using in vivo experiments, and in vitro results do not always reflect the in vivo situation. Nevertheless, detailed investigations on the expression profile of the M1-like and M2-like macrophages should provide further insights and be topics of future examinations. Interestingly, a recent study has demonstrated that IFNγ priming of macrophages via epigenetic and transcriptional changes leads to decreased recruitment of leukocytes and therefore resolved inflammation [69]. Since T cells can secrete IFNγ, among others, it seems possible that the absence of IFNγ release from γδ T cells in the depleted mice could further account for the observed increase in leukocyte number.

Depletion of γδ T cells using the anti-γδ TCR mAb clone UC7-13D5 has been performed in many different experimental setups [70–75]. In addition to the depletion of γδ T cells, it is conceivable that side effects were induced by the administration of the antibody, which contribute to the observed findings in γδ T cell depleted mice. Indeed, it has been observed that treatment with the anti-γδ TCR mAb clone UC7-13D5 led to a slight and short-term increase in the percentage of αβ T lymphocytes, which, however, returned to normal levels within the first days [76]. Furthermore, changes in IFNγ production or in the activity of cytotoxic T cells and natural killer cells observed in other studies indicate that γδ T cell depletion may have led to similar side effects also in our experimental setting [77,78]. Finally, it is known that the binding of anti-γδ TCR mAb to γδ T cells leads to the formation of antigen-antibody complexes, resulting in the production and release of cytokines via activation of the complement system and further binding to Fcγ receptors on immune cells [79–82]. Accordingly, further detailed studies are necessary to define whether the observed effects (found in femoral artery ligated but not sham-operated legs) are exclusively due to the lack of γδ T cells or due to unrecognized side effects caused by the depleting antibody, although we did not find major differences between untreated and isotype control treated mice.

Ligation of the femoral artery results in reduced blood flow to the lower leg, leading to ischemia, local tissue damage and fibrosis [5,10]. It is known that increased tissue damage represents an increased ischemic stimulus for enhanced angiogenesis [83]. Our results showed that the increased tissue damage in the γδ T cell depleted group, however, was associated with reduced capillarity and therefore decreased angiogenesis. Thus, the depletion of γδ T cells did not result in improved angiogenesis compared to the WT and ISO groups despite the increased ischemic tissue damage. In addition to the initiation of angiogenesis in the lower leg, in our murine hindlimb model, ligation of the femoral artery simultaneously induces arteriogenesis in the thigh. Pre-existing collateral vessels, connecting the profunda femoral artery to the femoral artery, begin to grow (arteriogenesis) and are responsible for the additional blood supply to the lower leg. In 2016, Chillo et al. described that improved arteriogenesis results in decreased ischemic tissue damage in the lower leg [83]. Thus, an influence of a potentially comprised arteriogenesis on the degree of ischemic tissue damage found in the gastrocnemius muscle tissue of γδ T cell depleted mice cannot be excluded.

In general, tissue ischemia results in the development of new capillaries. Two mechanisms of angiogenesis are known: (a) sprouting angiogenesis, which is the formation of new capillary branches from pre-existing capillaries through the migration and proliferation of ECs, and (b) intussusception, in which splitting of a single capillary results in the formation of two vessels [6–8]. In our studies, we demonstrated that the depletion of γδ T cells led to reduced angiogenesis by a decreased number of proliferating ECs and a decreased capillary to muscle fiber ratio. The reduced number of proliferating ECs (BrdU$^+$ ECs) indicates that sprouting angiogenesis was impaired in γδ T cell depleted mice. In addition, we found a reduced number of phospho-VEGFR-2 (Tyr1175) positive ECs in γδ T cell depleted mice. VEGFR-2 is considered the most important receptor for VEGF-A-mediated mitotic effects in ECs. Reduced activation of this receptor as reflected by reduced forms of VEGFR-2 phosphorylated at tyrosine 1175 points furthermore to reduced sprouting angiogenesis [84,85]. However, it also suggests that VEGF-A mediated mitotic signaling is impaired in γδ T cell depleted mice. However, intussusception, also referred to as splitting angiogenesis, might be affected as well. Dimova et al. showed in two experiments that mononuclear cells can contribute to the formation and stabilization of transluminal pillars, which is a prerequisite for the splitting of the preexisting vessels. Since lymphocytes belong to the mononuclear cells, it seems possible that the absence of γδ T cells in our experiment led to impaired intussusceptive angiogenesis. However, whether the mononuclear cells affecting splitting angiogenesis are actually monocytes or lymphocytes or other immune cells remains to be investigated [86,87].

In summary, we show that depletion of γδ T cells results in impaired angiogenesis and increased tissue damage in our murine hindlimb model of ischemia. Together with the increased infiltration of leukocytes, reflected by an increased number of neutrophils and predominantly pro-inflammatory M1-like polarized macrophages in γδ T cell depleted mice, our data indicate that γδ T cells play a crucial role in the context of angiogenesis and tissue regeneration.

Supplementary Materials: The following supporting information can be downloaded at: https://www.mdpi.com/article/10.3390/cells11091490/s1, Figure S1: Representative immunofluorescence images of sham-operated legs showing low leukocyte count without any difference in number in WT, ISO and γδ T cell depleted mice; Figure S2: Representative immunofluorescence images of sham-operated legs showing almost no neutrophiles or neutrophil extracellular traps (NETs) in WT, ISO and γδ T cell depleted mice; Figure S3: MRC1 negative macrophages (CD68$^+$/MRC1$^-$) show co-staining with TNF-α; Figure S4: MRC1 positive macrophages (CD68$^+$/MRC1$^+$) show co-staining with IL-10; Figure S5: Representative immunofluorescence images of sham-operated legs showing low numbers of macrophages in WT, ISO and γδ T cell depleted mice.

Author Contributions: Surgical interventions, K.K.; histology, C.A., P.G. and M.K.; conceptualization, C.A., M.L. and E.D.; methodology, C.A., K.K., P.G., M.K., M.L. and E.D.; software, C.A.; validation, C.A., K.K., P.G., M.K., M.L. and E.D.; formal analysis, C.A.; investigation, C.A., M.L. and E.D.; resources, C.A., K.K. and E.D.; data curation, C.A.; writing—original draft preparation, C.A.; writing—review and editing, C.A., K.K., P.G., M.K., M.L. and E.D.; visualization, C.A.; supervision, K.K., M.L. and E.D.; project administration, E.D.; funding acquisition, E.D. All authors have read and agreed to the published version of the manuscript.

Funding: This research was funded by the Lehre@LMU and the Förderprogramm für Forschung und Lehre (FöFoLe) from the Ludwig-Maximilians-Universität, Munich, Germany.

Institutional Review Board Statement: Not applicable.

Informed Consent Statement: Not applicable.

Data Availability Statement: The data presented in this study are available on request from the first author.

Acknowledgments: The authors thank C. Eder and D. van den Heuvel for their technical support and H. Arnholdt and A. L. Hansen for their support in text editing.

Conflicts of Interest: The authors declare no conflict of interest.

References

1. Timmis, A.; Townsend, N.; Gale, C.P.; Torbica, A.; Lettino, M.; Petersen, S.E.; Mossialos, E.A.; Maggioni, A.P.; Kazakiewicz, D.; May, H.T.; et al. European Society of Cardiology: Cardiovascular Disease Statistics 2019. *Eur. Heart J.* **2020**, *41*, 12–85. [CrossRef]
2. Preissner, K.T.; Fischer, S.; Deindl, E. Extracellular RNA as a Versatile DAMP and Alarm Signal That Influences Leukocyte Recruitment in Inflammation and Infection. *Front. Cell Dev. Biol.* **2020**, *8*, 619221. [CrossRef] [PubMed]
3. Natarelli, L.; Virgili, F.; Weber, C. SARS-CoV-2, Cardiovascular Diseases, and Noncoding RNAs: A Connected Triad. *Int. J. Mol. Sci.* **2021**, *22*, 12243. [CrossRef] [PubMed]
4. Bauersachs, R.; Zeymer, U.; Brière, J.B.; Marre, C.; Bowrin, K.; Huelsebeck, M. Burden of Coronary Artery Disease and Peripheral Artery Disease: A Literature Review. *Cardiovasc. Ther.* **2019**, *2019*, 8295054. [CrossRef]

5. Limbourg, A.; Korff, T.; Napp, L.C.; Schaper, W.; Drexler, H.; Limbourg, F.P. Evaluation of postnatal arteriogenesis and angiogenesis in a mouse model of hind-limb ischemia. *Nat. Protoc.* **2009**, *4*, 1737–1746. [CrossRef]
6. Carmeliet, P. Mechanisms of angiogenesis and arteriogenesis. *Nat. Med.* **2000**, *6*, 389–395. [CrossRef]
7. Egginton, S.; Zhou, A.L.; Brown, M.D.; Hudlicka, O. Unorthodox angiogenesis in skeletal muscle. *Cardiovasc. Res.* **2001**, *49*, 634–646. [CrossRef]
8. Mentzer, S.J.; Konerding, M.A. Intussusceptive angiogenesis: Expansion and remodeling of microvascular networks. *Angiogenesis* **2014**, *17*, 499–509. [CrossRef]
9. Carmeliet, P.; Jain, R.K. Angiogenesis in cancer and other diseases. *Nature* **2000**, *407*, 249–257. [CrossRef]
10. Adams, R.H.; Alitalo, K. Molecular regulation of angiogenesis and lymphangiogenesis. *Nat. Rev. Mol. Cell Biol.* **2007**, *8*, 464–478. [CrossRef]
11. Gaudry, M.; Bregerie, O.; Andrieu, V.; El Benna, J.; Pocidalo, M.A.; Hakim, J. Intracellular pool of vascular endothelial growth factor in human neutrophils. *Blood* **1997**, *90*, 4153–4161. [CrossRef] [PubMed]
12. Tecchio, C.; Cassatella, M.A. Neutrophil-derived cytokines involved in physiological and pathological angiogenesis. *Chem. Immunol. Allergy* **2014**, *99*, 123–137. [CrossRef] [PubMed]
13. Liang, W.; Ferrara, N. The Complex Role of Neutrophils in Tumor Angiogenesis and Metastasis. *Cancer Immunol. Res.* **2016**, *4*, 83–91. [CrossRef] [PubMed]
14. Aldabbous, L.; Abdul-Salam, V.; McKinnon, T.; Duluc, L.; Pepke-Zaba, J.; Southwood, M.; Ainscough, A.J.; Hadinnapola, C.; Wilkins, M.R.; Toshner, M.; et al. Neutrophil Extracellular Traps Promote Angiogenesis: Evidence From Vascular Pathology in Pulmonary Hypertension. *Arter. Thromb. Vasc. Biol.* **2016**, *36*, 2078–2087. [CrossRef]
15. Yuan, K.; Zheng, J.; Huang, X.; Zhang, Y.; Han, Y.; Hu, R.; Jin, X. Neutrophil extracellular traps promote corneal neovascularization-induced by alkali burn. *Int. Immunopharmacol.* **2020**, *88*, 106902. [CrossRef]
16. Lefrancais, E.; Mallavia, B.; Zhuo, H.; Calfee, C.S.; Looney, M.R. Maladaptive role of neutrophil extracellular traps in pathogen-induced lung injury. *JCI Insight* **2018**, *3*, e98178. [CrossRef] [PubMed]
17. Saffarzadeh, M.; Juenemann, C.; Queisser, M.A.; Lochnit, G.; Barreto, G.; Galuska, S.P.; Lohmeyer, J.; Preissner, K.T. Neutrophil extracellular traps directly induce epithelial and endothelial cell death: A predominant role of histones. *PLoS ONE* **2012**, *7*, e32366. [CrossRef]
18. Corliss, B.A.; Azimi, M.S.; Munson, J.M.; Peirce, S.M.; Murfee, W.L. Macrophages: An Inflammatory Link Between Angiogenesis and Lymphangiogenesis. *Microcirculation* **2016**, *23*, 95–121. [CrossRef]
19. Cursiefen, C.; Chen, L.; Borges, L.P.; Jackson, D.; Cao, J.; Radziejewski, C.; D'Amore, P.A.; Dana, M.R.; Wiegand, S.J.; Streilein, J.W. VEGF-A stimulates lymphangiogenesis and hemangiogenesis in inflammatory neovascularization via macrophage recruitment. *J. Clin. Investig.* **2004**, *113*, 1040–1050. [CrossRef]
20. Deshmane, S.L.; Kremlev, S.; Amini, S.; Sawaya, B.E. Monocyte chemoattractant protein-1 (MCP-1): An overview. *J. Interferon Cytokine Res.* **2009**, *29*, 313–326. [CrossRef]
21. Leibovich, S.J.; Polverini, P.J.; Shepard, H.M.; Wiseman, D.M.; Shively, V.; Nuseir, N. Macrophage-induced angiogenesis is mediated by tumour necrosis factor-alpha. *Nature* **1987**, *329*, 630–632. [CrossRef] [PubMed]
22. Jetten, N.; Verbruggen, S.; Gijbels, M.J.; Post, M.J.; De Winther, M.P.J.; Donners, M.M.P.C. Anti-inflammatory M2, but not pro-inflammatory M1 macrophages promote angiogenesis in vivo. *Angiogenesis* **2014**, *17*, 109–118. [CrossRef] [PubMed]
23. Hong, H.; Tian, X.Y. The Role of Macrophages in Vascular Repair and Regeneration after Ischemic Injury. *Int. J. Mol. Sci.* **2020**, *21*, 6328. [CrossRef] [PubMed]
24. Seraphim, P.M.; Leal, E.C.; Moura, J.; Goncalves, P.; Goncalves, J.P.; Carvalho, E. Lack of lymphocytes impairs macrophage polarization and angiogenesis in diabetic wound healing. *Life Sci.* **2020**, *254*, 117813. [CrossRef]
25. Yoo, S.A.; Kim, M.; Kang, M.C.; Kong, J.S.; Kim, K.M.; Lee, S.; Hong, B.K.; Jeong, G.H.; Lee, J.; Shin, M.G.; et al. Placental growth factor regulates the generation of T(H)17 cells to link angiogenesis with autoimmunity. *Nat. Immunol.* **2019**, *20*, 1348–1359. [CrossRef]
26. Dunk, C.; Smith, S.; Hazan, A.; Whittle, W.; Jones, R.L. Promotion of angiogenesis by human endometrial lymphocytes. *Immunol. Investig.* **2008**, *37*, 583–610. [CrossRef]
27. Rizov, M.; Andreeva, P.; Dimova, I. Molecular regulation and role of angiogenesis in reproduction. *Taiwan J. Obstet. Gynecol.* **2017**, *56*, 127–132. [CrossRef]
28. Jin, C.; Lagoudas, G.K.; Zhao, C.; Bullman, S.; Bhutkar, A.; Hu, B.; Ameh, S.; Sandel, D.; Liang, X.S.; Mazzilli, S.; et al. Commensal Microbiota Promote Lung Cancer Development via γδ T Cells. *Cell* **2019**, *176*, 998–1013.e1016. [CrossRef]
29. Morita, C.T.; Beckman, E.M.; Bukowski, J.F.; Tanaka, Y.; Band, H.; Bloom, B.R.; Golan, D.E.; Brenner, M.B. Direct presentation of nonpeptide prenyl pyrophosphate antigens to human gamma delta T cells. *Immunity* **1995**, *3*, 495–507. [CrossRef]
30. Groh, V.; Steinle, A.; Bauer, S.; Spies, T. Recognition of stress-induced MHC molecules by intestinal epithelial gammadelta T cells. *Science* **1998**, *279*, 1737–1740. [CrossRef]
31. Das, H.; Groh, V.; Kuijl, C.; Sugita, M.; Morita, C.T.; Spies, T.; Bukowski, J.F. MICA engagement by human Vgamma2Vdelta2 T cells enhances their antigen-dependent effector function. *Immunity* **2001**, *15*, 83–93. [CrossRef]
32. Groh, V.; Wu, J.; Yee, C.; Spies, T. Tumour-derived soluble MIC ligands impair expression of NKG2D and T-cell activation. *Nature* **2002**, *419*, 734–738. [CrossRef] [PubMed]

33. Wrobel, P.; Shojaei, H.; Schittek, B.; Gieseler, F.; Wollenberg, B.; Kalthoff, H.; Kabelitz, D.; Wesch, D. Lysis of a broad range of epithelial tumour cells by human gamma delta T cells: Involvement of NKG2D ligands and T-cell receptor- versus NKG2D-dependent recognition. *Scand. J. Immunol.* **2007**, *66*, 320–328. [CrossRef] [PubMed]
34. Rincon-Orozco, B.; Kunzmann, V.; Wrobel, P.; Kabelitz, D.; Steinle, A.; Herrmann, T. Activation of V gamma 9V delta 2 T cells by NKG2D. *J. Immunol.* **2005**, *175*, 2144–2151. [CrossRef] [PubMed]
35. Ghadially, H.; Brown, L.; Lloyd, C.; Lewis, L.; Lewis, A.; Dillon, J.; Sainson, R.; Jovanovic, J.; Tigue, N.J.; Bannister, D.; et al. MHC class I chain-related protein A and B (MICA and MICB) are predominantly expressed intracellularly in tumour and normal tissue. *Br. J. Cancer* **2017**, *116*, 1208–1217. [CrossRef]
36. Wang, J. Neutrophils in tissue injury and repair. *Cell Tissue Res.* **2018**, *371*, 531–539. [CrossRef]
37. Gong, Y.; Koh, D.-R. Neutrophils promote inflammatory angiogenesis via release of preformed VEGF in an in vivo corneal model. *Cell Tissue Res.* **2010**, *339*, 437–448. [CrossRef]
38. Ardi, V.C.; Kupriyanova, T.A.; Deryugina, E.I.; Quigley, J.P. Human neutrophils uniquely release TIMP-free MMP-9 to provide a potent catalytic stimulator of angiogenesis. *Proc. Natl. Acad. Sci. USA* **2007**, *104*, 20262–20267. [CrossRef]
39. Christoffersson, G.; Vågesjö, E.; Vandooren, J.; Lidén, M.; Massena, S.; Reinert, R.B.; Brissova, M.; Powers, A.C.; Opdenakker, G.; Phillipson, M. VEGF-A recruits a proangiogenic MMP-9-delivering neutrophil subset that induces angiogenesis in transplanted hypoxic tissue. *Blood* **2012**, *120*, 4653–4662. [CrossRef]
40. Scapini, P.; Nesi, L.; Morini, M.; Tanghetti, E.; Belleri, M.; Noonan, D.; Presta, M.; Albini, A.; Cassatella, M.A. Generation of biologically active angiostatin kringle 1-3 by activated human neutrophils. *J. Immunol.* **2002**, *168*, 5798–5804. [CrossRef]
41. Ai, S.; Cheng, X.W.; Inoue, A.; Nakamura, K.; Okumura, K.; Iguchi, A.; Murohara, T.; Kuzuya, M. Angiogenic activity of bFGF and VEGF suppressed by proteolytic cleavage by neutrophil elastase. *Biochem. Biophys. Res. Commun.* **2007**, *364*, 395–401. [CrossRef] [PubMed]
42. Chavakis, T.; Cines, D.B.; Rhee, J.S.; Liang, O.D.; Schubert, U.; Hammes, H.P.; Higazi, A.A.; Nawroth, P.P.; Preissner, K.T.; Bdeir, K. Regulation of neovascularization by human neutrophil peptides (alpha-defensins): A link between inflammation and angiogenesis. *FASEB J.* **2004**, *18*, 1306–1308. [CrossRef] [PubMed]
43. Funken, D.; Yu, Y.; Feng, X.; Imvised, T.; Gueler, F.; Prinz, I.; Madadi-Sanjani, O.; Ure, B.M.; Kuebler, J.F.; Klemann, C. Lack of gamma delta T cells ameliorates inflammatory response after acute intestinal ischemia reperfusion in mice. *Sci. Rep.* **2021**, *11*, 18628. [CrossRef]
44. Mittal, M.; Siddiqui, M.R.; Tran, K.; Reddy, S.P.; Malik, A.B. Reactive oxygen species in inflammation and tissue injury. *Antioxid. Redox. Signal.* **2014**, *20*, 1126–1167. [CrossRef] [PubMed]
45. Papayannopoulos, V. Neutrophil extracellular traps in immunity and disease. *Nat. Rev. Immunol.* **2018**, *18*, 134–147. [CrossRef]
46. Brinkmann, V.; Reichard, U.; Goosmann, C.; Fauler, B.; Uhlemann, Y.; Weiss, D.S.; Weinrauch, Y.; Zychlinsky, A. Neutrophil extracellular traps kill bacteria. *Science* **2004**, *303*, 1532–1535. [CrossRef]
47. Wong, S.L.; Demers, M.; Martinod, K.; Gallant, M.; Wang, Y.; Goldfine, A.B.; Kahn, C.R.; Wagner, D.D. Diabetes primes neutrophils to undergo NETosis, which impairs wound healing. *Nat. Med.* **2015**, *21*, 815–819. [CrossRef]
48. Du Cheyne, C.; Tay, H.; De Spiegelaere, W. The complex TIE between macrophages and angiogenesis. *Anat. Histol. Embryol.* **2020**, *49*, 585–596. [CrossRef]
49. Scapini, P.; Morini, M.; Tecchio, C.; Minghelli, S.; Di Carlo, E.; Tanghetti, E.; Albini, A.; Lowell, C.; Berton, G.; Noonan, D.M.; et al. CXCL1/Macrophage Inflammatory Protein-2-Induced Angiogenesis In Vivo Is Mediated by Neutrophil-Derived Vascular Endothelial Growth Factor-A. *J. Immunol.* **2004**, *172*, 5034–5040. [CrossRef]
50. Rani, M.; Zhang, Q.; Oppeltz, R.F.; Schwacha, M.G. Gamma delta T cells regulate inflammatory cell infiltration of the lung after trauma-hemorrhage. *Shock* **2015**, *43*, 589–597. [CrossRef]
51. Seignez, C.; Phillipson, M. The multitasking neutrophils and their involvement in angiogenesis. *Curr. Opin. Hematol.* **2017**, *24*, 3–8. [CrossRef] [PubMed]
52. Wang, J.; Hossain, M.; Thanabalasuriar, A.; Gunzer, M.; Meininger, C.; Kubes, P. Visualizing the function and fate of neutrophils in sterile injury and repair. *Science* **2017**, *358*, 111–116. [CrossRef] [PubMed]
53. Ponomarev, E.D.; Dittel, B.N. Gamma delta T cells regulate the extent and duration of inflammation in the central nervous system by a Fas ligand-dependent mechanism. *J. Immunol.* **2005**, *174*, 4678–4687. [CrossRef] [PubMed]
54. Murdoch, J.R.; Gregory, L.G.; Lloyd, C.M. γδT cells regulate chronic airway inflammation and development of airway remodelling. *Clin. Exp. Allergy* **2014**, *44*, 1386–1398. [CrossRef]
55. Oishi, Y.; Manabe, I. Macrophages in inflammation, repair and regeneration. *Int. Immunol.* **2018**, *30*, 511–528. [CrossRef] [PubMed]
56. Murray, P.J. Macrophage Polarization. *Annu. Rev. Physiol.* **2017**, *79*, 541–566. [CrossRef] [PubMed]
57. Mosser, D.M.; Edwards, J.P. Exploring the full spectrum of macrophage activation. *Nat. Rev. Immunol.* **2008**, *8*, 958–969. [CrossRef]
58. Liu, S.; Chen, J.; Shi, J.; Zhou, W.; Wang, L.; Fang, W.; Zhong, Y.; Chen, X.; Chen, Y.; Sabri, A.; et al. M1-like macrophage-derived exosomes suppress angiogenesis and exacerbate cardiac dysfunction in a myocardial infarction microenvironment. *Basic Res. Cardiol.* **2020**, *115*, 22. [CrossRef]

59. Palmieri, E.M.; Menga, A.; Martín-Pérez, R.; Quinto, A.; Riera-Domingo, C.; De Tullio, G.; Hooper, D.C.; Lamers, W.H.; Ghesquière, B.; McVicar, D.W.; et al. Pharmacologic or Genetic Targeting of Glutamine Synthetase Skews Macrophages toward an M1-like Phenotype and Inhibits Tumor Metastasis. *Cell Rep.* **2017**, *20*, 1654–1666. [CrossRef]
60. Martins, L.; Gallo, C.C.; Honda, T.S.B.; Alves, P.T.; Stilhano, R.S.; Rosa, D.S.; Koh, T.J.; Han, S.W. Skeletal muscle healing by M1-like macrophages produced by transient expression of exogenous GM-CSF. *Stem Cell Res. Ther.* **2020**, *11*, 473. [CrossRef]
61. Lucas, T.; Waisman, A.; Ranjan, R.; Roes, J.; Krieg, T.; Müller, W.; Roers, A.; Eming, S.A. Differential roles of macrophages in diverse phases of skin repair. *J. Immunol.* **2010**, *184*, 3964–3977. [CrossRef] [PubMed]
62. Besner, G.E.; Klagsbrun, M. Macrophages secrete a heparin-binding inhibitor of endothelial cell growth. *Microvasc. Res.* **1991**, *42*, 187–197. [CrossRef]
63. Falcone, D.J.; Khan, K.M.; Layne, T.; Fernandes, L. Macrophage formation of angiostatin during inflammation. A byproduct of the activation of plasminogen. *J. Biol. Chem.* **1998**, *273*, 31480–31485. [CrossRef] [PubMed]
64. Zajac, E.; Schweighofer, B.; Kupriyanova, T.A.; Juncker-Jensen, A.; Minder, P.; Quigley, J.P.; Deryugina, E.I. Angiogenic capacity of M1- and M2-polarized macrophages is determined by the levels of TIMP-1 complexed with their secreted proMMP-9. *Blood* **2013**, *122*, 4054–4067. [CrossRef]
65. Willenborg, S.; Lucas, T.; van Loo, G.; Knipper, J.A.; Krieg, T.; Haase, I.; Brachvogel, B.; Hammerschmidt, M.; Nagy, A.; Ferrara, N.; et al. CCR2 recruits an inflammatory macrophage subpopulation critical for angiogenesis in tissue repair. *Blood* **2012**, *120*, 613–625. [CrossRef]
66. Dort, J.; Fabre, P.; Molina, T.; Dumont, N.A. Macrophages Are Key Regulators of Stem Cells during Skeletal Muscle Regeneration and Diseases. *Stem. Cells Int.* **2019**, *2019*, 4761427. [CrossRef]
67. Moore, E.M.; West, J.L. Harnessing Macrophages for Vascularization in Tissue Engineering. *Ann. Biomed. Eng.* **2019**, *47*, 354–365. [CrossRef]
68. Gordon, S.; Taylor, P.R. Monocyte and macrophage heterogeneity. *Nat. Rev. Immunol.* **2005**, *5*, 953–964. [CrossRef]
69. Hoeksema, M.A.; Scicluna, B.P.; Boshuizen, M.C.; van der Velden, S.; Neele, A.E.; Van den Bossche, J.; Matlung, H.L.; van den Berg, T.K.; Goossens, P.; de Winther, M.P. IFN-γ priming of macrophages represses a part of the inflammatory program and attenuates neutrophil recruitment. *J. Immunol.* **2015**, *194*, 3909–3916. [CrossRef]
70. Kühl, A.A.; Pawlowski, N.N.; Grollich, K.; Loddenkemper, C.; Zeitz, M.; Hoffmann, J.C. Aggravation of intestinal inflammation by depletion/deficiency of gammadelta T cells in different types of IBD animal models. *J. Leukoc. Biol.* **2007**, *81*, 168–175. [CrossRef]
71. Wu, H.; Wang, Y.M.; Wang, Y.; Hu, M.; Zhang, G.Y.; Knight, J.F.; Harris, D.C.; Alexander, S.I. Depletion of gammadelta T cells exacerbates murine adriamycin nephropathy. *J. Am. Soc. Nephrol.* **2007**, *18*, 1180–1189. [CrossRef] [PubMed]
72. Maeda, Y.; Reddy, P.; Lowler, K.P.; Liu, C.; Bishop, D.K.; Ferrara, J.L. Critical role of host gammadelta T cells in experimental acute graft-versus-host disease. *Blood* **2005**, *106*, 749–755. [CrossRef] [PubMed]
73. Wang, T.; Gao, Y.; Scully, E.; Davis, C.T.; Anderson, J.F.; Welte, T.; Ledizet, M.; Koski, R.; Madri, J.A.; Barrett, A.; et al. Gamma delta T cells facilitate adaptive immunity against West Nile virus infection in mice. *J. Immunol.* **2006**, *177*, 1825–1832. [CrossRef] [PubMed]
74. Shibata, K.; Yamada, H.; Hara, H.; Kishihara, K.; Yoshikai, Y. Resident Vdelta1+ gammadelta T cells control early infiltration of neutrophils after Escherichia coli infection via IL-17 production. *J. Immunol.* **2007**, *178*, 4466–4472. [CrossRef]
75. Pöllinger, B.; Junt, T.; Metzler, B.; Walker, U.A.; Tyndall, A.; Allard, C.; Bay, S.; Keller, R.; Raulf, F.; Di Padova, F.; et al. Th17 cells, not IL-17+ γδ T cells, drive arthritic bone destruction in mice and humans. *J. Immunol.* **2011**, *186*, 2602–2612. [CrossRef]
76. Kobayashi, Y.; Kawai, K.; Ito, K.; Honda, H.; Sobue, G.; Yoshikai, Y. Aggravation of murine experimental allergic encephalomyelitis by administration of T-cell receptor gammadelta-specific antibody. *J. Neuroimmunol.* **1997**, *73*, 169–174. [CrossRef]
77. Williams, D.M.; Grubbs, B.G.; Schachter, J.; Magee, D.M. Gamma interferon levels during Chlamydia trachomatis pneumonia in mice. *Infect. Immun.* **1993**, *61*, 3556–3558. [CrossRef]
78. Seo, N.; Tokura, Y.; Takigawa, M.; Egawa, K. Depletion of IL-10- and TGF-beta-producing regulatory gamma delta T cells by administering a daunomycin-conjugated specific monoclonal antibody in early tumor lesions augments the activity of CTLs and NK cells. *J. Immunol.* **1999**, *163*, 242–249.
79. Porter, R.R.; Reid, K.B. Activation of the complement system by antibody-antigen complexes: The classical pathway. *Adv. Protein Chem.* **1979**, *33*, 1–71. [CrossRef]
80. Dodds, A.W.; Sim, R.B.; Porter, R.R.; Kerr, M.A. Activation of the first component of human complement (C1) by antibody-antigen aggregates. *Biochem. J.* **1978**, *175*, 383–390. [CrossRef]
81. Acharya, D.; Li, X.R.L.; Heineman, R.E.; Harrison, R.E. Complement Receptor-Mediated Phagocytosis Induces Proinflammatory Cytokine Production in Murine Macrophages. *Front. Immunol.* **2019**, *10*, 3049. [CrossRef] [PubMed]
82. Rönnelid, J.; Ahlin, E.; Nilsson, B.; Nilsson-Ekdahl, K.; Mathsson, L. Immune complex-mediated cytokine production is regulated by classical complement activation both in vivo and in vitro. *Adv. Exp. Med. Biol.* **2008**, *632*, 187–201. [PubMed]
83. Chillo, O.; Kleinert, E.C.; Lautz, T.; Lasch, M.; Pagel, J.I.; Heun, Y.; Troidl, K.; Fischer, S.; Caballero-Martinez, A.; Mauer, A.; et al. Perivascular Mast Cells Govern Shear Stress-Induced Arteriogenesis by Orchestrating Leukocyte Function. *Cell Rep.* **2016**, *16*, 2197–2207. [CrossRef] [PubMed]

84. Li, B.; Zhang, Y.; Yin, R.; Zhong, W.; Chen, R.; Yan, J. Activating CD137 Signaling Promotes Sprouting Angiogenesis via Increased VEGFA Secretion and the VEGFR2/Akt/eNOS Pathway. *Mediat. Inflamm.* **2020**, *2020*, 1649453. [CrossRef]
85. Kim, D.Y.; Park, J.A.; Kim, Y.; Noh, M.; Park, S.; Lie, E.; Kim, E.; Kim, Y.M.; Kwon, Y.G. SALM4 regulates angiogenic functions in endothelial cells through VEGFR2 phosphorylation at Tyr1175. *FASEB J.* **2019**, *33*, 9842–9857. [CrossRef]
86. Dimova, I.; Hlushchuk, R.; Makanya, A.; Styp-Rekowska, B.; Ceausu, A.; Flueckiger, S.; Lang, S.; Semela, D.; Le Noble, F.; Chatterjee, S.; et al. Inhibition of Notch signaling induces extensive intussusceptive neo-angiogenesis by recruitment of mononuclear cells. *Angiogenesis* **2013**, *16*, 921–937. [CrossRef]
87. Dimova, I.; Karthik, S.; Makanya, A.; Hlushchuk, R.; Semela, D.; Volarevic, V.; Djonov, V. SDF-1/CXCR4 signalling is involved in blood vessel growth and remodelling by intussusception. *J. Cell Mol. Med.* **2019**, *23*, 3916–3926. [CrossRef]

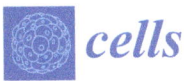

Review

Crosstalk between Interleukin-1β and Type I Interferons Signaling in Autoinflammatory Diseases

Philippe Georgel

Laboratoire d'ImmunoRhumatologie Moléculaire, Institut National de la Santé et de la Recherche Médicale (INSERM) UMR_S 1109, Institut Thématique Interdisciplinaire (ITI) de Médecine de Précision de Strasbourg, Transplantex NG, Faculté de Médecine, Fédération Hospitalo-Universitaire OMICARE, Fédération de Médecine Translationnelle de Strasbourg (FMTS), Université de Strasbourg, 67085 Strasbourg, France; pgeorgel@unistra.fr

Abstract: Interleukin-1β (IL-1β) and type I interferons (IFNs) are major cytokines involved in autoinflammatory/autoimmune diseases. Separately, the overproduction of each of these cytokines is well described and constitutes the hallmark of inflammasomopathies and interferonopathies, respectively. While their interaction and the crosstalk between their downstream signaling pathways has been mostly investigated in the frame of infectious diseases, little information on their interconnection is still available in the context of autoinflammation promoted by sterile triggers. In this review, we will examine the respective roles of IL-1β and type I IFNs in autoinflammatory/rheumatic diseases and analyze their potential connections in the pathophysiology of some of these diseases, which could reveal novel therapeutic opportunities.

Keywords: inflammation; type I interferons; interleukin-1β; crosstalk

Citation: Georgel, P. Crosstalk between Interleukin-1β and Type I Interferons Signaling in Autoinflammatory Diseases. *Cells* **2021**, *10*, 1134. https://doi.org/10.3390/cells10051134

Academic Editors: Silvia Fischer and Elisabeth Deindl

Received: 28 March 2021
Accepted: 6 May 2021
Published: 8 May 2021

Publisher's Note: MDPI stays neutral with regard to jurisdictional claims in published maps and institutional affiliations.

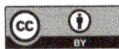

Copyright: © 2021 by the author. Licensee MDPI, Basel, Switzerland. This article is an open access article distributed under the terms and conditions of the Creative Commons Attribution (CC BY) license (https://creativecommons.org/licenses/by/4.0/).

1. Introduction

Numerous reports have documented the roles of IL-1β and type I interferons (IFNs) in the defense mechanisms that are engaged upon bacterial (such as *M. tuberculosis* [1]) and viral [2] infections. Type I (and type III) IFNs exert powerful antiviral activities that have been extensively described [3,4], while those mediated by IL-1β are more scarcely defined [5]. Furthermore, the interplay of these cytokines and their downstream signaling pathways has also been largely explored during infectious diseases [6], COVID-19 being the most recent example [7].

These cytokines are produced following the activation of dedicated pattern-recognition receptors (PRRs) [8] in response to specific pathogens and the associated molecular patterns (PAMPs) that they express. Interestingly, the same PRRs (nucleotide-binding oligomerization domain-like receptors—NLRs, Toll-like receptors—TLR or AIM2-like receptors—ALRs) are also activated upon the detection of danger signals (DAMPs [9–11]) produced in sterile conditions. In this case, inflammation, instead of creating the appropriate conditions to clear off an invading pathogen, generates tissue damage and evolves towards detrimental endpoints for the host. First, this review will provide some examples of autoimmune/autoinflammatory diseases that are caused by the deregulated expression of type I IFNs and IL-1β. Indeed, these cytokines are major mediators of inflammation and can be incriminated in many cytokinopathies [12], which are diseases caused by alterations in a single gene affecting cytokines expression. Several examples of interferonopathies and inflammasomopathies will illustrate these cases. Additionally, type I IFNs and IL-1β perturbations can also result from interactions between many genes and the host environment. Lupus, a disease in which patients exhibit an "IFN signature" [13] (i.e., overexpression of a subset of IFN-stimulated genes) and Alzheimer's disease, during which IL-1β is known to be overexpressed [14], will serve as examples for such complex (multigenic/multifactorial) diseases in which these cytokines are involved. Next, we will analyze several cases where reciprocal interactions between them have been observed, and the therapeutic perspectives that have been derived from these observations. Multiple sclerosis, a disease treated with IFN-β (among other therapeutic options) and which is also characterized by increased IL-1β expression, will be described. In parallel, gout and rheumatoid arthritis (RA) are joint inflammatory diseases in which reducing IL-1β overexpression can represent an efficient therapeutic opportunity. Interestingly, promoting type I IFNs expression recently appeared as an attractive way to dampen IL-1β production in animal models for gout and RA [15,16]. These examples in which type I IFNs and IL-1β exert a reciprocal control will reveal novel options to treat patients suffering from these inflammatory diseases, whose general features are given in Table 1. Finally, innovative cell culture methods designed to investigate and aimed at deciphering these interactions between cytokines at the molecular and cellular levels will be discussed in a prospective chapter.

Table 1. Type I IFNs- and IL-1β-mediated pathologies discussed in this review.

Disease	Type	Genetic Defect	Cytokine Profile	Treatment
STING-associated vasculopathy with onset in infancy (SAVI)	interferonopathy	STING gain-of-function	exessive type I IFN secretion	corticosteroids jakinhibs (clinical trials)
Systemic Lupus Erythematosus (SLE)	rheumatic autoimmune/autoinflammatory disease	multifactorial disease	IFN signature (overexpression of IFN-stimulated genes)	corticosteroids Immunosuppressants (e.g., methotrexate) biologics (e.g., antiB-cell mAb)
Familial Mediterranean Fever (FMF)	inflammasomopathy	mutations in MEFV (Mediterranean fever, also named PYRIN)	constitutive IL-1β secretion	colchicin biologics (IL-1β receptor antagonist, anti IL-1β mAb)
Alzheimer's disease (AD)	Neurodegenerative disease	multifactorial disease	excessive IL-1β, IL-6 and TNF secretion	Cholinesterase inhibitors N-methyl D-aspartate (NMDA) antagonists anti amyloid-β mAb (clinical trials)
Gout	rheumatic autoinflammatory disease	multifactorial disease	excessive IL-1β secretion	colchicin biologics (IL-1β receptor antagonist, anti IL-1β mAb)
Rheumatoid Arthritis (RA)	rheumatic autoimmune/autoinflammatory disease	multifactorial disease	TNF overexpression IL-1β overexpression IFN signature (overexpression of IFN-stimulated genes)	corticosteroids Immunosuppressants (e.g., methotrexate) biologics (e.g., anti TNF mAb)
Multiple sclerosis (MS)	inflammatory, neurodegenerative disease	multifactorial disease	increased IFNγ, IL-12, IL-17 secretion/activation	IFN-β biologics (e.g., antiB-cell mAb)

2. Type I IFNs in Autoinflammation

Since their initial discovery in 1957 [17], type I IFNs have been essentially considered beneficial with regards to their unique antiviral activities [18]. More recently, however, it appeared that the deregulated and inappropriate expression of these cytokines could be harmful. Indeed, in the absence of any obvious viral trigger, the overexpression of type I IFNs was noted in patients suffering from inflammatory disorders [19], some of which were caused by single-gene mutations (monogenic diseases), while others are classified within complex diseases, i.e., requiring environmental factors and many specific genetic alterations to promote pathogenic features. *STING*-associated vasculopathy with onset in infancy (SAVI) belongs to the first category of ailments and is caused by a gain-of-function mutation in the *STING* gene; this gene encodes a protein that is at the cross-roads between the cGAS (cyclic GMP-AMP synthase, an exogenous DNA sensor) and the interferon regulatory factors (IRFs)-3 and -7, which induce type I IFN transcription [20]. In these patients, TANK-binding kinase (TBK1) is constitutively activated in the absence of viral RNA, leading to spontaneous and massive type I IFN production. Fortunately, Janus kinase inhibitors might be promising drugs to block the signaling pathway downstream of the type I IFNs receptor (IFNAR) and provide relief to a subset of patients with SAVI syndrome [21]. In past years, many additional genetic origins of type I interferonopathies were elucidated following whole-exome sequencing in patients and controls in families affected by these rare symptoms [22,23].

On the other hand, systemic lupus erythematosus (SLE), with the exception of childhood-onset SLE, is a complex disease driven by a combination of genetic, epigenetic and environmental factors [24]. Of note, a hallmark of SLE is the so-called "IFN signature", describing the overexpression of IFN-stimulated genes (ISGs) in circulating mononuclear blood cells or target tissues [25]. Of note, the level of ISGs expression appears correlated with disease severity [26]. Interestingly, ISGs overexpression is also observed in other inflammatory diseases, such as rheumatoid arthritis [13]. More recently, single-cell RNAseq technology enabled a precise description of gene expression in SLE patients that appeared to form a more heterogeneous population than previously suspected [27]. Such stratification of patients with multiOMICs technologies already sets the grounds for more targeted, individualized therapies [28]. In the frame of the present review, it is noteworthy to observe that, in addition to type I IFNs, IL-1 family member expression can also be used as a biomarker in SLE patients [29]. Finally, severe complications occurring in lupus patients, such as macrophage activation syndrome or pericarditis, have been successfully reduced with anakinra, an IL-1b antagonist [30,31], showing that both IFNs-I and IL-1 participate in lupus pathogenesis, at least in a subset of patients.

3. IL-1β in Autoinflammation

Similar to type I IFN-dependent diseases, many inflammatory syndromes result from uncontrolled IL-1β expression. Among them, inflammasomopathies are a group of monogenic diseases caused by hereditary defects in inflammasomes components. Inflammasomes are intracellular multiprotein complexes composed of a sensor (detecting pathogen-associated molecules, such as peptidoglycans from Gram-positive bacteria or sterile components, such as silicate or urate crystals), an adaptor (ASC for apoptosis-associated speck-like protein containing a caspase recruitment domain) and the Caspase 1. Following multimerization of this complex, activated Caspase 1 cleaves pro IL-1β into its mature, bioactive form, which is exported out of the cell through pores formed by GasderminD [32]. The prototypical inflammasomopathy with periodic fever is familial mediterranean fever (FMF), a disease caused by mutations in the *MEFV* (mediterranean fever) gene encoding the protein PYRIN, which is part of the inflammasome complex. Gain-of-function mutations in the *MEFV* gene lead to increased Caspase 1 activation and IL-1β levels [33]. The development of IL-1β antagonists has considerably improved the management of these patients [34].

In addition to these monogenic inflammatory diseases, emerging evidence suggests that IL-1β is also involved in complex neurological disorders, such as Alzheimer's disease (AD) [35]. Indeed, AD occurrence depends on many factors, such as age, comorbidities, genetics and education level. However, a strong correlation between AD and reactive oxygen species (ROS) production has been evidenced, where ROS are major inducers of NLRP3-dependent IL-1β production [36], including in neurons [37]. Importantly, this observation has led to novel therapeutic options for neurodegenerative disorders affecting an increasing number of patients worldwide.

4. Interplay between Type I IFNs and IL-1β in Inflammatory/Autoimmune Diseases

Whilst interferonopathies and inflammasomopathies may appear as very divergent or even antagonistic inflammatory diseases (although an overlap can be observed in some instances, as mentioned in the previous chapters), the pathogenesis of some inflammatory conditions clearly involves both type I IFNs and IL-1β. Multiple sclerosis (MS) belongs to this category, since IL-1β is strongly implicated in this inflammatory, neurodegenerative disease [38], and IFN-β is still a classical first-line therapy [39], although rituximab (an anti-CD20 monoclonal antibody designed to induce B cell ablation) was shown recently as a promising option [40]. Low STING-dependent type I IFNs expression in peripheral blood mononuclear cells (PBMC) isolated from MS patients [41] is in agreement with these observations.

The mechanism by which IFN-β exerts its anti-inflammatory actions has been partially elucidated [42]. It is now very clear that type I IFNs promote IFNAR-dependent *IL-1Ra* (encoding an antagonist of the IL-1β receptor) and *IL-10* gene expressions. Furthermore, type I IFNs and IL-10 were recently shown to negatively regulate the activation of the NLRP3 inflammasome in a STAT3-dependent manner [43–45]. These data support the notion that IL-1β and type I IFNs exert antagonistic activities that have been experimentally tested in various inflammatory settings (collagen-induced arthritis, allotransplant rejection), whereby the beneficial administration of type I IFNs has been documented.

Reduced expression of *NLRP3* was also shown to participate in the anti-inflammatory benefits of type I IFNs in MS [46,47]. This observation also likely accounts for the spectacular therapeutic potential of imiquimod, a TLR7 agonist and strong inducer of type I IFNs, which we observed in a mouse model of acute uratic inflammation [15]. Importantly, our work using this mouse model of gout as well as RA models [16] enabled us to develop a framework in which complex cellular interactions are required to account for the counter-regulatory effects mediated by type I IFNs on IL-1β [48]. Future work using elaborate cell culture systems will be necessary to decipher this cellular dialog, as discussed below. Surprisingly, the regulatory roles of IL-1β on type I IFNs and ISGs expression are more scarcely documented [49], and these experimental cell culture experiments would also be useful to explore this issue. In this regard, the recent observation that IL-1β promotes type I IFN and ISGs expression in bone marrow-derived dendritic cells (BMDC) appears of particular interest [6]. A schematic network of type I IFNs and IL-1β interactions is depicted in Figure 1.

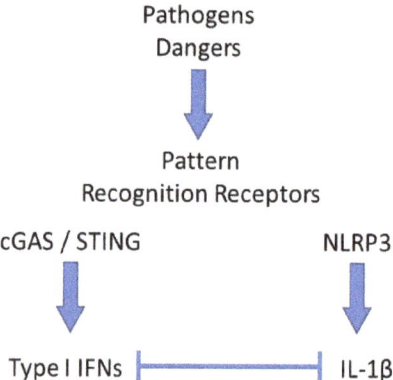

Figure 1. Schematic network of interactions between type I IFNs and IL-1β. Pathogens- or danger-associated molecular patterns (PAMPs, DAMPs) interact with their cognate pattern recognition receptor (PRRs). In the example shown here, DNA binding and activation of the cGAS/STING pathway leads to type I interferons (IFNs) secretion, while monosodium urate (MSU) crystals activate the NLRP3 inflammasome, which induces IL-1β release. In most cases, both cytokines exert antagonistic activities, mutually repressing their expression levels by various mechanisms.

5. Therapeutic Consequences

As mentioned above, some overlap may exist between IL-1β and type I IFNs in various inflammatory settings, opening novel therapeutic opportunities.

5.1. Targeting Type I IFNs in Il-1β-Dependent Diseases

Type I IFNs-based therapies were developed long ago and were particularly useful in hepatitis C virus-infected patients, despite considerable side effects [50]. In this regard, our strategy to perform epicutanieous application of a cream containing imiquimod, a powerful promoter of IFN synthesis to treat inflamed joints of RA or gout mice, appeared as a promising approach to avoid adverse reactions [15,16]. Importantly, we observed a drastic reduction in neutrophils in the cellular infiltrate following imiquimod application, which also certainly participates in the reduced local inflammation through the limitation of ROS production. Topical imiquimod has been used for 20 years in humans to treat genital warts and skin carcinoma [51]; its pharmacokinetics and precautions for use are well known. Therefore, we believe that our pre-clinical studies advocate for using this drug to treat joint inflammation in RA or gout patients, as well as localized skin inflammation, showing evidence of a massive neutrophilic infiltrate (neutrophilic dermatoses). On the other hand, strategies presently in use or under development aim at reducing the IFN-dependent signaling pathway, for instance, in SLE patients with anifrolumab, a monoclonal antibody targeting the type I IFN receptor subunit 1 [52]. Other tools to reduce IFN signaling are the Janus kinase (JAK) inhibitors (jakinhibs), a novel family of compounds effective in myeloproliferative or autoimmune (such as RA) diseases [53]. Given their antagonism, a rise in IL-1β can be expected in patients with reduced type I IFN production as a result of treatment with anifrolumab or jakinhibs, which might require specific attention, and possibly the need for additional anti-IL-1β therapy.

5.2. Targeting IL-1β in Interferonopathies

Jakinhibs are the most promising therapeutic opportunities for patients afflicted by type I interferonopathies [54]. As mentioned above, following IL-1β expression levels might be critical in these critically ill patients.

In addition, IL-1β inhibition might also represent a useful strategy in various inflammatory diseases, including interferonopathies. Indeed, this cytokine is also expressed in the central nervous system, where it mediates pain [55]. Supporting this notion is the observation that psoriatic arthritis (PsA) patients treated with anti-TNF antibodies still experience pain, while joint inflammation is concomitantly reduced [56]. In these patients, and possibly in others treated with TNF inhibitors or more generally experiencing pain as a result of inflammatory reactions, there might be room for IL-1β blockers (canakinumab, anakinra). Finally, it is interesting to note that experiments in the experimental autoimmune encephalomyelitis (EAE) mouse model support the therapeutic potential of IL-1 blockade in MS [57], an approach that has been tested in a very limited number of patients suffering colchicine-resistant familial mediterranean fever (FMF, an inflammasomopathy) and MS [58]. Strikingly, MS symptoms were markedly reduced in these patients.

Altogether, these observations indicate that the management of patients suffering inflammatory symptoms might require a combination of drugs targeting various players involved in the pathogenesis of these diseases. Future work aiming at a better characterization of the interplay between these players is needed to provide more efficient and targeted therapeutic approaches. Some insights aiming at this goal are suggested in the perspectives and conclusions of the present review.

6. Perspectives

Although several molecular interactions between type I IFNs and IL-1β have been described (transcriptional induction of *IL-1Ra* and *IL-10* genes upon IFN-β treatment [42]; and reciprocally, increased transcription of *IFN-β* and *ISGs* following IL-1β addition in the culture medium of BMDCs [6]), most studies have been performed in cell cultures where one cell type only has been investigated (dendritic cell, monocytes/macrophages, etc.). This constitutes a fundamental weakness, since these cytokines are produced by different cell types (neutrophils [59], eosinophils [60]) interacting in a specific microenvironment. To gain access to more physiological interactions at the cellular and molecular levels, co-cultures, either in two-dimension systems (Boyden chambers) or even using more complex organoids, need to be developed [61]. As seen in Figure 2, considering only type I IFNs (IFN-α/β) and IL-1β and the five main immune cell types that are able to produce them, upon the TLR7-dependent stimulation (with imiquimod, IMQ) of pDCs, an already complex network of interactions is created, in which the reciprocal effects of these cytokines are presently totally unknown and certainly quite different from what can be observed in monotypic cell cultures. Producing mixed cultures in Boyden chambers (which has been previously performed [62]) could be a good starting point, in which each cell type (for instance, pDC and macrophages, or pDC and neutrophils) could be investigated separately after cell sorting with high-throughput technologies (RNAseq) and analyzed morphologically (apoptosis, NETosis, polarization) in various conditions driving cytokine (type I IFNs or IL-1β) synthesis. Such approaches might be instrumental to better characterize, at the cellular level, the recently described interaction between IL-1β-dependent mitochondrial DNA release and cGAS/STING-dependent type I IFNs secretion [63]. In the future, spheroids or organoids might add complexity to the system by adding support cells such as keratinocytes or fibrocytes and extracellular matrix components.

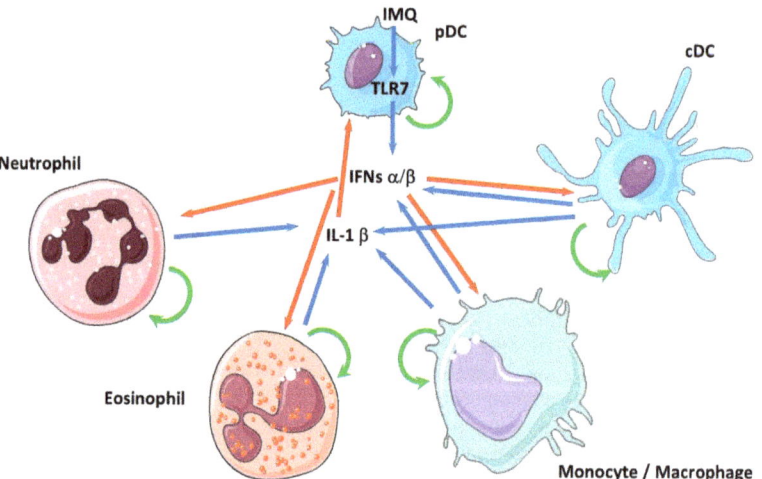

Figure 2. The complex network of interactions between type I IFNs, IL-1β and the cells that produce them. Simplified representation of the potential interactions between plasmacytoid (pDC) or conventional (cDC) dendritic cell, macrophages/monocytes, neutrophils and eosinophils upon, for example, imiquimod (IMQ) stimulation acting via TLR7 in pDCs. Blue arrows denote cytokine expression, red arrows indicate that these cytokines exert an effect (activation or inhibition) on target cells and green arrows represent retro-control of the cytokines on the cells that produce them.

7. Conclusions

We have merely touched on the complexity of inflammation here by analyzing the reciprocal interactions of two cytokines. Despite the paramount importance of IL-1β and type I IFNs in autoinflammatory diseases, many other cytokines, among which TNF are self-evident, can certainly not be neglected. In 2006, Bancherau and Pascual published a seminal paper in which they extended the Th1/Th2 concept into a "compass of immunity and immunopathology" organized into two perpendicular axes: one defined by the reciprocal interactions of IFN-α and TNF and the other by IL-4 and IFN-γ [64]. According to this model, SLE was identified by an overexpression of IFN-α. Fifteen years later, high-throughput technologies have evidenced the heterogeneity of patients suffering from complex diseases such as SLE or RA, which are now defined as pathotypes [65]. Because some cytokines are direct drivers of immunopathology and because the quantification of most cytokines is easily feasible with multiplex technology, we suggest that providing an extensive profiling of cytokines (in the blood or the affected tissue if accessible), a "cytokinome" as suggested by others [66], would be a useful tool to better define patients sub-groups by comparison with a reference of healthy subjects [67]. This approach, illustrated by the "multidimensional compass" illustrated in Figure 3, would also be instrumental in defining the best therapeutic option for a patient, following its impact on the normalization of its cytokine profile and eventually adjusting it. In this example, two RA patients are identified by increased TNF expression compared to a control group (with the reference cytokinome resulting from a set of healthy donors) with variables (age, sex, etc.) matching the patients. However, following anti-TNF therapy, each exhibited a different outcome. In patient 1, the normalization of TNF levels was accompanied by increased IFN-α/β secretion and paradoxical psoriasis (a recently described possible consequence of anti-TNF antibodies [68]), which might require appropriate management (jakinhibs, eventually). On the other hand, patient 2, in which the same treatment also enabled a marked reduction in the circulating TNF level and improvement of joint inflammation, responded by an additional strong decrease in IL-1β expression (as previously described [69]), putting him at risk of developing various microbial infections and therefore requiring specific monitoring in the future. These hypothetical cases indicate that the determination of the cytokinome and its evolution upon treatment might bring substantial benefits to patients with inflammatory diseases.

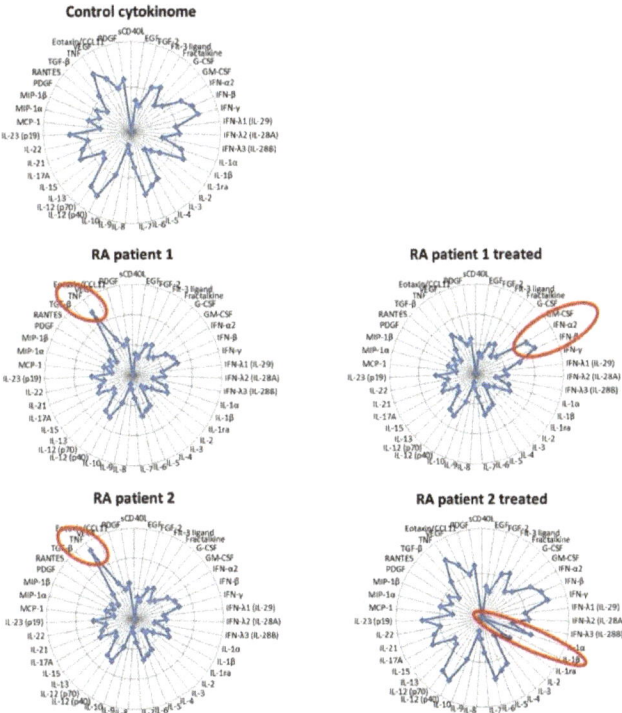

Figure 3. The multidimensional compass of inflammation. Radar plot showing the hypothetical expression levels of 43 cytokines/chemokines in the Control and two RA patients before and after anti-TNF therapy.

Funding: This work was supported by the Agence Nationale de la Recherche (ANR)-ANR-11-LABX-0070_TRANSPLANTEX, the Institut National de la Santé et de la Recherche Médicale (INSERM), MSD-Avenir grant AUTOGEN, the University of Strasbourg (including IDEX UNISTRA), the European regional development fund (European Union) INTERREG V programs, TRIDIAG and PERSONALIS and Fédération Hospitalo-Universitaire (FHU) OMICARE.

Institutional Review Board Statement: Not applicable.

Informed Consent Statement: Not applicable.

Data Availability Statement: Not applicable.

Acknowledgments: PG thanks Seiamak Bahram (Strasbourg University, France) and Stephan Bluml (Vienna University, Austria) for the critical reading of the manuscript.

Conflicts of Interest: The author declares no conflict of interest.

References

1. Ma, J.; Zhao, S.; Gao, X.; Wang, R.; Liu, J.; Zhou, X.; Zhou, Y. The Roles of Inflammasomes in Host Defense against *Mycobacterium tuberculosis*. *Pathogens* **2021**, *10*, 120. [CrossRef]
2. Schoggins, J.W. Recent advances in antiviral interferon-stimulated gene biology. *F1000Research* **2018**, *7*, 309. [CrossRef]
3. Lazear, H.M.; Schoggins, J.W.; Diamond, M.S. Shared and Distinct Functions of Type I and Type III Interferons. *Immunity* **2019**, *50*, 907–923. [CrossRef]
4. Li, S.-F.; Gong, M.-J.; Zhao, F.-R.; Shao, J.-J.; Xie, Y.-L.; Zhang, Y.-G.; Chang, H.-Y. Type I Interferons: Distinct Biological Activities and Current Applications for Viral Infection. *Cell. Physiol. Biochem.* **2018**, *51*, 2377–2396. [CrossRef]
5. Orzalli, M.H.; Smith, A.; Jurado, K.A.; Iwasaki, A.; Garlick, J.A.; Kagan, J.C. An Antiviral Branch of the IL-1 Signaling Pathway Restricts Immune-Evasive Virus Replication. *Mol. Cell* **2018**, *71*, 825–840. [CrossRef] [PubMed]
6. Aarreberg, L.D.; Wilkins, C.; Ramos, H.J.; Green, R.; Davis, M.A.; Chow, K.; Gale, M. Interleukin-1beta Signaling in Dendritic Cells Induces Antiviral Interferon Responses. *mBio* **2018**, *9*, 2.
7. Jamilloux, Y.; Henry, T.; Belot, A.; Viel, S.; Fauter, M.; El Jammal, T.; Walzer, T.; François, B.; Sève, P. Should we stimulate or suppress immune responses in COVID-19? Cytokine and anti-cytokine interventions. *Autoimmun. Rev.* **2020**, *19*, 102567. [CrossRef] [PubMed]
8. Kawai, T.; Akira, S. The roles of TLRs, RLRs and NLRs in pathogen recognition. *Int. Immunol.* **2009**, *21*, 317–337. [CrossRef]
9. Land, W.G. The Role of Damage-Associated Molecular Patterns in Human Diseases: Part I—Promoting inflammation and immunity. *Sultan Qaboos Univ. Med. J.* **2015**, *15*, e9–e21.
10. Land, W.G. The Role of Damage-Associated Molecular Patterns (DAMPs) in Human Diseases: Part II: DAMPs as diagnostics, prognostics and therapeutics in clinical medicine. *Sultan Qaboos Univ. Med. J.* **2015**, *15*, e157–e170. [PubMed]
11. Gong, T.; Liu, L.; Jiang, W.; Zhou, R. DAMP-sensing receptors in sterile inflammation and inflammatory diseases. *Nat. Rev. Immunol.* **2020**, *20*, 95–112. [CrossRef]
12. Moghaddas, F.; Masters, S.L. Monogenic autoinflammatory diseases: Cytokinopathies. *Cytokine* **2015**, *74*, 237–246. [CrossRef] [PubMed]
13. Szymczak, F.; Colli, M.L.; Mamula, M.J.; Evans-Molina, C.; Eizirik, D.L. Gene expression signatures of target tissues in type 1 diabetes, lupus erythematosus, multiple sclerosis, and rheumatoid arthritis. *Sci. Adv.* **2021**, *7*, eabd7600. [CrossRef] [PubMed]
14. Batista, A.F.; Rody, T.; Forny-Germano, L.; Cerdeiro, S.; Bellio, M.; Ferreira, S.T.; Munoz, D.P.; De Felice, F.G. Interleukin-1beta mediates alterations in mitochondrial fusion/fission proteins and memory impairment induced by amyloid-beta oligomers. *J. Neuroinflam.* **2021**, *18*, 54. [CrossRef]
15. Mariotte, A.; De Cauwer, A.; Po, C.; Abou-Faycal, C.; Pichot, A.; Paul, N.; Aouadi, I.; Carapito, R.; Frisch, B.; Macquin, C.; et al. A mouse model of MSU-induced acute inflammation in vivo suggests imiquimod-dependent targeting of Il-1beta as relevant therapy for gout patients. *Theranostics* **2020**, *10*, 2158–2171. [CrossRef]
16. Nehmar, R.; Alsaleh, G.; Voisin, B.; Flacher, V.; Mariotte, A.; Saferding, V.; Puchner, A.; Niederreiter, B.; Vandamme, T.; Schabbauer, G.; et al. Therapeutic Modulation of Plasmacytoid Dendritic Cells in Experimental Arthritis. *Arthritis Rheumatol.* **2017**, *69*, 2124–2135. [CrossRef] [PubMed]
17. Isaacs, A.; Lindenmann, J. Virus interference. I. The interferon. *Proc. R. Soc. Lond. Ser. B Boil. Sci.* **1957**, *147*, 258–267.
18. Duncan, C.J.; Randall, R.E.; Hambleton, S. Genetic Lesions of Type I Interferon Signalling in Human Antiviral Immunity. *Trends Genet.* **2021**, *37*, 46–58. [CrossRef] [PubMed]
19. Reich, N.C. Too much of a good thing: Detrimental effects of interferon. *Semin. Immunol.* **2019**, *43*, 101282. [CrossRef] [PubMed]
20. Melki, I.; Rose, Y.; Uggenti, C.; Van Eyck, L.; Frémond, M.-L.; Kitabayashi, N.; Rice, G.I.; Jenkinson, E.M.; Boulai, A.; Jeremiah, N.; et al. Disease-associated mutations identify a novel region in human STING necessary for the control of type I interferon signaling. *J. Allergy Clin. Immunol.* **2017**, *140*, 543–552.e5. [CrossRef]

21. Volpi, S.; Insalaco, A.; Caorsi, R.; Santori, E.; Messia, V.; Sacco, O.; Terheggen-Lagro, S.; Cardinale, F.; Scarselli, A.; Pastorino, C.; et al. Efficacy and Adverse Events During Janus Kinase Inhibitor Treatment of SAVI Syndrome. *J. Clin. Immunol.* **2019**, *39*, 476–485. [CrossRef]
22. Kretschmer, S.; Lee-Kirsch, M.A. Type I interferon-mediated autoinflammation and autoimmunity. *Curr. Opin. Immunol.* **2017**, *49*, 96–102. [CrossRef]
23. Savic, S.; Caseley, E.A.; McDermott, M.F. Moving towards a systems-based classification of innate immune-mediated diseases. *Nat. Rev. Rheumatol.* **2020**, *16*, 222–237. [CrossRef]
24. Gupta, S.; Kaplan, M.J. Bite of the wolf: Innate immune responses propagate autoimmunity in lupus. *J. Clin. Investig.* **2021**, *131*, e144918. [CrossRef] [PubMed]
25. Bennett, L.; Palucka, A.K.; Arce, E.; Cantrell, V.; Borvak, J.; Banchereau, J.; Pascual, V. Interferon and Granulopoiesis Signatures in Systemic Lupus Erythematosus Blood. *J. Exp. Med.* **2003**, *197*, 711–723. [CrossRef]
26. Mai, L.; Asaduzzaman, A.; Noamani, B.; Fortin, P.R.; Gladman, D.D.; Touma, Z.; Urowitz, M.B.; Wither, J. The baseline interferon signature predicts disease severity over the subsequent 5 years in systemic lupus erythematosus. *Arthritis Res.* **2021**, *23*, 29. [CrossRef]
27. Nehar-Belaid, D.; Hong, S.; Marches, R.; Chen, G.; Bolisetty, M.; Baisch, J.; Walters, L.; Punaro, M.; Rossi, R.J.; Chung, C.-H.; et al. Mapping systemic lupus erythematosus heterogeneity at the single-cell level. *Nat. Immunol.* **2020**, *21*, 1094–1106. [CrossRef] [PubMed]
28. Morand, E.F.; Furie, R.; Tanaka, Y.; Bruce, I.N.; Askanase, A.D.; Richez, C.; Bae, S.-C.; Brohawn, P.Z.; Pineda, L.; Berglind, A.; et al. Trial of Anifrolumab in Active Systemic Lupus Erythematosus. *N. Engl. J. Med.* **2020**, *382*, 211–221. [CrossRef] [PubMed]
29. Italiani, P.; Manca, M.L.; Angelotti, F.; Melillo, D.; Pratesi, F.; Puxeddu, I.; Boraschi, D.; Migliorini, P. IL-1 family cytokines and soluble receptors in systemic lupus erythematosus. *Arthritis Res.* **2018**, *20*, 27. [CrossRef]
30. Cafarelli, F.; Coladonato, L.; Lopalco, G.; Cacciapaglia, F.; Cantarini, L.; Iannone, F. Successful treatment with anakinra of refractory pericarditis in systemic lupus erythematosus. *Clin. Exp. Rheumatol.* **2020**, *39*, 227.
31. Kubler, L.; Bittmann, I.; Kuipers, J.G. Macrophage activation syndrome triggered by active systemic lupus erythematosus: Successful treatment by interleukin-1 inhibition (anakinra). *Z. Rheumatol.* **2020**, *79*, 1040–1045. [CrossRef] [PubMed]
32. Malik, A.; Kanneganti, T.-D. Inflammasome activation and assembly at a glance. *J. Cell Sci.* **2017**, *130*, 3955–3963. [CrossRef]
33. Sönmez, H.E.; Özen, S. A clinical update on inflammasopathies. *Int. Immunol.* **2017**, *29*, 393–400. [CrossRef] [PubMed]
34. Malcova, H.; Strizova, Z.; Milota, T.; Striz, I.; Sediva, A.; Cebecauerova, D.; Horvath, R. IL-1 Inhibitors in the Treatment of Monogenic Periodic Fever Syndromes: From the Past to the Future Perspectives. *Front. Immunol.* **2021**, *11*, 619257. [CrossRef] [PubMed]
35. Pennisi, M.; Crupi, R.; Di Paola, R.; Ontario, M.L.; Bella, R.; Calabrese, E.J.; Crea, R.; Cuzzocrea, S.; Calabrese, V. Inflammasomes, hormesis, and antioxidants in neuroinflammation: Role of NRLP3 in Alzheimer disease. *J. Neurosci. Res.* **2017**, *95*, 1360–1372. [CrossRef]
36. Camilli, G.; Bohm, M.; Piffer, A.C.; Lavenir, R.; Williams, D.L.; Neven, B.; Grateau, G.; Georgin-Lavialle, S.; Quintin, J. beta-Glucan-induced reprogramming of human macrophages inhibits NLRP3 inflammasome activation in cryopyrinopathies. *J. Clin. Investig.* **2020**, *130*, 4561–4573. [CrossRef]
37. Dilger, R.N.; Johnson, R.W. Aging, microglial cell priming, and the discordant central inflammatory response to signals from the peripheral immune system. *J. Leukoc. Biol.* **2008**, *84*, 932–939. [CrossRef] [PubMed]
38. Musella, A.; Fresegna, D.; Rizzo, F.R.; Gentile, A.; De Vito, F.; Caioli, S.; Guadalupi, L.; Bruno, A.; Dolcetti, E.; Buttari, F.; et al. 'Prototypical' proinflammatory cytokine (IL-1) in multiple sclerosis: Role in pathogenesis and therapeutic targeting. *Expert Opin. Targets* **2020**, *24*, 37–46. [CrossRef]
39. McGinley, P.M.; Goldschmidt, C.H.; Rae-Grant, A.D. Diagnosis and Treatment of Multiple Sclerosis: A Review. *JAMA* **2021**, *325*, 765–779. [CrossRef]
40. Chisari, C.G.; Sgarlata, E.; Arena, S.; Toscano, S.; Luca, M.; Patti, F. Rituximab for the treatment of multiple sclerosis: A review. *J. Neurol.* **2021**, 1–25.
41. Masanneck, L.; Eichler, S.; Vogelsang, A.; Korsen, M.; Wiendl, H.; Budde, T.; Meuth, S.G. The STING-IFN-beta-Dependent Axis Is Markedly Low in Patients with Relapsing-Remitting Multiple Sclerosis. *Int. J. Mol. Sci.* **2020**, *21*, 9249. [CrossRef] [PubMed]
42. Guarda, G.; Braun, M.; Staehli, F.; Tardivel, A.; Mattmann, C.; Förster, I.; Farlik, M.; Decker, T.; Du Pasquier, R.A.; Romero, P.; et al. Type I Interferon Inhibits Interleukin-1 Production and Inflammasome Activation. *Immunity* **2011**, *34*, 213–223. [CrossRef] [PubMed]
43. Mayer-Barber, K.D.; Yan, B. Clash of the Cytokine Titans: Counter-regulation of interleukin-1 and type I interferon-mediated inflammatory responses. *Cell. Mol. Immunol.* **2017**, *14*, 22–35. [CrossRef] [PubMed]
44. Ludigs, K.; Parfenov, V.; Du Pasquier, R.A.; Guarda, G. Type I IFN-mediated regulation of IL-1 production in inflammatory disorders. *Cell. Mol. Life Sci.* **2012**, *69*, 3395–3418. [CrossRef] [PubMed]
45. Van Kempen, T.S.; Wenink, M.H.; Leijten, E.F.; Radstake, T.R.; Boes, M. Perception of self: Distinguishing autoimmunity from autoinflammation. *Nat. Rev. Rheumatol.* **2015**, *11*, 483–492. [CrossRef] [PubMed]
46. Malhotra, S.; Costa, C.; Eixarch, H.; Keller, C.W.; Amman, L.; Martínez-Banaclocha, H.; Midaglia, L.; Sarró, E.; Machín-Díaz, I.; Villar, L.M.; et al. NLRP3 inflammasome as prognostic factor and therapeutic target in primary progressive multiple sclerosis patients. *Brain* **2020**, *143*, 1414–1430. [CrossRef]

47. Piancone, F.; Saresella, M.; Marventano, I.; La Rosa, F.; Santangelo, M.A.; Caputo, D.; Mendozzi, L.; Rovaris, M.; Clerici, M. Monosodium Urate Crystals Activate the Inflammasome in Primary Progressive Multiple Sclerosis. *Front. Immunol.* **2018**, *9*, 983. [CrossRef]
48. Nehmar, R.; Mariotte, A.; De Cauwer, A.; Sibilia, J.; Bahram, S.; Georgel, P. Therapeutic Perspectives for Interferons and Plasmacytoid Dendritic Cells in Rheumatoid Arthritis. *Trends Mol. Med.* **2018**, *24*, 338–347. [CrossRef]
49. Kohase, M.; Zhang, Y.; Lin, J.X.; Yamazaki, S.; Sehgal, P.B.; Vilček, J. Interleukin-1 can inhibit interferon-beta synthesis and its antiviral action: Comparison with tumor necrosis factor. *J. Interferon. Res.* **1988**, *8*, 559–570. [CrossRef]
50. SSlim, J.; Afridi, M.S. Managing Adverse Effects of Interferon-Alfa and Ribavirin in Combination Therapy for HCV. *Infect. Dis. Clin. N. Am.* **2012**, *26*, 917–929. [CrossRef] [PubMed]
51. Wagstaff, J.A.; Perry, C.M. Topical imiquimod: A review of its use in the management of anogenital warts, actinic keratoses, basal cell carcinoma and other skin lesions. *Drugs* **2007**, *67*, 2187–2210. [CrossRef]
52. Tanaka, Y.; Tummala, R. Anifrolumab, a monoclonal antibody to the type I interferon receptor subunit 1, for the treatment of systemic lupus erythematosus: An overview from clinical trials. *Mod. Rheumatol.* **2021**, *31*, 1–12. [CrossRef] [PubMed]
53. Clere-Jehl, R.; Mariotte, A.; Meziani, F.; Bahram, S.; Georgel, P.; Helms, J. JAK–STAT Targeting Offers Novel Therapeutic Opportunities in Sepsis. *Trends Mol. Med.* **2020**, *26*, 987–1002. [CrossRef]
54. Melki, I.; Frémond, M.-L. Type I Interferonopathies: From a Novel Concept to Targeted Therapeutics. *Curr. Rheumatol. Rep.* **2020**, *22*, 32. [CrossRef] [PubMed]
55. Mailhot, B.; Christin, M.; Tessandier, N.; Sotoudeh, C.; Bretheau, F.; Turmel, R.; Pellerin, È.; Wang, F.; Bories, C.; Joly-Beauparlant, C.; et al. Neuronal interleukin-1 receptors mediate pain in chronic inflammatory diseases. *J. Exp. Med.* **2020**, *217*. [CrossRef] [PubMed]
56. Conaghan, P.G.; Alten, R.; Deodhar, A.; Sullivan, E.; Blackburn, S.; Tian, H.; Gandhi, K.; Jugl, S.M.; Strand, V. Relationship of pain and fatigue with health-related quality of life and work in patients with psoriatic arthritis on TNFi: Results of a multi-national real-world study. *RMD Open* **2020**, *6*, e001240. [CrossRef] [PubMed]
57. Lin, C.C.; Edelson, B.T. New Insights into the Role of IL-1 beta in Experimental Autoimmune Encephalomyelitis and Multiple Sclerosis. *J. Immunol.* **2017**, *198*, 4553–4560. [CrossRef]
58. Ozdogan, H.; Ugurlu, S.; Uygunoglu, U.; Tutuncu, M.; Gul, A.; Akman, G.; Siva, A. The efficacy of anti- IL-1 treatment in three patients with coexisting familial Mediterranean fever and multiple sclerosis. *Mult. Scler. Relat. Disord.* **2020**, *45*, 102332. [CrossRef]
59. Iula, L.; Keitelman, I.A.; Sabbione, F.; Fuentes, F.; Guzman, M.; Galletti, J.G.; Gerber, P.P.; Ostrowski, M.; Geffner, J.R.; Jancic, C.C.; et al. Autophagy Mediates Interleukin-1β Secretion in Human Neutrophils. *Front. Immunol.* **2018**, *9*, 269. [CrossRef] [PubMed]
60. Esnault, S.; Kelly, E.A.; Nettenstrom, L.M.; Cook, E.B.; Seroogy, C.M.; Jarjour, N.N. Human eosinophils release IL-1ß and increase expression of IL-17A in activated CD4+T lymphocytes. *Clin. Exp. Allergy* **2012**, *42*, 1756–1764. [CrossRef]
61. Bassi, G.; Grimaudo, M.; Panseri, S.; Montesi, M. Advanced Multi-Dimensional Cellular Models as Emerging Reality to Reproduce In Vitro the Human Body Complexity. *Int. J. Mol. Sci.* **2021**, *22*, 1195. [CrossRef] [PubMed]
62. Becker, J.; Kinast, V.; Döring, M.; Lipps, C.; Duran, V.; Spanier, J.; Tegtmeyer, P.-K.; Wirth, D.; Cicin-Sain, L.; Alcamí, A.; et al. Human monocyte-derived macrophages inhibit HCMV spread independent of classical antiviral cytokines. *Virulence* **2018**, *9*, 1669–1684. [CrossRef] [PubMed]
63. Aarreberg, L.D.; Esser-Nobis, K.; Driscoll, C.; Shuvarikov, A.; Roby, J.A.; Gale, M., Jr. Interleukin-1β Induces mtDNA Release to Activate Innate Immune Signaling via cGAS-STING. *Mol. Cell* **2019**, *74*, 801–815. [CrossRef] [PubMed]
64. Banchereau, J.; Pascual, V. Type I Interferon in Systemic Lupus Erythematosus and Other Autoimmune Diseases. *Immunity* **2006**, *25*, 383–392. [CrossRef]
65. Lliso-Ribera, G.; Humby, F.; Lewis, M.; Nerviani, A.; Mauro, D.; Rivellese, F.; Kelly, S.; Hands, R.; Bene, F.; Ramamoorthi, N.; et al. Synovial tissue signatures enhance clinical classification and prognostic/treatment response algorithms in early inflammatory arthritis and predict requirement for subsequent biological therapy: Results from the pathobiology of early arthritis cohort (PEAC). *Ann. Rheum. Dis.* **2019**, *78*, 1642–1652.
66. Costantini, S.; Castello, G.; Colonna, G. Human Cytokinome: A new challenge for systems biology. *Bioinformation* **2010**, *5*, 166–167. [CrossRef]
67. Brzustewicz, E.; Bzoma, I.; Daca, A.; Szarecka, M.; Bykowska, M.S.; Witkowski, J.M.; Bryl, E. Heterogeneity of the cytokinome in undifferentiated arthritis progressing to rheumatoid arthritis and its change in the course of therapy. Move toward personalized medicine. *Cytokine* **2017**, *97*, 1–13. [CrossRef] [PubMed]
68. Conrad, C.; Di Domizio, J.; Mylonas, A.; Belkhodja, C.; DeMaria, O.; Navarini, A.A.; Lapointe, A.-K.; French, L.E.; Vernez, M.; Gilliet, M. TNF blockade induces a dysregulated type I interferon response without autoimmunity in paradoxical psoriasis. *Nat. Commun.* **2018**, *9*, 25. [CrossRef]
69. Brennan, F.; Jackson, A.; Chantry, D.; Maini, R.; Feldmann, M. Inhibitory effect of TNF alpha antibodies on synovial cell interleukin-1 production in rheumatoid arthritis. *Lancet* **1989**, *2*, 244–247. [CrossRef]

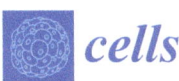

Review

It's All in the PAN: Crosstalk, Plasticity, Redundancies, Switches, and Interconnectedness Encompassed by PANoptosis Underlying the Totality of Cell Death-Associated Biological Effects

Jessica M. Gullett, Rebecca E. Tweedell and Thirumala-Devi Kanneganti *

Department of Immunology, St. Jude Children's Research Hospital, Memphis, TN 38105, USA; jessica.gullett@stjude.org (J.M.G.); rebecca.tweedell@stjude.org (R.E.T.)
* Correspondence: thirumala-devi.kanneganti@stjude.org; Tel.: +1-(901)-595-3634; Fax: +1-(901)-595-5766

Abstract: The innate immune system provides the first line of defense against cellular perturbations. Innate immune activation elicits inflammatory programmed cell death in response to microbial infections or alterations in cellular homeostasis. Among the most well-characterized programmed cell death pathways are pyroptosis, apoptosis, and necroptosis. While these pathways have historically been defined as segregated and independent processes, mounting evidence shows significant crosstalk among them. These molecular interactions have been described as 'crosstalk', 'plasticity', 'redundancies', 'molecular switches', and more. Here, we discuss the key components of cell death pathways and note several examples of crosstalk. We then explain how the diverse descriptions of crosstalk throughout the literature can be interpreted through the lens of an integrated inflammatory cell death concept, PANoptosis. The totality of biological effects in PANoptosis cannot be individually accounted for by pyroptosis, apoptosis, or necroptosis alone. We also discuss PANoptosomes, which are multifaceted macromolecular complexes that regulate PANoptosis. We consider the evidence for PANoptosis, which has been mechanistically characterized during influenza A virus, herpes simplex virus 1, *Francisella novicida*, and *Yersinia* infections, as well as in response to altered cellular homeostasis, in inflammatory diseases, and in cancers. We further discuss the role of IRF1 as an upstream regulator of PANoptosis and conclude by reexamining historical studies which lend credence to the PANoptosis concept. Cell death has been shown to play a critical role in infections, inflammatory diseases, neurodegenerative diseases, cancers, and more; therefore, having a holistic understanding of cell death is important for identifying new therapeutic strategies.

Keywords: PANoptosis; PANoptosome; pyroptosis; apoptosis; necroptosis; inflammatory cell death; inflammasome; inflammation; innate immunity; infection; NLR; caspase; IRF1; ZBP1; RIPK1; RIPK3; MLKL; NLRP3; AIM2; Pyrin; caspase-1; ASC; caspase-8; caspase-3; caspase-7; crosstalk; plasticity; redundancy

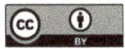

1. Introduction

The innate immune system is the first line of defense against infection and cellular insults; innate immune receptors can recognize the molecular signatures of pathogens, called pathogen-associated molecular patterns (PAMPs), as well as components released by damaged cells, called damage-associated molecular patterns (DAMPs). The innate immune system activates genetically defined programmed cell death pathways in response to microbial infections or alterations in cellular homeostasis; among the most well characterized of these programmed cell death responses are pyroptosis, apoptosis, and necroptosis. Though canonically proposed as segregated cellular processes responding to individualized PAMPs and DAMPs, mounting evidence shows significant interactions between the components of pyroptosis, apoptosis, and necroptosis. Historically, the literature on cell death and innate immune signaling has used different terms to describe these interactions, such as 'crosstalk', 'plasticity', 'redundancies', and 'molecular switches'. Consideration of the totality of biological effects from cell death in multiple studies has led to the conceptualization of PANoptosis [1–20], an inflammatory cell death pathway that integrates components from other cell death pathways. PANoptosis is implicated in driving innate immune responses and inflammation and cannot be individually accounted for by pyroptosis, apoptosis, or necroptosis alone. PANoptosis is regulated by PANoptosomes, multifaceted macromolecular complexes. Here, we review the key components of programmed cell death pathways and highlight the plasticity among pyroptosis, apoptosis, and necroptosis. We then discuss the conceptualization of PANoptosis, which continues to evolve over time based on data, and examine the current evidence supporting this concept.

Key Components in Inflammatory Programmed Cell Death Pathways

Among the most comprehensively studied cell death processes to date are pyroptosis, apoptosis, and necroptosis [21,22]. Each occurs in response to cellular insults, but they differ in terms of their molecular machinery. Pyroptosis is a lytic form of proinflammatory cell death that was originally described as a caspase-1-mediated death [23]. Pyroptotic cell death typically involves the formation of the inflammasome, a supramolecular platform that is composed of a sensor, adaptor protein ASC, and caspase-1 [24]. The five most well-known inflammasomes, which are named after their corresponding sensor based on the genetic characterization of sensors and triggers, are the NLR family inflammasomes, NLRP1 [24], NLRP3 [25–27], and NAIP/NLRC4 [28–30], as well as those formed by other sensors containing pyrin domains, such as Pyrin [31] and AIM2 [32,33]. Sensor activation polymerizes the adaptor protein ASC into prion-like structures referred to as ASC specks [34–36], which recruit caspase-1 to allow its autoproteolysis and activation [24,37]. Activated caspase-1 cleaves inflammatory cytokines IL-1β and IL-18 [38] as well as the pore-forming molecule gasdermin D (GSDMD) [39]. The GSDMD-mediated pores allow the release of the inflammatory cytokines [40–44] along with other inflammatory molecules such as HMGB1, which serve as DAMPs and further propagate an innate immune inflammatory response. GSDMD is also activated by caspase-11 (mice) and caspase-4/5 (humans) in the process of non-canonical inflammasome activation [39–41,44,45]. In addition to requiring cleavage for activation, GSDMD is also regulated at the transcriptional level by IFN regulatory factor 2 (IRF2), with a compensatory role for IRF1, in murine bone marrow-derived macrophages (BMDMs) [46]; in human cells IRF2 does not regulate GSDMD expression but does regulate caspase-4-mediated cell death, and IRF1 acts cooperatively in this process in response to IFN-γ [47].

Apoptosis is a form of programmed cell death originally described as a 'mechanism of controlled cell deletion' characterized by its distinct morphological membrane blebbing and subsequent cell shrinkage [48]. It proceeds through either an extrinsic or intrinsic pathway, though both result in the activation of the same executioner caspases. The intrinsic pathway forms an APAF1-mediated apoptosome in response to homeostatic disruptions, such as DNA damage or loss of mitochondrial stability [49]. This multiprotein complex includes APAF1, cytochrome c, and the initiator caspase caspase-9 which, upon cleavage, activates the downstream effector/executioner caspases, caspase-3 and -7 [50,51]. Extrinsic apoptosis occurs after ligand binding to death receptors, such as Fas and TNF-α receptor (TNFR), on the cell surface; downstream of death receptor binding, FADD translocates to the receptor, which recruits caspase-8. Caspase-8 is the key extrinsic apoptotic initiator caspase which cleaves downstream caspases, caspase-3 and -7, to execute cell death [52,53]. Caspase-8 can also induce activation of intrinsic apoptosis by activating the proapoptotic molecule Bid [54–56], which translocates to the mitochondria to facilitate pore formation by BAX/BAK and induce mitochondrial outer membrane permeabilization (MOMP) and apoptosome formation [57,58].

Necroptosis, another lytic form of cell death, occurs in response to caspase-8 inhibition and is RIPK3- and MLKL-dependent [22,59–61]. The apoptotic caspase-8 typically blocks necroptosis by cleaving RIPK3, CYLD, and RIPK1 [62–64]. Necroptosis can be initiated in response to the activation of toll-like receptors (TLRs), death receptors, or through interferon (IFN) signaling [65]. A well-characterized necroptosis response is induced by TNF-α. Its binding to TNFR induces signaling that activates RIPK1 to become phosphorylated and, along with TRADD, FADD, and caspase-8, form complex II [66]. When caspase-8 is inhibited, RIPK1 interacts with RIPK3 to form a cell death-inducing necrosome. The RIPK1-RIPK3 complex promotes phosphorylation of MLKL, causing its oligomerization. The MLKL multimer then translocates to the plasma membrane, where it interacts with phospholipids and forms pores [67,68]. In addition to MLKL phosphorylation by RIPK3, MLKL activity is also regulated by other post-translational modifications, such as ubiquitylation, which is necessary for higher-order oligomerization [69].

Within each of these cell death pathways, there are several regulators and auxiliary components. For example, additional inflammasome components have been identified that are involved in its regulation and activation, such as NEK7 [70–73] and DDX3X [74], as well as transcription factors such as IRF1 [75], IRF2 [46,47], and IRF8 [76]. Additionally, NINJ1 has been identified as a critical component for plasma membrane rupture [77]. There are also variations in the signaling cascades that exist within each programmed cell death pathway, making the complexity of these cellular processes, including regulatory components, cell- and trigger-specific responses, and time-dependent responses, limitless. Additional components and layers of complexity have been extensively reviewed elsewhere [22,78,79].

2. Evidence of Crosstalk at the Molecular Level

Understanding the activation and execution of inflammatory cell death pathways has been an active area of research, particularly given the clinical relevance of cell death pathways in infections, inflammatory diseases, cancers, and beyond [2,4,5,7–9,11–13,16,18–20]. As a result of these studies, several examples of crosstalk and flexibility have been identified between the molecular components of programmed cell death pathways. Here, we will limit our discussion to genetically defined examples over time.

At their core, apoptosis and necroptosis are intricately molecularly linked, given that TNF-induced caspase-8 activation drives apoptosis while inhibition of caspase-8 during this process drives necroptosis [80]. The rescue of caspase-8-deficient embryos by the loss of RIPK3 or MLKL has long been documented [81–84], and enzymatically active caspase-8 is critical in the regulation and balance of apoptosis and necroptosis [85,86].

Beyond the intrinsic connection between apoptosis and necroptosis, caspase-1, an essential component of inflammasomes, cleaves apoptosis-associated caspase-7 during *Salmonella* infection (NLRC4 inflammasome trigger) as well as in response to LPS + ATP stimulation (NLRP3 inflammasome trigger) [17]. The pyroptotic caspase-1 also cleaves apoptotic PARP1 in response to inflammasome-activating triggers [6], and loss of caspase-1 during *Salmonella* infection leads to activation of apoptotic proteins instead [87]. In addition, cells lacking pyroptotic caspase-1 and caspase-11 have reduced mitochondrial damage in response to inflammasome-activating triggers such as the NLRP3-activating LPS + ATP treatment or AIM2-activating dsDNA transfection [88], suggesting additional crosstalk between inflammasomes and apoptotic processes. Reciprocally, the apoptotic caspase-8 serves as a regulatory component of pyroptotic inflammasomes [19]. Fluorescence microscopy has shown the colocalization of caspase-8 and ASC in both pyroptosis-deficient and pyroptosis-sufficient cells in response to infections [12,89–91]. Additionally, caspase-8, along with FADD, is required to both prime and activate canonical (ligand-induced) and noncanonical (*E. coli*- or *Citrobacter rodentium*-induced) NLRP3 inflammasomes [19]. Caspase-8 can be recruited during NLRC4 and NLRP1b inflammasome formation [91–93] and at ASC specks involving multiple inflammasome sensors, such as NLRP3 and NLRC4 or AIM2 and Pyrin [12,94]; FADD can also be recruited to these ASC specks in response to FlaTox, a combination of the bacterial PAMPs *Bacillus anthracis* protective antigen and the N-terminus of lethal factor fused to *Legionella pneumophila* flagellin [93]. However, caspase-8 is not required for *Salmonella*-induced cell death at 2, 6, and 24 h post-infection using an MOI of 1 or 10 [91], showcasing the variability of the roles of caspase-8 within the programmed cell death response.

Crosstalk has also been identified between cell death molecules by studying the totality of biological effects in disease processes. For example, inflammatory bone disease in mice carrying the *Pstpip2*^{cmo} mutation persists despite deletion of caspase-1 or combined deletion of caspase-8/RIPK3 (deletion of caspase-8 alone is embryonically lethal [84]); the inflammation is only rescued by the combined deletion of NLRP3 or caspase-1 with caspase-8/RIPK3 [16,18], highlighting the functional redundancies of pyroptotic molecules NLRP3 and caspase-1 with the apoptosis-necroptosis modulator caspase-8. In the context of infection, influenza A virus (IAV) induces activation of pyroptotic, apoptotic, and necroptotic proteins, and loss of RIPK3 protects against much of the cell death, but combined deletion of caspase-8 and RIPK3 is necessary to further reduce cell death [9], providing additional mechanistic evidence of overlaps in the functions of molecules involved in cell death activation.

Beyond caspase-8 and RIPK3, the necroptotic molecule MLKL has also been implicated in crosstalk between cell death pathways. For example, ASC oligomerization to induce NLRP3 inflammasome activation can occur in response to treatment with TLR3 ligands and zVAD, but the ASC oligomerization is blocked in MLKL-deficient cells [95]. As oligomerized MLKL forms pores in the plasma membrane, a cascade of cellular consequences begins, including the efflux of potassium ions. This necroptosis-induced ionic efflux has been shown to activate the NLRP3 inflammasome [96,97]. Together, these data show how necroptosis and inflammasomes (pyroptosis) are interconnected.

Given the recently identified role of gasdermins in cell death, it has also been found that gasdermins mediate crosstalk between cell death pathways. GSDMD was initially identified as an executioner of pyroptotic cell death in response to caspase-1, caspase-4/-5 (human) or caspase-11 (mouse) cleavage [39,45]. Caspase-8 can also cleave GSDMD to activate pore formation and cell death during *Yersinia* infection [3,98–100]. Further studies have found that GSDMD can also be processed by the apoptosis-inducing caspase-3 in such a manner that renders GSDMD inactive, suppressing pyroptosis [101]. However, inflammasome and GSDMD activation in response to Shiga toxin 2 and LPS are also associated with increased mitochondrial ROS [102], and GSDMD can form pores in the mitochondrial membrane to release canonically proapoptotic molecules and activate caspase-3 in a BAK/BAX-independent manner [103,104]. Other members of the gasdermin family are also increasingly implicated in cell death crosstalk. Microarray and subsequent pathway analysis of inner ear samples from day-0 postnatal mice showed that the gene set involved in apoptosis is downregulated in mice lacking *Gsdme* as compared with wild-type controls [105]. Furthermore, GSDME can be cleaved by caspase-3, an apoptotic cell death effector, and can induce pyroptotic death [106,107]. In THP-1 cells lacking GSDMD, GSDME allows the release of IL-1β in response to nigericin, Val-boroPro, or *Salmonella* infection, though limited cell death was observed with endogenous GSDME expression levels in these cells [108]. In murine cells, NLRP3 inflammasome activation in GSDMD-deficient cells results in IL-1β and IL-18 release through caspase-8/-3 and GSDME activation [109]. GSDME serves in a feed-forward loop to promote caspase-3 activation by forming pores in the mitochondrial membrane and inducing the release of cytochrome c in response to traditional intrinsic and extrinsic apoptotic stimuli; overexpression studies have shown similar results with GSDMA [103]. Beyond these connections, in cells lacking pyroptosis via GSDMD-deficiency, caspase-1 can cleave caspase-3 and Bid to promote apoptotic cell death in response to inflammasome triggers such as LPS priming and poly(dA:dT) transfection, or during *Salmonella* infection [110,111]. Furthermore, the APAF1-apoptosome has been shown to interact with caspase-11 when cells are challenged with bile acid; the result is caspase-3 cleavage and the execution of pyroptotic death in a GSDME-mediated process [112]. Other pore-forming molecules may also be involved in this crosstalk, as pannexin-1 activation downstream of caspase-8 or -9 activation leads to NLRP3 inflammasome formation in a GSDMD- and GSDME-independent process [113].

3. Prototypical Examples of PANoptosis

The depth and breadth of literature encompassing innate immune signaling and programmed cell death is impressive. Repeatedly, the literature acknowledges instances of crosstalk between components of pyroptosis, apoptosis, and necroptosis. This crosstalk occurs in context-dependent manners and is sometimes referred to as 'plasticity' or 'redundancy', with cell death components often labeled as 'molecular switches'. The overwhelming amount of evidence for the interconnectedness between cell death pathways has led to the conceptualization of PANoptosis as an inflammatory cell death pathway. The totality of biological effects in PANoptosis cannot be individually accounted for by pyroptosis, apoptosis, or necroptosis alone [2–20]. PANoptosis has been increasingly implicated in infectious and inflammatory diseases as well as in cancers and cancer therapies [2–5,7–16,18,20,114–118]. Here, we will focus on the most mechanistically well-characterized examples of PANoptosis and PANoptosomes [3,7,9–12,20] (Figure 1).

As the conceptualization of PANoptosis implies, PANoptosis involves the activation of several molecules previously characterized as mediators of independent cell death pathways. For instance, Z-DNA-binding protein 1 (ZBP1) was previously known to induce necrosis in response to a mutant form of MCMV expressing a tetra-alanine RHIM substitution in vIRA (M45*mut*RHIM) [119] and was shown to interact with the necroptotic molecules RIPK1 and RIPK3 [120], but more recent evidence has shown that ZBP1 acts as a cytosolic innate immune sensor for endogenous nucleic acids or during IAV infection to induce activation of the NLRP3 inflammasome, caspase-1, caspase-8, caspase-3, caspase-7 [7,9,11], and MLKL [7,11,121]. Molecularly, ZBP1 mediates the formation of a multiprotein ZBP1-PANoptosome complex, containing ZBP1, RIPK3, RIPK1, caspase-8, caspase-6, ASC, and NLRP3 [10,11]. To date, this complex has been characterized by immunoprecipitation [7,10,11], and immunofluorescence has also shown colocalization of caspase-8 and RIPK3 with ASC specks in individual cells during IAV infection [122]. Further studies, including biochemical analyses and cryo-EM evaluation, are needed to fully understand how components come together in individual cells. The ZBP1-PANoptosome complex can also be implicated in tumorigenesis, where ADAR1 acts as a negative regulator to prevent the interaction between ZBP1 and RIPK3 and promote tumorigenesis. Limiting the interaction between ADAR1 and ZBP1 by sequestering ADAR1 in the nucleus, through treatment with nuclear transport inhibitors (KPT-330) in conjunction with IFN, potentiates PANoptosis and limits tumorigenesis [7].

Additionally, the inflammasome sensor AIM2 also initiates the formation of PANoptosome complexes during herpes simplex virus 1 (HSV1) and *Francisella novicida* infections. This PANoptosome, termed the AIM2-PANoptosome, contains AIM2, ZBP1, Pyrin, ASC, caspase-1, caspase-8, RIPK3, RIPK1, and FADD [12]. PANoptosomes have also been identified by immunoprecipitation during *Yersinia* infection, where RIPK1, RIPK3, caspase-8, FADD, ASC, and NLRP3 can be co-immunoprecipitated [3]. In the context of *Yersinia* infection, RIPK1 is necessary for activation of caspase-1, GSDMD, caspase-8, caspase-3, and caspase-7, but it negatively regulates the activation of MLKL, highlighting the multifaceted modulation of cell death effectors that can occur within PANoptosis [3]. PANoptosis has also been observed in response to TAK1 inhibition in macrophages, which can occur as a result of *Yersinia* infection due to its effector YopJ or in response to genetic mutations or treatment with TAK1 inhibitors [5,20,98,100]. In the case of TAK1-deficient macrophages, spontaneous PANoptosis occurs and is characterized by the activation of the NLRP3 inflammasome, caspase-1, caspase-3, caspase-8, and MLKL [5,20]; stimulation with LPS in TAK1-deficient macrophages induces colocalization of RIPK1, ASC, and caspase-8 in a RIPK1 kinase-independent manner [20].

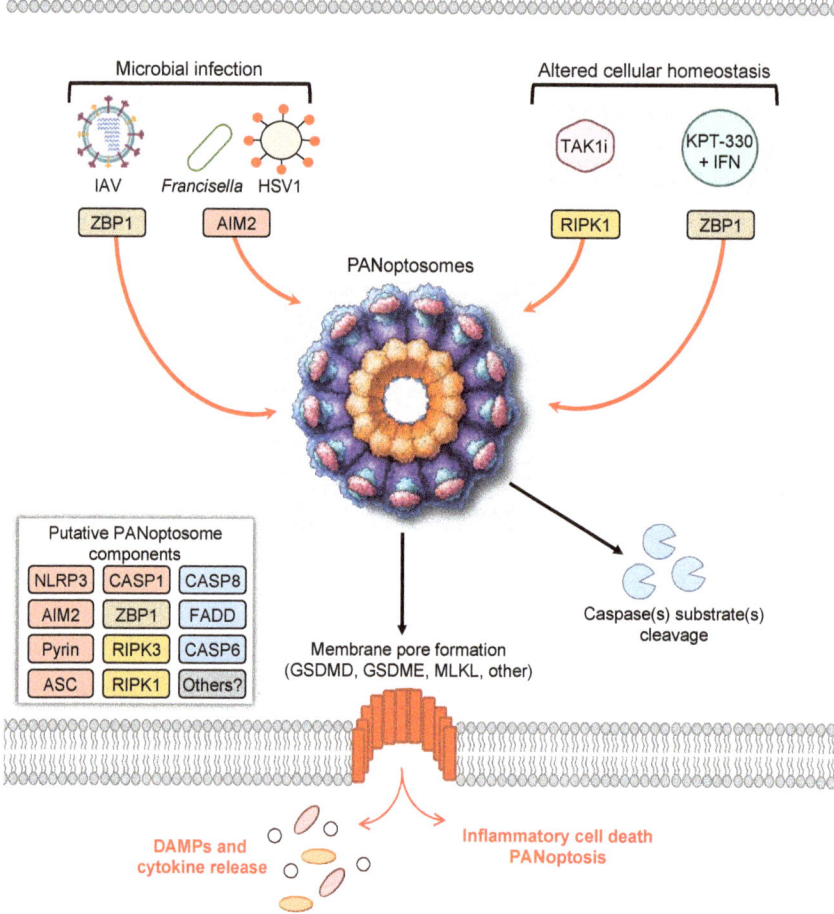

Figure 1. PANoptosis and PANoptosome formation. Upon exposure to cellular insults, such as microbial infection or altered cellular homeostasis, sensors can detect the perturbation and activate PANoptosis. Prototypical examples of PANoptosis are depicted here. Sensor activation can lead to the formation of a multiprotein complex, the PANoptosome. PANoptosomes have the potential to bring together diverse components from previously segregated cell death pathways. These may be dynamic complexes, and their protein composition may vary in trigger- and time-dependent manners. Potential PANoptosome components putatively include inflammasome sensors, such as nucleotide-binding oligomerization domain-like receptor family pyrin domain-containing 3 (NLRP3), absent in melanoma 2 (AIM2), Pyrin, Z-DNA-binding protein 1 (ZBP1), or others; apoptosis-associated speck-like protein containing a caspase activation and recruitment domain (ASC); caspase-1 (CASP1); receptor-interacting serine/threonine protein kinase 3 (RIPK3); RIPK1; caspase-8 (CASP8); Fas-associated protein with death domain (FADD); and/or caspase-6 (CASP6). PANoptosis involves membrane pore formation for the execution of cell death to release cytokines, such as IL-1β and IL-18, and DAMPs. Figure created with https://biorender.com/ (accessed on 17 March 2022).

4. PANoptosis Regulation via IRF1

As with other cell death pathways, PANoptosis must be tightly regulated to control the execution of cell death. IRF1, a molecule long recognized for its roles in regulating cell death [123,124], is a key upstream regulator of PANoptosis. In the absence of IRF1 during IAV infection, ZBP1 protein expression, along with NLRP3 inflammasome, caspase-1, caspase-8, caspase-3, and MLKL activation, are all reduced [75]. In the context of colorectal tumorigenesis, IRF1 facilitates the activation of PANoptosis to limit tumorigenesis [8]. PANoptosis has also been observed to be driven by IRF1 in response to the combination of TNF and IFN-γ. TNF and IFN-γ release can occur physiologically during cytokine storm syndromes, including during SARS-CoV-2 infection [2], and together they induce PANoptosis through the JAK/IRF1 signaling axis [2,4]; this observation has led to a mechanistic definition for cytokine storm as a life-threatening condition caused by excessive production of cytokines mediated by PANoptosis [125]. Additionally, the AIM2 inflammasome has also been shown to be regulated by IRF1 during *Francisella* infection [126], suggesting a possible regulatory role of IRF1 in PANoptosis mediated by the AIM2-PANoptosome, although this remains to be investigated.

5. A Rose by Any Other Name

Given the extensive history characterizing innate immune signaling and cell death molecules, complexes, and processes, it is important to revisit previous studies to potentially connect key concepts. The recent expansion of studies on PANoptosis further combined with a fresh look at the full body of literature in the cell death field suggests that the concept of PANoptosis has been hiding in plain sight (Tables 1 and 2). Many researchers have reported instances of cell death crosstalk, functional redundancy, or interconnectedness [127], all of which sets the foundation for PANoptosis. As one key example, a wealth of literature exists on the apoptotic caspase-8 and how its loss or impaired functionality modulates multiple programmed cell death pathways and their plasticity in development and disease [62,128–132]. Mice expressing a catalytically inactive version of caspase-8, i.e., $Casp8^{C362A/C362A}$, are embryonically lethal [130]. Cells carrying $Casp8^{C362A/C362A}$ form ASC specks, induce activation of the inflammatory caspase substrate GSDMD, and activate apoptotic caspases, caspase-3 and caspase-7, to mediate cell death. While embryonic lethality in mice carrying $Casp8^{C362A/C362A}$ can be partially rescued by deleting pyroptotic caspase-1 or ASC, mice with combined deletions of caspase-1/-11/RIPK3 have the best survival outcome [130], suggesting that multiple cell death pathways are responsible for the embryonic lethality. Similar results are observed in mice carrying another enzymatically inactive caspase-8 mutation, $Casp8^{C362S/C362S}$, where lethality is rescued by combined deletion of MLKL/ASC or MLKL/caspase-1 [128], suggesting that the apoptotic caspase-8 can play a scaffolding role, and multiple cell death effectors are involved in the cell death in mice carrying catalytically inactive caspase-8. On the one hand, mice carrying a non-cleavable version of caspase-8 ($Casp8^{D387A/D387A}$ [$Casp8^{DA/DA}$] or homozygous $Casp8^{D212A/D218A/D225A/D387A}$ [$Casp8^{4DA/4DA}$]) are viable and normal [62,129,132], while, on the other hand, $Casp8^{DA/DA}Mlkl^{-/-}$ and $Casp8^{DA/DA}Ripk3^{-/-}$ mice develop extensive inflammation. This inflammation can be rescued by deletion of one allele of FASL, FADD, or RIPK1 [129], implicating apoptotic and necroptotic molecules in this inflammation. Furthermore, cell type-specific deletions of caspase-8 have identified additional connections. Mice lacking intestinal epithelial cell (IEC) caspase-8 develop colitis and ileitis which can be rescued by deletion of MLKL. Colitis and ileitis also occur in mice lacking FADD in IECs, with cell death mediated by MLKL and caspase-8-dependent activation of GSDMD. Upstream, loss of ZBP1 is sufficient to prevent ileitis in both mice with caspase-8- and FADD-deficient IECs [131]. Collectively, these results align well with the PANoptosis concept, where there is a totality of biological effects in the phenotype that do not fit within pyroptosis, apoptosis, or necroptosis alone.

Table 1. Totality of cell death in cellular responses.

Trigger	PANoptosome Sensor	Regulator	Pyroptosis Genotype	Cell Death?	Apoptosis Genotype	Cell Death?	Necroptosis Genotype	Cell Death?	PANoptosis Genotype	Cell Death?
IAV [9–11,133]	ZBP1	IRF1	Nlrp3$^{-/-}$	✓	Casp8$^{DA/DA}$	✓	Ripk3$^{-/-}$	D	Fadd$^{-/-}$Ripk3$^{-/-}$	D
			Casp1/11$^{-/-}$	✓	Casp6$^{-/-}$	D	Mlkl$^{-/-}$	✓	Casp8$^{-/-}$Ripk3$^{-/-}$	X
							Ripk1^{K45A}	✓	Casp1/11$^{-/-}$Casp8$^{-/-}$Ri	X
KPT + IFN [7]	ZBP1	IRF1	Nlrp3$^{-/-}$	✓	Casp3$^{-/-}$	✓	Ripk3$^{-/-}$	D	Casp8$^{-/-}$Ripk3$^{-/-}$	X
			Asc$^{-/-}$	✓	Casp7$^{-/-}$	✓	Mlkl$^{-/-}$	✓		
			Casp1$^{-/-}$	✓						
			Casp11$^{-/-}$	✓						
Francisella [12,134]	AIM2	IRF1	Aim2$^{-/-}$	X			Ripk3$^{-/-}$	D	Casp8$^{-/-}$Ripk3$^{-/-}$	X
			Casp1/11$^{-/-}$	X						
			Asc$^{-/-}$	X						
			Mefv$^{-/-}$	D						
			Nlrp3$^{-/-}$	✓						
			Nlrc4$^{-/-}$	✓						
HSV1 [12]	AIM2		Aim2$^{-/-}$	X			Ripk3$^{-/-}$	D	Casp8$^{-/-}$Ripk3$^{-/-}$	X
			Mefv$^{-/-}$	D						
			Nlrp3$^{-/-}$	✓						
			Nlrc4$^{-/-}$	✓						
Yersinia [3]	RIPK1		Casp1/11$^{-/-}$	✓	Casp3$^{-/-}$	✓	Ripk3$^{-/-}$	✓	Casp8$^{-/-}$Ripk3$^{-/-}$	D
			Gsdmd$^{-/-}$	✓	Casp7$^{-/-}$	✓	Ripk1$^{-/-}$	D	Casp1/11$^{-/-}$Casp8$^{-/-}$Ri	X
							Mlkl$^{-/-}$	✓		
TNF + IFN-γ [8]		IRF1	Casp1/11$^{-/-}$	✓	Casp3$^{-/-}$	D	Ripk3$^{-/-}$	✓	Casp8$^{-/-}$Ripk3$^{-/-}$	X
			Casp1$^{-/-}$	✓	Casp7$^{-/-}$	✓			Fadd$^{-/-}$Ripk3$^{-/-}$	X
			Casp11$^{-/-}$	✓						

Table 1. *Cont.*

Trigger	PANoptosome Sensor	Regulator	Pyroptosis		Apoptosis		Necroptosis		PANoptosis	
			Genotype	Cell Death?	Genotype	Cell Death?	Genotype	Cell Death?	Genotype	Cell Death?
MHV [15]			$Nlrp3^{-/-}$	I			$Ripk3^{-/-}$	D	$Casp8^{-/-}Ripk3^{-/-}$	X
			$Casp1/11^{-/-}$	I						
			$Aim2^{-/-}$	✓					$Casp1/11^{-/-}Casp8^{-/-}Ripk3^{-/-}$	X
			$Nlrc4^{-/-}$	✓						
			$Casp11^{-/-}$	✓						
Salmonella [10,30,135,136]			$Nlrc4^{-/-}$	D					$Casp8^{-/-}Ripk3^{-/-}$	✓
			$Casp1/11^{-/-}$	D					$Casp1/11^{-/-}Casp8^{-/-}Ripk3^{-/-}$	X
			$Casp11^{-/-}$	D						
			$Asc^{-/-}$	D						
Pseudomonas [137–139]			$Nlrc4^{-/-}$	D					$Casp1/11^{-/-}Casp8^{-/-}Ripk3^{-/-}$	X
			$Asc^{-/-}$	✓						
			$Casp1^{-/-}$	X						

Studies have consistently identified cell death crosstalk, plasticity, redundancy, interconnection, and molecular switches in evaluations of disease and cellular phenotypes. The totality of biological effects in these studies cannot be individually accounted for by pyroptosis, apoptosis, or necroptosis alone, leading to the conceptualization of PANoptosis. This table focuses on cell death in murine bone marrow-derived macrophages as a model. For genotypes representing a disruption in each programmed cell death pathway, the presence or absence of cell death (Cell death?) is denoted for each. ✓, cell death occurs at levels similar to those seen in wild-type cells; **I**, increased cell death as compared with wild-type; **D**, decreased cell death as compared with wild-type; **X**, no cell death.

Table 2. Totality of cell death in disease phenotypes.

Model	Pathology	Pyroptosis		Apoptosis		Necroptosis		PANoptosis	
		Genotype	Disease?	Genotype	Disease?	Genotype	Disease?	Genotype	Disease?
Pstpip2cmo [16,18,140,141]	Osteomyelitis	Nlrp3−/−	✓	Casp8−/−Ripk3−/− a	✓	Ripk3−/−	✓	Nlrp3−/−Casp8−/−Ripk3−/−	X
		Casp1−/−	✓					Casp1−/−Casp8−/−Ripk3−/−	X
Sharpincpdm [142–146]	Dermatitis	Nlrp3−/−	D	Bid−/−	D	Mlkl−/−	D	Ripk3−/−Fadd−/−	X
		Casp1/11−/−	D			Ripk3−/−	D	Ripk3−/−TraddIE-KO	X
						Ripk1K45A	X	Casp8−/−Ripk3−/−	X b
Ptpn6spin [147,148]	Dermatosis	Nlrp3−/−	✓	Casp8−/−Ripk3−/− a	✓	Ripk3−/−	✓	Casp8−/−Ripk1−/−Ripk3−/−	X
		Casp1−/−	✓			Mlkl−/−	✓		
						Ripk1K45A	D		
Hoil deficiency [149]	Embryonic lethality			Casp8−/−	✓	Ripk3−/−	D	Casp8−/−Mlkl−/−	D
				Casp8−/−Ripk3−/− a	D c	Mlkl−/−	D	Casp8−/−Ripk1−/−	X
						Ripk1K45A	D	Ripk3−/−	X
Caspase-8 deficiency [62,81–84,131]	Embryonic lethality			Casp8−/−	✓	Ripk1D138N	D	Casp8−/−Ripk3−/−	X
								Casp8−/−Mlkl−/−	X
Casp8C362A [130]	Embryonic lethality	Nlrp3−/−Mlkl−/−	✓	Fadd−/−Mlkl−/−	D	Mlkl−/−	✓	Casp1/11−/−Ripk3−/−	X
		Casp1−/−Mlkl−/−	✓						
		Casp11−/−Mlkl−/−	D						
		Asc−/−Mlkl−/−	D						
LPS shock [2,150]	Lethality	Asc−/−	✓			Ripk3−/−	D	Casp8−/−Ripk3−/−	X
		Casp11−/−	D					Casp8−/−Ripk3K51A	X
								Casp8−/−Ripk3−/−Ripk1−/−	X
TNF + IFN-γ shock [2]	Lethality					Ripk3−/−	✓	Casp8−/−Ripk3−/−	X
FlaTox injection [151,152]	Hypothermia	Nlc4−/−	X	Casp8−/−Ripk3−/− a	✓	Ripk3−/−	✓	Casp1−/−Casp8−/−Ripk3−/−	D
		Asc−/−	D						X
		Casp1−/−	D					Asc−/−Casp8−/−Ripk3−/−	X
		Casp1/11−/−	D						
		Gsdmd−/−	D						

[a] Casp8−/−Ripk3−/− genotype is considered as an apoptosis deletion only when the phenotype is the same as the Ripk3−/− genotype, showing that the added deletion of apoptotic caspase-8 does not affect the phenotype. [b] Sharpincpdm Casp8+/−Ripk3−/− mice could be born but did not survive to weaning. [c] Hoil−/−Casp8−/−Ripk3−/− mice succumb at late gestation through a process that appears to be independent of cell death, while Hoil−/−Casp8+/−Ripk3−/− mice undergo cell death-induced loss of yolk sac vascularization to contribute to lethality. Disease phenotypes in mouse models are associated with many different cell death molecules. Deletion of specific combinations can alleviate disease. The totality of biological effects in these studies cannot be individually accounted for by pyroptosis, apoptosis, or necroptosis alone, leading to the conceptualization of PANoptosis. For genotypes representing a disruption in each programmed cell death pathway, the presence or absence of disease (Disease?) is denoted for each. ✓, disease or lethality occurs at levels similar to those seen in wild-type animals; D, decreased disease or lethality as compared with wild-type; X, no disease or lethality (rescued).

Many other in vivo disease phenotypes can be assessed through the PANoptosis lens. For instance, the osteomyelitic disease observed in mice carrying a *Pstpip2*^{cmo} mutation is likely associated with PANoptosis. The bone disease in these mice is driven by aberrant production of IL-1β and is associated with inflammasome activation and cell death. Given the clear role of inflammasome-mediated cytokine release in the disease, it seemed likely that deletion of pyroptotic molecules, such as NLRP3 or caspase-1, would rescue the disease. However, this was not the case. Only mice lacking combinations of cell death molecules, including NLRP3/caspase-8/RIPK3 or caspase-1/-8/RIPK3, are protected from disease [16,18]. Similar results are observed in the *Sharpin*^{cpdm} mouse model, where mutations in SHARPIN, a linear ubiquitin chain assembly complex component critical for TNF signaling activation, result in skin inflammation. In these mice, deletion of NLRP3 or caspase-1 [142] or MLKL alone [143] delays, but does not prevent, the skin inflammation, while combined deletion of FADD/RIPK3 in epidermal cells rescues the inflammation [144]. Additionally, footpad inflammation in mice carrying the *Ptpn6*^{spin} mutation is not rescued by single deletions of caspase-1, NLRP3, RIPK3, MLKL, or the combined deletion of caspase-8/RIPK3 [147,148]. The inflammatory disease in these mice, which resembles neutrophilic dermatosis in humans, is mediated by the RIPK1/IL-1α signaling axis, but combined deletion of caspase-8/RIPK3/RIPK1 is needed to prevent the inflammation [148]. Furthermore, innate immunity and programmed cell death have been connected to neurodegenerative diseases such as Alzheimer's disease (AD). Elevated levels of proinflammatory cytokines that can be released by cell death, such as TNF-α and IL-1β, are found in the brains and serum of people with AD and can cause neuroinflammation and AD-related pathologies [153]. The potential for PANoptosis is shown in studies with amyloid precursor protein/presenilin 1 (APP/PS1) transgenic mice carrying kinase-dead RIPK1 (*Ripk1*^{D138N}). A deficiency in functional RIPK1 results in reduced disease and decreased proinflammatory IL-1β release [154], linking necroptotic and pyroptotic molecules in this model. Given the multifaceted nature of the cell death in many in vivo disease phenotypes, it is likely that many others could also be considered within the PANoptosis concept.

Several infection models have also demonstrated cell death crosstalk and interconnectivity that can be considered within the PANoptosis concept. As discussed above, ZBP1-mediated cell death during IAV infection is the prototypical example of PANoptosis. In initial studies, IAV-induced cell death was often viewed as redundant or thought to concurrently activate multiple cell death pathways [75,121,155], but later work elucidated the molecular mechanisms of ZBP1-PANoptosome formation and established the complex [11]. ZBP1-mediated PANoptosis has also been implicated in tumorigenesis [7] and fungal infections with *Candida albicans* and *Aspergillus fumigatus* [14]. In response to other viruses, PANoptosis mediated through AIM2-PANoptosome formation has also been characterized during HSV1 infection [12]. Additionally, during hepatitis C virus infection, fluorescence microscopy has shown concurrent caspase-1 and caspase-3 activation [156], suggesting simultaneous activation of these molecules in individual cells, which could be explained by PANoptosis.

Bacterial pathogens have also been found to induce cell death where the molecular phenotypes observed do not fall within pyroptosis, apoptosis, or necroptosis activation alone, suggesting PANoptosis is occurring. In response to FlaTox, mice lacking either the combination of caspase-1/RIPK3 or the combination of caspase-8/RIPK3 still experience pathology, while combined loss of caspase-1/-8/RIPK3 provides protection [151]. Similarly, co-deletion of ASC or caspase-8/RIPK3 with caspase-1/-11 phenocopies NLRC4 deletion during challenge with flagellin or infection with *Legionella* [92,151]. In *Salmonella* infection, 'flexible' cell death has been observed, and it has been reported that components of different cell death pathways interact. *Salmonella*-induced NLRC4 inflammasome activation drives cell death to clear bacteria from the host, and mice deficient in RIPK3 and caspase-1 are moderately impaired in their ability to clear the bacteria, while bacterial clearance in mice deficient in RIPK3, caspase-1, and caspase-8 is significantly more impaired [151]. Subsequent studies have shown that cells deficient in caspase-1/-11 or caspase-8/RIPK3 still undergo cell death in response to the infection, while cells deficient in caspase-1/-11/-8/RIPK3 [10] or cells deficient in caspase-1/-11/-12/-8/RIPK3 [135] are protected from cell death. Infection with *Bacillus anthracis* also activates multiple cell death effectors, including caspase-1, -8, and -3. Deletion of RIPK3 is not sufficient to protect cells from death during this infection, while the combined deletion of caspase-8/RIPK3 does prevent cell death [157]. Additionally, *Pseudomonas aeruginosa* induces cell death characterized by activation of caspase-1, GSDMD, caspase-8, -3, -7, and MLKL. While deletion of the pyroptotic sensors NLRP3 and NLRC4 together significantly reduces cell death in response to *P. aeruginosa*, combined deletion of caspase-1/-11/-8/RIPK3 provides full protection from cell death [137]. As each of these phenotypes cannot be explained by activation of pyroptosis, apoptosis, or necroptosis alone, they may fit in the category of PANoptosis.

Having PANoptosis as a component of the innate immune response is likely advantageous on the organismal level. Inhibiting cell death effectors is a commonly used pathogen defense strategy [158–160], and PANoptosis allows the cell to utilize multiple routes of cell death if one or more key cell death effectors is inhibited. Biologically, the redundancy displayed by PANoptosis ensures a fail-safe mechanism for cell death, thereby increasing the likelihood of organismal survival. During *Yersinia* infection, the bacteria secrete YopJ, a bacterial effector that inhibits TAK1-dependent inflammatory signaling [98,100]. However, in response to the inhibition of TAK1, host cells undergo cell death characterized by activation of the NLRP3 inflammasome, caspase-1, -3, -7, and MLKL [5]. Recently, *Yersinia* infection was found to activate PANoptosis, with infection inducing the formation of a PANoptosome containing RIPK1, RIPK3, caspase-8, ASC, FADD, and NLRP3 [3]. *Shigella flexneri* also uses its effector molecules, OspC1 to inhibit caspase-8 and OspD3 to inhibit RIPK1/RIPK3, in an attempt to evade the cell death crosstalk [161], which could give this bacterium a strategy to prevent PANoptosis.

6. Discussion and Future Directions

Experimental design often restricts how we test the innate immune response, limiting our ability to fully determine connections between molecular processes. The host response is likely more complex than we understand, but we can appreciate that the host must be able to recognize and respond to a variety of danger signals and cellular insults to execute the appropriate cellular response. It would likely be evolutionarily advantageous for a barrage of cellular insults to be neutralized using an integrated immune response, such as that stemming from PANoptosis. Therefore, it is important to be inclusive and consider the totality of biological effects in PANoptosis when studying cell death. These phenotypes may be missed when focusing on a single cell death pathway due to functional redundancies and overlaps between molecules. Additionally, the activation of molecular executioner signatures of pyroptosis, apoptosis, and necroptosis are not required simultaneously in an individual cell for a cell death process to fit within the PANoptosis concept. Furthermore, there are certainly conditions where pyroptosis, apoptosis, or necroptosis alone carries out the cell death, such as pyroptosis in wild-type cells exposed to LPS + ATP or necroptosis in wild-type cells exposed to TNF + zVAD. Only by studying the totality of the effects of programmed cell death in physiologically relevant models can we identify the important differences between these instances and PANoptosis.

Multiple PANoptosome complexes have been associated with PANoptosis to date [3,7,9–12,20], and additional work is required to fully understand these complexes. Their molecular composition may be flexible and dynamic. In the case of other cell death-inducing complexes, such as the NLRP3 inflammasome, there are canonical and non-canonical iterations; the same may also be true for PANoptosomes. Canonical PANoptosomes may contain caspase-8, RIPK3, and inflammasome components, as has been observed during IAV, HSV1, *Francisella*, and *Yersinia* infections [3,10–12], while non-canonical PANoptosomes may contain caspase-8 and RIPK3 as major molecules, as is likely the case during TNF + IFN-γ stimulation [2,4]. More work is needed to continue to evaluate these complexes, the dynamics of their formation, and their regulation. Furthermore, in addition to the ZBP1- and AIM2-PANoptosome complexes that have been molecularly characterized based on their upstream sensors, it is likely that many other sensor-specific PANoptosomes exist and form in response to infections and conditions of altered cellular homeostasis that have not yet been tested. This has been found with inflammasomes and will likely be a conserved phenomenon. Whether sensors are strictly intracellular, or cell surface receptors are also involved, is also currently unknown.

The complexity of tissue- and cell-specific responses, in relation to PANoptosis, should also be considered and further investigated. PANoptosis is a fluid process due to the many ways cell death can be executed. Some routes of cell death may be favored in certain tissues or cell types. Additionally, the PANoptotic response may be executed differently in various cell types based on differences in gene expression of key cell death molecules that exist among cells. It is also worth noting that many cancers are largely associated with dysregulation of apoptosis, further highlighting pathway specificity in some contexts. Understanding the subtle nuances which make each tissue and cell type unique may be useful in determining how PANoptosis occurs in order to harness this process for therapeutic purposes.

Furthermore, there is a need to mechanistically understand the regulation of PANoptosis, as this could be the key to developing new clinical therapeutics for human cancers and diseases. IRF1 has been implicated as a central upstream regulator [2,4,8,75], and other components of this pathway should be elucidated. Inhibiting certain molecular components of cell death may enhance the activation of others, as has been observed previously [15,137], and this requires careful consideration during the drug design process. Perhaps targeting one aspect of cell death will result in subpar clinical therapies due to the redundancy of PANoptotic molecules.

PANoptosis has been implicated across the disease spectrum, including in cerebral ischemia [114]; bacterial, viral, and fungal infections [3,9–15], including oral infections [115,116]; inflammatory diseases [2,5,16,18,20]; cancers [4,7,8]; and cancer therapies [4,7,117,118]. It will be important to improve our understanding of this pathway and identify how previous descriptions of crosstalk, plasticity, redundancies, molecular switches, and interconnectedness among cell death processes fit within this inclusive concept to gain a holistic picture of cell death. Only when we identify all the ingredients in the PAN can we begin to effectively target these molecules and develop novel therapeutics to save lives and improve patient outcomes.

Author Contributions: Writing—original draft, J.M.G. and R.E.T.; writing—review and editing, J.M.G., R.E.T. and T.-D.K. All authors have read and agreed to the published version of the manuscript.

Funding: Work from the Kanneganti laboratory is supported by the National Institutes of Health (AI101935, AI124346, AI160179, AR056296, and CA253095 to T.-D.K.) and the American Lebanese Syrian Associated Charities (to T.-D.K.). The content is solely the responsibility of the authors and does not necessarily represent the official views of the National Institutes of Health.

Institutional Review Board Statement: Not applicable.

Informed Consent Statement: Not applicable.

Data Availability Statement: Not applicable.

Acknowledgments: We apologize to our colleagues in the field whose work could not be cited owing to space limitations. We thank all the members of the Kanneganti laboratory for their comments and suggestions. We also thank XVIVO for assistance with scientific illustrations.

Conflicts of Interest: The authors declare no conflict of interest.

References

1. Malireddi, R.K.S.; Kesavardhana, S.; Kanneganti, T.D. ZBP1 and TAK1: Master Regulators of NLRP3 Inflammasome/Pyroptosis, Apoptosis, and Necroptosis (PAN-optosis). *Front. Cell. Infect. Microbiol.* **2019**, *9*, 406. [CrossRef] [PubMed]
2. Karki, R.; Sharma, B.R.; Tuladhar, S.; Williams, E.P.; Zalduondo, L.; Samir, P.; Zheng, M.; Sundaram, B.; Banoth, B.; Malireddi, R.K.S.; et al. Synergism of TNF-alpha and IFN-gamma Triggers Inflammatory Cell Death, Tissue Damage, and Mortality in SARS-CoV-2 Infection and Cytokine Shock Syndromes. *Cell* **2021**, *184*, 149–168.e117. [CrossRef] [PubMed]
3. Malireddi, R.K.S.; Kesavardhana, S.; Karki, R.; Kancharana, B.; Burton, A.R.; Kanneganti, T.D. RIPK1 Distinctly Regulates Yersinia-Induced Inflammatory Cell Death, PANoptosis. *Immunohorizons* **2020**, *4*, 789–796. [CrossRef] [PubMed]
4. Malireddi, R.K.S.; Karki, R.; Sundaram, B.; Kancharana, B.; Lee, S.; Samir, P.; Kanneganti, T.D. Inflammatory Cell Death, PANoptosis, Mediated by Cytokines in Diverse Cancer Lineages Inhibits Tumor Growth. *Immunohorizons* **2021**, *5*, 568–580. [CrossRef] [PubMed]
5. Malireddi, R.K.S.; Gurung, P.; Mavuluri, J.; Dasari, T.K.; Klco, J.M.; Chi, H.; Kanneganti, T.D. TAK1 restricts spontaneous NLRP3 activation and cell death to control myeloid proliferation. *J. Exp. Med.* **2018**, *215*, 1023–1034. [CrossRef]
6. Malireddi, R.K.; Ippagunta, S.; Lamkanfi, M.; Kanneganti, T.D. Cutting edge: Proteolytic inactivation of poly(ADP-ribose) polymerase 1 by the Nlrp3 and Nlrc4 inflammasomes. *J. Immunol.* **2010**, *185*, 3127–3130. [CrossRef]
7. Karki, R.; Sundaram, B.; Sharma, B.R.; Lee, S.; Malireddi, R.K.S.; Nguyen, L.N.; Christgen, S.; Zheng, M.; Wang, Y.; Samir, P.; et al. ADAR1 restricts ZBP1-mediated immune response and PANoptosis to promote tumorigenesis. *Cell Rep.* **2021**, *37*, 109858. [CrossRef]
8. Karki, R.; Sharma, B.R.; Lee, E.; Banoth, B.; Malireddi, R.K.S.; Samir, P.; Tuladhar, S.; Mummareddy, H.; Burton, A.R.; Vogel, P.; et al. Interferon regulatory factor 1 regulates PANoptosis to prevent colorectal cancer. *JCI Insight* **2020**, *5*, e136720. [CrossRef]
9. Kuriakose, T.; Man, S.M.; Subbarao Malireddi, R.K.; Karki, R.; Kesavardhana, S.; Place, D.E.; Neale, G.; Vogel, P.; Kanneganti, T.D. ZBP1/DAI is an innate sensor of influenza virus triggering the NLRP3 inflammasome and programmed cell death pathways. *Sci. Immunol.* **2016**, *1*, aag2045. [CrossRef]
10. Christgen, S.; Zheng, M.; Kesavardhana, S.; Karki, R.; Malireddi, R.K.S.; Banoth, B.; Place, D.E.; Briard, B.; Sharma, B.R.; Tuladhar, S.; et al. Identification of the PANoptosome: A Molecular Platform Triggering Pyroptosis, Apoptosis, and Necroptosis (PANoptosis). *Front. Cell. Infect. Microbiol.* **2020**, *10*, 237. [CrossRef]
11. Zheng, M.; Karki, R.; Vogel, P.; Kanneganti, T.D. Caspase-6 is a key regulator of innate immunity, inflammasome activation and host defense. *Cell* **2020**, *181*, 674–687.e13. [CrossRef]
12. Lee, S.; Karki, R.; Wang, Y.; Nguyen, L.N.; Kalathur, R.C.; Kanneganti, T.D. AIM2 forms a complex with pyrin and ZBP1 to drive PANoptosis and host defence. *Nature* **2021**, *597*, 415–419. [CrossRef]
13. Kesavardhana, S.; Malireddi, R.K.S.; Burton, A.R.; Porter, S.N.; Vogel, P.; Pruett-Miller, S.M.; Kanneganti, T.D. The Zα2 domain of ZBP1 is a molecular switch regulating influenza-induced PANoptosis and perinatal lethality during development. *J. Biol. Chem.* **2020**, *295*, 8325–8330. [CrossRef] [PubMed]
14. Banoth, B.; Tuladhar, S.; Karki, R.; Sharma, B.R.; Briard, B.; Kesavardhana, S.; Burton, A.; Kanneganti, T.D. ZBP1 promotes fungi-induced inflammasome activation and pyroptosis, apoptosis, and necroptosis (PANoptosis). *J. Biol. Chem.* **2020**, *295*, 18276–18283. [CrossRef] [PubMed]
15. Zheng, M.; Williams, E.P.; Malireddi, R.K.S.; Karki, R.; Banoth, B.; Burton, A.; Webby, R.; Channappanavar, R.; Jonsson, C.B.; Kanneganti, T.D. Impaired NLRP3 inflammasome activation/pyroptosis leads to robust inflammatory cell death via caspase-8/RIPK3 during coronavirus infection. *J. Biol. Chem.* **2020**, *295*, 14040–14052. [CrossRef] [PubMed]
16. Lukens, J.R.; Gurung, P.; Vogel, P.; Johnson, G.R.; Carter, R.A.; McGoldrick, D.J.; Bandi, S.R.; Calabrese, C.R.; Walle, L.V.; Lamkanfi, M.; et al. Dietary modulation of the microbiome affects autoinflammatory disease. *Nature* **2014**, *516*, 246–249. [CrossRef] [PubMed]
17. Lamkanfi, M.; Kanneganti, T.D.; Van Damme, P.; Vanden Berghe, T.; Vanoverberghe, I.; Vandekerckhove, J.; Vandenabeele, P.; Gevaert, K.; Nunez, G. Targeted peptidecentric proteomics reveals caspase-7 as a substrate of the caspase-1 inflammasomes. *Mol. Cell. Proteom.* **2008**, *7*, 2350–2363. [CrossRef]
18. Gurung, P.; Burton, A.; Kanneganti, T.D. NLRP3 inflammasome plays a redundant role with caspase 8 to promote IL-1β–mediated osteomyelitis. *Proc. Natl. Acad. Sci. USA* **2016**, *113*, 4452–4457. [CrossRef]
19. Gurung, P.; Anand, P.K.; Malireddi, R.K.; Vande Walle, L.; Van Opdenbosch, N.; Dillon, C.P.; Weinlich, R.; Green, D.R.; Lamkanfi, M.; Kanneganti, T.D. FADD and caspase-8 mediate priming and activation of the canonical and noncanonical Nlrp3 inflammasomes. *J. Immunol.* **2014**, *192*, 1835–1846. [CrossRef]
20. Malireddi, R.K.S.; Gurung, P.; Kesavardhana, S.; Samir, P.; Burton, A.; Mummareddy, H.; Vogel, P.; Pelletier, S.; Burgula, S.; Kanneganti, T.D. Innate immune priming in the absence of TAK1 drives RIPK1 kinase activity-independent pyroptosis, apoptosis, necroptosis, and inflammatory disease. *J. Exp. Med.* **2020**, *217*, e20191644. [CrossRef]
21. Kesavardhana, S.; Malireddi, R.K.S.; Kanneganti, T.D. Caspases in Cell Death, Inflammation, and Pyroptosis. *Annu. Rev. Immunol.* **2020**, *38*, 567–595. [CrossRef] [PubMed]
22. Galluzzi, L.; Vitale, I.; Aaronson, S.A.; Abrams, J.M.; Adam, D.; Agostinis, P.; Alnemri, E.S.; Altucci, L.; Amelio, I.; Andrews, D.W.; et al. Molecular mechanisms of cell death: Recommendations of the Nomenclature Committee on Cell Death 2018. *Cell Death Differ.* **2018**, *25*, 486–541. [CrossRef] [PubMed]
23. Cookson, B.T.; Brennan, M.A. Pro-inflammatory programmed cell death. *Trends Microbiol.* **2001**, *9*, 113–114. [CrossRef]

24. Martinon, F.; Burns, K.; Tschopp, J. The inflammasome: A molecular platform triggering activation of inflammatory caspases and processing of proIL-beta. *Mol. Cell* **2002**, *10*, 417–426. [CrossRef]
25. Kanneganti, T.D.; Ozoren, N.; Body-Malapel, M.; Amer, A.; Park, J.H.; Franchi, L.; Whitfield, J.; Barchet, W.; Colonna, M.; Vandenabeele, P.; et al. Bacterial RNA and small antiviral compounds activate caspase-1 through cryopyrin/Nalp3. *Nature* **2006**, *440*, 233–236. [CrossRef] [PubMed]
26. Mariathasan, S.; Weiss, D.S.; Newton, K.; McBride, J.; O'Rourke, K.; Roose-Girma, M.; Lee, W.P.; Weinrauch, Y.; Monack, D.M.; Dixit, V.M. Cryopyrin activates the inflammasome in response to toxins and ATP. *Nature* **2006**, *440*, 228–232. [CrossRef]
27. Martinon, F.; Petrilli, V.; Mayor, A.; Tardivel, A.; Tschopp, J. Gout-associated uric acid crystals activate the NALP3 inflammasome. *Nature* **2006**, *440*, 237–241. [CrossRef]
28. Franchi, L.; Amer, A.; Body-Malapel, M.; Kanneganti, T.D.; Ozoren, N.; Jagirdar, R.; Inohara, N.; Vandenabeele, P.; Bertin, J.; Coyle, A.; et al. Cytosolic flagellin requires Ipaf for activation of caspase-1 and interleukin 1beta in salmonella-infected macrophages. *Nat. Immunol.* **2006**, *7*, 576–582. [CrossRef]
29. Miao, E.A.; Alpuche-Aranda, C.M.; Dors, M.; Clark, A.E.; Bader, M.W.; Miller, S.I.; Aderem, A. Cytoplasmic flagellin activates caspase-1 and secretion of interleukin 1beta via Ipaf. *Nat. Immunol.* **2006**, *7*, 569–575. [CrossRef]
30. Mariathasan, S.; Newton, K.; Monack, D.M.; Vucic, D.; French, D.M.; Lee, W.P.; Roose-Girma, M.; Erickson, S.; Dixit, V.M. Differential activation of the inflammasome by caspase-1 adaptors ASC and Ipaf. *Nature* **2004**, *430*, 213–218. [CrossRef]
31. Xu, H.; Yang, J.; Gao, W.; Li, L.; Li, P.; Zhang, L.; Gong, Y.N.; Peng, X.; Xi, J.J.; Chen, S.; et al. Innate immune sensing of bacterial modifications of Rho GTPases by the Pyrin inflammasome. *Nature* **2014**, *513*, 237–241. [CrossRef] [PubMed]
32. Fernandes-Alnemri, T.; Yu, J.W.; Datta, P.; Wu, J.; Alnemri, E.S. AIM2 activates the inflammasome and cell death in response to cytoplasmic DNA. *Nature* **2009**, *458*, 509–513. [CrossRef] [PubMed]
33. Hornung, V.; Ablasser, A.; Charrel-Dennis, M.; Bauernfeind, F.; Horvath, G.; Caffrey, D.R.; Latz, E.; Fitzgerald, K.A. AIM2 recognizes cytosolic dsDNA and forms a caspase-1-activating inflammasome with ASC. *Nature* **2009**, *458*, 514–518. [CrossRef] [PubMed]
34. Cai, X.; Chen, J.; Xu, H.; Liu, S.; Jiang, Q.X.; Halfmann, R.; Chen, Z.J. Prion-like polymerization underlies signal transduction in antiviral immune defense and inflammasome activation. *Cell* **2014**, *156*, 1207–1222. [CrossRef] [PubMed]
35. Lu, A.; Magupalli, V.G.; Ruan, J.; Yin, Q.; Atianand, M.K.; Vos, M.R.; Schröder, G.F.; Fitzgerald, K.A.; Wu, H.; Egelman, E.H. Unified polymerization mechanism for the assembly of ASC-dependent inflammasomes. *Cell* **2014**, *156*, 1193–1206. [CrossRef]
36. Masumoto, J.; Taniguchi, S.; Ayukawa, K.; Sarvotham, H.; Kishino, T.; Niikawa, N.; Hidaka, E.; Katsuyama, T.; Higuchi, T.; Sagara, J. ASC, a novel 22-kDa protein, aggregates during apoptosis of human promyelocytic leukemia HL-60 cells. *J. Biol. Chem.* **1999**, *274*, 33835–33838. [CrossRef]
37. Sborgi, L.; Ravotti, F.; Dandey, V.P.; Dick, M.S.; Mazur, A.; Reckel, S.; Chami, M.; Scherer, S.; Huber, M.; Böckmann, A.; et al. Structure and assembly of the mouse ASC inflammasome by combined NMR spectroscopy and cryo-electron microscopy. *Proc. Natl. Acad. Sci. USA* **2015**, *112*, 13237–13242. [CrossRef]
38. Dinarello, C.A. Immunological and inflammatory functions of the interleukin-1 family. *Annu. Rev. Immunol.* **2009**, *27*, 519–550. [CrossRef]
39. Shi, J.; Zhao, Y.; Wang, K.; Shi, X.; Wang, Y.; Huang, H.; Zhuang, Y.; Cai, T.; Wang, F.; Shao, F. Cleavage of GSDMD by inflammatory caspases determines pyroptotic cell death. *Nature* **2015**, *526*, 660–665. [CrossRef]
40. He, W.T.; Wan, H.; Hu, L.; Chen, P.; Wang, X.; Huang, Z.; Yang, Z.H.; Zhong, C.Q.; Han, J. Gasdermin D is an executor of pyroptosis and required for interleukin-1beta secretion. *Cell Res.* **2015**, *25*, 1285–1298. [CrossRef]
41. Aglietti, R.A.; Estevez, A.; Gupta, A.; Ramirez, M.G.; Liu, P.S.; Kayagaki, N.; Ciferri, C.; Dixit, V.M.; Dueber, E.C. GsdmD p30 elicited by caspase-11 during pyroptosis forms pores in membranes. *Proc. Natl. Acad. Sci. USA* **2016**, *113*, 7858–7863. [CrossRef] [PubMed]
42. Ding, J.; Wang, K.; Liu, W.; She, Y.; Sun, Q.; Shi, J.; Sun, H.; Wang, D.C.; Shao, F. Pore-forming activity and structural autoinhibition of the gasdermin family. *Nature* **2016**, *535*, 111–116. [CrossRef] [PubMed]
43. Liu, X.; Zhang, Z.; Ruan, J.; Pan, Y.; Magupalli, V.G.; Wu, H.; Lieberman, J. Inflammasome-activated gasdermin D causes pyroptosis by forming membrane pores. *Nature* **2016**, *535*, 153–158. [CrossRef] [PubMed]
44. Sborgi, L.; Ruhl, S.; Mulvihill, E.; Pipercevic, J.; Heilig, R.; Stahlberg, H.; Farady, C.J.; Muller, D.J.; Broz, P.; Hiller, S. GSDMD membrane pore formation constitutes the mechanism of pyroptotic cell death. *EMBO J.* **2016**, *35*, 1766–1778. [CrossRef]
45. Kayagaki, N.; Stowe, I.B.; Lee, B.L.; O'Rourke, K.; Anderson, K.; Warming, S.; Cuellar, T.; Haley, B.; Roose-Girma, M.; Phung, Q.T.; et al. Caspase-11 cleaves gasdermin D for non-canonical inflammasome signalling. *Nature* **2015**, *526*, 666–671. [CrossRef]
46. Kayagaki, N.; Lee, B.L.; Stowe, I.B.; Kornfeld, O.S.; O'Rourke, K.; Mirrashidi, K.M.; Haley, B.; Watanabe, C.; Roose-Girma, M.; Modrusan, Z.; et al. IRF2 transcriptionally induces GSDMD expression for pyroptosis. *Sci. Signal.* **2019**, *12*, eaax4917. [CrossRef]
47. Benaoudia, S.; Martin, A.; Puig Gamez, M.; Gay, G.; Lagrange, B.; Cornut, M.; Krasnykov, K.; Claude, J.B.; Bourgeois, C.F.; Hughes, S.; et al. A genome-wide screen identifies IRF2 as a key regulator of caspase-4 in human cells. *EMBO Rep.* **2019**, *20*, e48235. [CrossRef]
48. Kerr, J.F.; Wyllie, A.H.; Currie, A.R. Apoptosis: A basic biological phenomenon with wide-ranging implications in tissue kinetics. *Br. J. Cancer* **1972**, *26*, 239–257. [CrossRef]
49. Zou, H.; Henzel, W.J.; Liu, X.; Lutschg, A.; Wang, X. Apaf-1, a human protein homologous to C. elegans CED-4, participates in cytochrome c-dependent activation of caspase-3. *Cell* **1997**, *90*, 405–413. [CrossRef]
50. Kim, H.E.; Du, F.; Fang, M.; Wang, X. Formation of apoptosome is initiated by cytochrome c-induced dATP hydrolysis and subsequent nucleotide exchange on Apaf-1. *Proc. Natl. Acad. Sci. USA* **2005**, *102*, 17545–17550. [CrossRef]

51. Li, P.; Nijhawan, D.; Budihardjo, I.; Srinivasula, S.M.; Ahmad, M.; Alnemri, E.S.; Wang, X. Cytochrome c and dATP-dependent formation of Apaf-1/caspase-9 complex initiates an apoptotic protease cascade. *Cell* **1997**, *91*, 479–489. [CrossRef]
52. Boldin, M.P.; Goncharov, T.M.; Goltsev, Y.V.; Wallach, D. Involvement of MACH, a novel MORT1/FADD-interacting protease, in Fas/APO-1- and TNF receptor-induced cell death. *Cell* **1996**, *85*, 803–815. [CrossRef]
53. Muzio, M.; Chinnaiyan, A.M.; Kischkel, F.C.; O'Rourke, K.; Shevchenko, A.; Ni, J.; Scaffidi, C.; Bretz, J.D.; Zhang, M.; Gentz, R.; et al. FLICE, a novel FADD-homologous ICE/CED-3-like protease, is recruited to the CD95 (Fas/APO-1) death–inducing signaling complex. *Cell* **1996**, *85*, 817–827. [CrossRef]
54. Gross, A.; Yin, X.M.; Wang, K.; Wei, M.C.; Jockel, J.; Milliman, C.; Erdjument-Bromage, H.; Tempst, P.; Korsmeyer, S.J. Caspase cleaved BID targets mitochondria and is required for cytochrome c release, while BCL-XL prevents this release but not tumor necrosis factor-R1/Fas death. *J. Biol. Chem.* **1999**, *274*, 1156–1163. [CrossRef]
55. Luo, X.; Budihardjo, I.; Zou, H.; Slaughter, C.; Wang, X. Bid, a Bcl2 interacting protein, mediates cytochrome c release from mitochondria in response to activation of cell surface death receptors. *Cell* **1998**, *94*, 481–490. [CrossRef]
56. Li, H.; Zhu, H.; Xu, C.J.; Yuan, J. Cleavage of BID by caspase 8 mediates the mitochondrial damage in the Fas pathway of apoptosis. *Cell* **1998**, *94*, 491–501. [CrossRef]
57. Wei, M.C.; Lindsten, T.; Mootha, V.K.; Weiler, S.; Gross, A.; Ashiya, M.; Thompson, C.B.; Korsmeyer, S.J. tBID, a membrane-targeted death ligand, oligomerizes BAK to release cytochrome c. *Genes Dev.* **2000**, *14*, 2060–2071. [CrossRef]
58. Kuwana, T.; Mackey, M.R.; Perkins, G.; Ellisman, M.H.; Latterich, M.; Schneiter, R.; Green, D.R.; Newmeyer, D.D. Bid, Bax, and lipids cooperate to form supramolecular openings in the outer mitochondrial membrane. *Cell* **2002**, *111*, 331–342. [CrossRef]
59. Gong, Y.; Fan, Z.; Luo, G.; Yang, C.; Huang, Q.; Fan, K.; Cheng, H.; Jin, K.; Ni, Q.; Yu, X.; et al. The role of necroptosis in cancer biology and therapy. *Mol Cancer* **2019**, *18*, 100. [CrossRef]
60. Nailwal, H.; Chan, F.K. Necroptosis in anti-viral inflammation. *Cell Death Differ.* **2019**, *26*, 4–13. [CrossRef]
61. Kang, T.B.; Ben-Moshe, T.; Varfolomeev, E.E.; Pewzner-Jung, Y.; Yogev, N.; Jurewicz, A.; Waisman, A.; Brenner, O.; Haffner, R.; Gustafsson, E.; et al. Caspase-8 serves both apoptotic and nonapoptotic roles. *J. Immunol.* **2004**, *173*, 2976–2984. [CrossRef] [PubMed]
62. Newton, K.; Wickliffe, K.E.; Dugger, D.L.; Maltzman, A.; Roose-Girma, M.; Dohse, M.; Kőműves, L.; Webster, J.D.; Dixit, V.M. Cleavage of RIPK1 by caspase-8 is crucial for limiting apoptosis and necroptosis. *Nature* **2019**, *574*, 428–431. [CrossRef] [PubMed]
63. O'Donnell, M.A.; Perez-Jimenez, E.; Oberst, A.; Ng, A.; Massoumi, R.; Xavier, R.; Green, D.R.; Ting, A.T. Caspase 8 inhibits programmed necrosis by processing CYLD. *Nat. Cell Biol.* **2011**, *13*, 1437–1442. [CrossRef] [PubMed]
64. Feng, S.; Yang, Y.; Mei, Y.; Ma, L.; Zhu, D.E.; Hoti, N.; Castanares, M.; Wu, M. Cleavage of RIP3 inactivates its caspase-independent apoptosis pathway by removal of kinase domain. *Cell. Signal.* **2007**, *19*, 2056–2067. [CrossRef] [PubMed]
65. Grootjans, S.; Vanden Berghe, T.; Vandenabeele, P. Initiation and execution mechanisms of necroptosis: An overview. *Cell Death Differ.* **2017**, *24*, 1184–1195. [CrossRef] [PubMed]
66. Vandenabeele, P.; Galluzzi, L.; Vanden Berghe, T.; Kroemer, G. Molecular mechanisms of necroptosis: An ordered cellular explosion. *Nat. Rev. Mol. Cell Biol.* **2010**, *11*, 700–714. [CrossRef]
67. Sun, L.; Wang, H.; Wang, Z.; He, S.; Chen, S.; Liao, D.; Wang, L.; Yan, J.; Liu, W.; Lei, X.; et al. Mixed lineage kinase domain-like protein mediates necrosis signaling downstream of RIP3 kinase. *Cell* **2012**, *148*, 213–227. [CrossRef]
68. Zhao, J.; Jitkaew, S.; Cai, Z.; Choksi, S.; Li, Q.; Luo, J.; Liu, Z.G. Mixed lineage kinase domain-like is a key receptor interacting protein 3 downstream component of TNF-induced necrosis. *Proc. Natl. Acad. Sci. USA* **2012**, *109*, 5322–5327. [CrossRef]
69. Garcia, L.R.; Tenev, T.; Newman, R.; Haich, R.O.; Liccardi, G.; John, S.W.; Annibaldi, A.; Yu, L.; Pardo, M.; Young, S.N.; et al. Ubiquitylation of MLKL at lysine 219 positively regulates necroptosis-induced tissue injury and pathogen clearance. *Nat. Commun.* **2021**, *12*, 3364. [CrossRef]
70. Sharif, H.; Wang, L.; Wang, W.L.; Magupalli, V.G.; Andreeva, L.; Qiao, Q.; Hauenstein, A.V.; Wu, Z.; Núñez, G.; Mao, Y.; et al. Structural mechanism for NEK7-licensed activation of NLRP3 inflammasome. *Nature* **2019**, *570*, 338–343. [CrossRef]
71. Shi, H.; Wang, Y.; Li, X.; Zhan, X.; Tang, M.; Fina, M.; Su, L.; Pratt, D.; Bu, C.H.; Hildebrand, S.; et al. NLRP3 activation and mitosis are mutually exclusive events coordinated by NEK7, a new inflammasome component. *Nat. Immunol.* **2016**, *17*, 250–258. [CrossRef] [PubMed]
72. Schmid-Burgk, J.L.; Chauhan, D.; Schmidt, T.; Ebert, T.S.; Reinhardt, J.; Endl, E.; Hornung, V. A Genome-wide CRISPR (Clustered Regularly Interspaced Short Palindromic Repeats) Screen Identifies NEK7 as an Essential Component of NLRP3 Inflammasome Activation. *J. Biol. Chem.* **2016**, *291*, 103–109. [CrossRef] [PubMed]
73. He, Y.; Zeng, M.Y.; Yang, D.; Motro, B.; Nunez, G. NEK7 is an essential mediator of NLRP3 activation downstream of potassium efflux. *Nature* **2016**, *530*, 354–357. [CrossRef] [PubMed]
74. Samir, P.; Kesavardhana, S.; Patmore, D.M.; Gingras, S.; Malireddi, R.K.S.; Karki, R.; Guy, C.S.; Briard, B.; Place, D.E.; Bhattacharya, A.; et al. DDX3X acts as a live-or-die checkpoint in stressed cells by regulating NLRP3 inflammasome. *Nature* **2019**, *573*, 590–594. [CrossRef] [PubMed]
75. Kuriakose, T.; Zheng, M.; Neale, G.; Kanneganti, T.D. IRF1 Is a Transcriptional Regulator of ZBP1 Promoting NLRP3 Inflammasome Activation and Cell Death during Influenza Virus Infection. *J. Immunol.* **2018**, *200*, 1489–1495. [CrossRef]
76. Karki, R.; Lee, E.; Place, D.; Samir, P.; Mavuluri, J.; Sharma, B.R.; Balakrishnan, A.; Malireddi, R.K.S.; Geiger, R.; Zhu, Q.; et al. IRF8 Regulates Transcription of Naips for NLRC4 Inflammasome Activation. *Cell* **2018**, *173*, 920–933.e13. [CrossRef]

77. Kayagaki, N.; Kornfeld, O.S.; Lee, B.L.; Stowe, I.B.; O'Rourke, K.; Li, Q.; Sandoval, W.; Yan, D.; Kang, J.; Xu, M.; et al. NINJ1 mediates plasma membrane rupture during lytic cell death. *Nature* 2021, *591*, 131–136. [CrossRef]
78. Christgen, S.; Place, D.E.; Kanneganti, T.D. Toward targeting inflammasomes: Insights into their regulation and activation. *Cell Res.* 2020, *30*, 315–327. [CrossRef]
79. Bertheloot, D.; Latz, E.; Franklin, B.S. Necroptosis, pyroptosis and apoptosis: An intricate game of cell death. *Cell Mol. Immunol.* 2021, *18*, 1106–1121. [CrossRef]
80. Holler, N.; Zaru, R.; Micheau, O.; Thome, M.; Attinger, A.; Valitutti, S.; Bodmer, J.L.; Schneider, P.; Seed, B.; Tschopp, J. Fas triggers an alternative, caspase-8-independent cell death pathway using the kinase RIP as effector molecule. *Nat. Immunol.* 2000, *1*, 489–495. [CrossRef]
81. Oberst, A.; Dillon, C.P.; Weinlich, R.; McCormick, L.L.; Fitzgerald, P.; Pop, C.; Hakem, R.; Salvesen, G.S.; Green, D.R. Catalytic activity of the caspase-8-FLIP(L) complex inhibits RIPK3-dependent necrosis. *Nature* 2011, *471*, 363–367. [CrossRef] [PubMed]
82. Kaiser, W.J.; Upton, J.W.; Long, A.B.; Livingston-Rosanoff, D.; Daley-Bauer, L.P.; Hakem, R.; Caspary, T.; Mocarski, E.S. RIP3 mediates the embryonic lethality of caspase-8-deficient mice. *Nature* 2011, *471*, 368–372. [CrossRef] [PubMed]
83. Alvarez-Diaz, S.; Dillon, C.P.; Lalaoui, N.; Tanzer, M.C.; Rodriguez, D.A.; Lin, A.; Lebois, M.; Hakem, R.; Josefsson, E.C.; O'Reilly, L.A.; et al. The Pseudokinase MLKL and the Kinase RIPK3 Have Distinct Roles in Autoimmune Disease Caused by Loss of Death-Receptor-Induced Apoptosis. *Immunity* 2016, *45*, 513–526. [CrossRef] [PubMed]
84. Varfolomeev, E.E.; Schuchmann, M.; Luria, V.; Chiannilkulchai, N.; Beckmann, J.S.; Mett, I.L.; Rebrikov, D.; Brodianski, V.M.; Kemper, O.C.; Kollet, O.; et al. Targeted disruption of the mouse Caspase 8 gene ablates cell death induction by the TNF receptors, Fas/Apo1, and DR3 and is lethal prenatally. *Immunity* 1998, *9*, 267–276. [CrossRef]
85. Lalaoui, N.; Boyden, S.E.; Oda, H.; Wood, G.M.; Stone, D.L.; Chau, D.; Liu, L.; Stoffels, M.; Kratina, T.; Lawlor, K.E.; et al. Mutations that prevent caspase cleavage of RIPK1 cause autoinflammatory disease. *Nature* 2020, *577*, 103–108. [CrossRef]
86. Chun, H.J.; Zheng, L.; Ahmad, M.; Wang, J.; Speirs, C.K.; Siegel, R.M.; Dale, J.K.; Puck, J.; Davis, J.; Hall, C.G.; et al. Pleiotropic defects in lymphocyte activation caused by caspase-8 mutations lead to human immunodeficiency. *Nature* 2002, *419*, 395–399. [CrossRef]
87. Puri, A.W.; Broz, P.; Shen, A.; Monack, D.M.; Bogyo, M. Caspase-1 activity is required to bypass macrophage apoptosis upon Salmonella infection. *Nat. Chem. Biol.* 2012, *8*, 745–747. [CrossRef]
88. Yu, J.; Nagasu, H.; Murakami, T.; Hoang, H.; Broderick, L.; Hoffman, H.M.; Horng, T. Inflammasome activation leads to Caspase-1-dependent mitochondrial damage and block of mitophagy. *Proc. Natl. Acad. Sci. USA* 2014, *111*, 15514–15519. [CrossRef]
89. Pierini, R.; Juruj, C.; Perret, M.; Jones, C.L.; Mangeot, P.; Weiss, D.S.; Henry, T. AIM2/ASC triggers caspase-8-dependent apoptosis in Francisella-infected caspase-1-deficient macrophages. *Cell Death Differ.* 2012, *19*, 1709–1721. [CrossRef]
90. Sagulenko, V.; Thygesen, S.J.; Sester, D.P.; Idris, A.; Cridland, J.A.; Vajjhala, P.R.; Roberts, T.L.; Schroder, K.; Vince, J.E.; Hill, J.M.; et al. AIM2 and NLRP3 inflammasomes activate both apoptotic and pyroptotic death pathways via ASC. *Cell Death Differ.* 2013, *20*, 1149–1160. [CrossRef]
91. Man, S.M.; Tourlomousis, P.; Hopkins, L.; Monie, T.P.; Fitzgerald, K.A.; Bryant, C.E. Salmonella infection induces recruitment of Caspase-8 to the inflammasome to modulate IL-1β production. *J. Immunol.* 2013, *191*, 5239–5246. [CrossRef] [PubMed]
92. Mascarenhas, D.P.A.; Cerqueira, D.M.; Pereira, M.S.F.; Castanheira, F.V.S.; Fernandes, T.D.; Manin, G.Z.; Cunha, L.D.; Zamboni, D.S. Inhibition of caspase-1 or gasdermin-D enable caspase-8 activation in the Naip5/NLRC4/ASC inflammasome. *PLoS Pathog.* 2017, *13*, e1006502. [CrossRef] [PubMed]
93. Van Opdenbosch, N.; Van Gorp, H.; Verdonckt, M.; Saavedra, P.H.V.; de Vasconcelos, N.M.; Goncalves, A.; Vande Walle, L.; Demon, D.; Matusiak, M.; Van Hauwermeiren, F.; et al. Caspase-1 Engagement and TLR-Induced c-FLIP Expression Suppress ASC/Caspase-8-Dependent Apoptosis by Inflammasome Sensors NLRP1b and NLRC4. *Cell Rep.* 2017, *21*, 3427–3444. [CrossRef] [PubMed]
94. Man, S.M.; Hopkins, L.J.; Nugent, E.; Cox, S.; Glück, I.M.; Tourlomousis, P.; Wright, J.A.; Cicuta, P.; Monie, T.P.; Bryant, C.E. Inflammasome activation causes dual recruitment of NLRC4 and NLRP3 to the same macromolecular complex. *Proc. Natl. Acad. Sci. USA* 2014, *111*, 7403–7408. [CrossRef]
95. Kang, S.; Fernandes-Alnemri, T.; Rogers, C.; Mayes, L.; Wang, Y.; Dillon, C.; Roback, L.; Kaiser, W.; Oberst, A.; Sagara, J.; et al. Caspase-8 scaffolding function and MLKL regulate NLRP3 inflammasome activation downstream of TLR3. *Nat. Commun.* 2015, *6*, 7515. [CrossRef]
96. Conos, S.A.; Chen, K.W.; De Nardo, D.; Hara, H.; Whitehead, L.; Nunez, G.; Masters, S.L.; Murphy, J.M.; Schroder, K.; Vaux, D.L.; et al. Active MLKL triggers the NLRP3 inflammasome in a cell-intrinsic manner. *Proc. Natl. Acad. Sci. USA* 2017, *114*, E961–E969. [CrossRef]
97. Gutierrez, K.D.; Davis, M.A.; Daniels, B.P.; Olsen, T.M.; Ralli-Jain, P.; Tait, S.W.; Gale, M., Jr.; Oberst, A. MLKL Activation Triggers NLRP3-Mediated Processing and Release of IL-1β Independently of Gasdermin-D. *J. Immunol.* 2017, *198*, 2156–2164. [CrossRef]
98. Sarhan, J.; Liu, B.C.; Muendlein, H.I.; Li, P.; Nilson, R.; Tang, A.Y.; Rongvaux, A.; Bunnell, S.C.; Shao, F.; Green, D.R.; et al. Caspase-8 induces cleavage of gasdermin D to elicit pyroptosis during Yersinia infection. *Proc. Natl. Acad. Sci. USA* 2018, *115*, E10888–E10897. [CrossRef]
99. Demarco, B.; Grayczyk, J.P.; Bjanes, E.; Le Roy, D.; Tonnus, W.; Assenmacher, C.A.; Radaelli, E.; Fettrelet, T.; Mack, V.; Linkermann, A.; et al. Caspase-8-dependent gasdermin D cleavage promotes antimicrobial defense but confers susceptibility to TNF-induced lethality. *Sci. Adv.* 2020, *6*, eabc3465. [CrossRef]
100. Orning, P.; Weng, D.; Starheim, K.; Ratner, D.; Best, Z.; Lee, B.; Brooks, A.; Xia, S.; Wu, H.; Kelliher, M.A.; et al. Pathogen blockade of TAK1 triggers caspase-8-dependent cleavage of gasdermin D and cell death. *Science* 2018, *362*, 1064–1069. [CrossRef]

101. Taabazuing, C.Y.; Okondo, M.C.; Bachovchin, D.A. Pyroptosis and apoptosis pathways engage in bidirectional crosstalk in monocytes and macrophages. *Cell Chem. Biol.* **2017**, *24*, 507–514. [CrossRef] [PubMed]
102. Platnich, J.M.; Chung, H.; Lau, A.; Sandall, C.F.; Bondzi-Simpson, A.; Chen, H.M.; Komada, T.; Trotman-Grant, A.C.; Brandelli, J.R.; Chun, J.; et al. Shiga Toxin/Lipopolysaccharide Activates Caspase-4 and Gasdermin D to Trigger Mitochondrial Reactive Oxygen Species Upstream of the NLRP3 Inflammasome. *Cell Rep.* **2018**, *25*, 1525–1536.e1527. [CrossRef] [PubMed]
103. Rogers, C.; Erkes, D.A.; Nardone, A.; Aplin, A.E.; Fernandes-Alnemri, T.; Alnemri, E.S. Gasdermin pores permeabilize mitochondria to augment caspase-3 activation during apoptosis and inflammasome activation. *Nat. Commun.* **2019**, *10*, 1689. [CrossRef] [PubMed]
104. de Vasconcelos, N.M.; Van Opdenbosch, N.; Van Gorp, H.; Parthoens, E.; Lamkanfi, M. Single-cell analysis of pyroptosis dynamics reveals conserved GSDMD-mediated subcellular events that precede plasma membrane rupture. *Cell Death Differ.* **2019**, *26*, 146–161. [CrossRef] [PubMed]
105. Op de Beeck, K.; Van Camp, G.; Thys, S.; Cools, N.; Callebaut, I.; Vrijens, K.; Van Nassauw, L.; Van Tendeloo, V.F.; Timmermans, J.P.; Van Laer, L. The DFNA5 gene, responsible for hearing loss and involved in cancer, encodes a novel apoptosis-inducing protein. *Eur. J. Hum. Genet.* **2011**, *19*, 965–973. [CrossRef]
106. Wang, Y.; Gao, W.; Shi, X.; Ding, J.; Liu, W.; He, H.; Wang, K.; Shao, F. Chemotherapy drugs induce pyroptosis through caspase-3 cleavage of a gasdermin. *Nature* **2017**, *547*, 99–103. [CrossRef]
107. Rogers, C.; Fernandes-Alnemri, T.; Mayes, L.; Alnemri, D.; Cingolani, G.; Alnemri, E.S. Cleavage of DFNA5 by caspase-3 during apoptosis mediates progression to secondary necrotic/pyroptotic cell death. *Nat. Commun.* **2017**, *8*, 14128. [CrossRef]
108. Zhou, B.; Abbott, D.W. Gasdermin E permits interleukin-1 beta release in distinct sublytic and pyroptotic phases. *Cell Rep.* **2021**, *35*, 108998. [CrossRef]
109. Wang, C.; Yang, T.; Xiao, J.; Xu, C.; Alippe, Y.; Sun, K.; Kanneganti, T.D.; Monahan, J.B.; Abu-Amer, Y.; Lieberman, J.; et al. NLRP3 inflammasome activation triggers gasdermin D-independent inflammation. *Sci. Immunol.* **2021**, *6*, eabj3859. [CrossRef]
110. Tsuchiya, K.; Nakajima, S.; Hosojima, S.; Thi Nguyen, D.; Hattori, T.; Manh Le, T.; Hori, O.; Mahib, M.R.; Yamaguchi, Y.; Miura, M.; et al. Caspase-1 initiates apoptosis in the absence of gasdermin D. *Nat. Commun.* **2019**, *10*, 2091. [CrossRef]
111. Heilig, R.; Dilucca, M.; Boucher, D.; Chen, K.W.; Hancz, D.; Demarco, B.; Shkarina, K.; Broz, P. Caspase-1 cleaves Bid to release mitochondrial SMAC and drive secondary necrosis in the absence of GSDMD. *Life Sci. Alliance* **2020**, *3*, e202000735. [CrossRef]
112. Xu, W.; Che, Y.; Zhang, Q.; Huang, H.; Ding, C.; Wang, Y.; Wang, G.; Cao, L.; Hao, H. Apaf-1 Pyroptosome Senses Mitochondrial Permeability Transition. *Cell Metab.* **2021**, *33*, 424–436.e410. [CrossRef] [PubMed]
113. Chen, K.W.; Demarco, B.; Heilig, R.; Shkarina, K.; Boettcher, A.; Farady, C.J.; Pelczar, P.; Broz, P. Extrinsic and intrinsic apoptosis activate pannexin-1 to drive NLRP3 inflammasome assembly. *EMBO J.* **2019**, *38*, e101638. [CrossRef] [PubMed]
114. Yan, W.T.; Yang, Y.D.; Hu, W.M.; Ning, W.Y.; Liao, L.S.; Lu, S.; Zhao, W.J.; Zhang, Q.; Xiong, K. Do pyroptosis, apoptosis, and necroptosis (PANoptosis) exist in cerebral ischemia? Evidence from cell and rodent studies. *Neural Regen. Res.* **2022**, *17*, 1761–1768. [CrossRef] [PubMed]
115. Jiang, W.; Deng, Z.; Dai, X.; Zhao, W. PANoptosis: A New Insight Into Oral Infectious Diseases. *Front. Immunol.* **2021**, *12*, 789610. [CrossRef]
116. Chi, D.; Lin, X.; Meng, Q.; Tan, J.; Gong, Q.; Tong, Z. Real-Time Induction of Macrophage Apoptosis, Pyroptosis, and Necroptosis by Enterococcus faecalis OG1RF and Two Root Canal Isolated Strains. *Front. Cell. Infect. Microbiol.* **2021**, *11*, 720147. [CrossRef]
117. Lin, J.F.; Hu, P.S.; Wang, Y.Y.; Tan, Y.T.; Yu, K.; Liao, K.; Wu, Q.N.; Li, T.; Meng, Q.; Lin, J.Z.; et al. Phosphorylated NFS1 weakens oxaliplatin-based chemosensitivity of colorectal cancer by preventing PANoptosis. *Signal Transduct. Target. Ther.* **2022**, *7*, 54. [CrossRef]
118. Song, M.; Xia, W.; Tao, Z.; Zhu, B.; Zhang, W.; Liu, C.; Chen, S. Self-assembled polymeric nanocarrier-mediated co-delivery of metformin and doxorubicin for melanoma therapy. *Drug Deliv.* **2021**, *28*, 594–606. [CrossRef]
119. Upton, J.W.; Kaiser, W.J.; Mocarski, E.S. DAI/ZBP1/DLM-1 complexes with RIP3 to mediate virus-induced programmed necrosis that is targeted by murine cytomegalovirus vIRA. *Cell Host Microbe* **2012**, *11*, 290–297. [CrossRef]
120. Kaiser, W.J.; Upton, J.W.; Mocarski, E.S. Receptor-interacting protein homotypic interaction motif-dependent control of NF-kappa B activation via the DNA-dependent activator of IFN regulatory factors. *J. Immunol.* **2008**, *181*, 6427–6434. [CrossRef]
121. Thapa, R.J.; Ingram, J.P.; Ragan, K.B.; Nogusa, S.; Boyd, D.F.; Benitez, A.A.; Sridharan, H.; Kosoff, R.; Shubina, M.; Landsteiner, V.J.; et al. DAI senses influenza A virus genomic RNA and activates RIPK3-dependent cell death. *Cell Host Microbe* **2016**, *20*, 674–681. [CrossRef] [PubMed]
122. Wang, Y.; Kanneganti, T.D. From pyroptosis, apoptosis and necroptosis to PANoptosis: A mechanistic compendium of programmed cell death pathways. *Comput. Struct. Biotechnol. J.* **2021**, *19*, 4641–4657. [CrossRef] [PubMed]
123. Tamura, T.; Ishihara, M.; Lamphier, M.S.; Tanaka, N.; Oishi, I.; Aizawa, S.; Matsuyama, T.; Mak, T.W.; Taki, S.; Taniguchi, T. An IRF-1-dependent pathway of DNA damage-induced apoptosis in mitogen-activated T lymphocytes. *Nature* **1995**, *376*, 596–599. [CrossRef] [PubMed]
124. Tanaka, N.; Ishihara, M.; Kitagawa, M.; Harada, H.; Kimura, T.; Matsuyama, T.; Lamphier, M.S.; Aizawa, S.; Mak, T.W.; Taniguchi, T. Cellular commitment to oncogene-induced transformation or apoptosis is dependent on the transcription factor IRF-1. *Cell* **1994**, *77*, 829–839. [CrossRef]
125. Karki, R.; Kanneganti, T.D. The 'cytokine storm': Molecular mechanisms and therapeutic prospects. *Trends Immunol.* **2021**, *42*, 681–705. [CrossRef]

126. Man, S.M.; Karki, R.; Malireddi, R.K.; Neale, G.; Vogel, P.; Yamamoto, M.; Lamkanfi, M.; Kanneganti, T.D. The transcription factor IRF1 and guanylate-binding proteins target activation of the AIM2 inflammasome by Francisella infection. *Nat. Immunol.* **2015**, *16*, 467–475. [CrossRef]
127. Vanden Berghe, T.; Kaiser, W.J.; Bertrand, M.J.; Vandenabeele, P. Molecular crosstalk between apoptosis, necroptosis, and survival signaling. *Mol. Cell. Oncol.* **2015**, *2*, e975093. [CrossRef]
128. Fritsch, M.; Gunther, S.D.; Schwarzer, R.; Albert, M.C.; Schorn, F.; Werthenbach, J.P.; Schiffmann, L.M.; Stair, N.; Stocks, H.; Seeger, J.M.; et al. Caspase-8 is the molecular switch for apoptosis, necroptosis and pyroptosis. *Nature* **2019**, *575*, 683–687. [CrossRef]
129. Tummers, B.; Mari, L.; Guy, C.S.; Heckmann, B.L.; Rodriguez, D.A.; Rühl, S.; Moretti, J.; Crawford, J.C.; Fitzgerald, P.; Kanneganti, T.D.; et al. Caspase-8-Dependent Inflammatory Responses Are Controlled by Its Adaptor, FADD, and Necroptosis. *Immunity* **2020**, *52*, 994–1006.e8. [CrossRef]
130. Newton, K.; Wickliffe, K.E.; Maltzman, A.; Dugger, D.L.; Reja, R.; Zhang, Y.; Roose-Girma, M.; Modrusan, Z.; Sagolla, M.S.; Webster, J.D.; et al. Activity of caspase-8 determines plasticity between cell death pathways. *Nature* **2019**, *575*, 679–682. [CrossRef]
131. Schwarzer, R.; Jiao, H.; Wachsmuth, L.; Tresch, A.; Pasparakis, M. FADD and Caspase-8 Regulate Gut Homeostasis and Inflammation by Controlling MLKL- and GSDMD-Mediated Death of Intestinal Epithelial Cells. *Immunity* **2020**, *52*, 978–993.e6. [CrossRef] [PubMed]
132. Kang, T.B.; Oh, G.S.; Scandella, E.; Bolinger, B.; Ludewig, B.; Kovalenko, A.; Wallach, D. Mutation of a self-processing site in caspase-8 compromises its apoptotic but not its nonapoptotic functions in bacterial artificial chromosome-transgenic mice. *J. Immunol.* **2008**, *181*, 2522–2532. [CrossRef] [PubMed]
133. Wang, Y.; Karki, R.; Zheng, M.; Kancharana, B.; Lee, S.; Kesavardhana, S.; Hansen, B.S.; Pruett-Miller, S.M.; Kanneganti, T.D. Cutting Edge: Caspase-8 Is a Linchpin in Caspase-3 and Gasdermin D Activation to Control Cell Death, Cytokine Release, and Host Defense during Influenza A Virus Infection. *J. Immunol.* **2021**, *207*, 2411–2416. [CrossRef] [PubMed]
134. Belhocine, K.; Monack, D.M. Francisella infection triggers activation of the AIM2 inflammasome in murine dendritic cells. *Cell Microbiol.* **2012**, *14*, 71–80. [CrossRef]
135. Doerflinger, M.; Deng, Y.; Whitney, P.; Salvamoser, R.; Engel, S.; Kueh, A.J.; Tai, L.; Bachem, A.; Gressier, E.; Geoghegan, N.D.; et al. Flexible Usage and Interconnectivity of Diverse Cell Death Pathways Protect against Intracellular Infection. *Immunity* **2020**, *53*, 533–547.e7. [CrossRef]
136. Broz, P.; Ruby, T.; Belhocine, K.; Bouley, D.M.; Kayagaki, N.; Dixit, V.M.; Monack, D.M. Caspase-11 increases susceptibility to Salmonella infection in the absence of caspase-1. *Nature* **2012**, *490*, 288–291. [CrossRef]
137. Sundaram, B.; Karki, R.; Kanneganti, T.D. NLRC4 Deficiency Leads to Enhanced Phosphorylation of MLKL and Necroptosis. *Immunohorizons* **2022**, *6*, 243–252. [CrossRef]
138. Sutterwala, F.S.; Mijares, L.A.; Li, L.; Ogura, Y.; Kazmierczak, B.I.; Flavell, R.A. Immune recognition of Pseudomonas aeruginosa mediated by the IPAF/NLRC4 inflammasome. *J. Exp. Med.* **2007**, *204*, 3235–3245. [CrossRef]
139. Miao, E.A.; Ernst, R.K.; Dors, M.; Mao, D.P.; Aderem, A. Pseudomonas aeruginosa activates caspase 1 through Ipaf. *Proc. Natl. Acad. Sci. USA* **2008**, *105*, 2562–2567. [CrossRef]
140. Ferguson, P.J.; Bing, X.; Vasef, M.A.; Ochoa, L.A.; Mahgoub, A.; Waldschmidt, T.J.; Tygrett, L.T.; Schlueter, A.J.; El-Shanti, H. A missense mutation in pstpip2 is associated with the murine autoinflammatory disorder chronic multifocal osteomyelitis. *Bone* **2006**, *38*, 41–47. [CrossRef]
141. Cassel, S.L.; Janczy, J.R.; Bing, X.; Wilson, S.P.; Olivier, A.K.; Otero, J.E.; Iwakura, Y.; Shayakhmetov, D.M.; Bassuk, A.G.; Abu-Amer, Y.; et al. Inflammasome-independent IL-1β mediates autoinflammatory disease in Pstpip2-deficient mice. *Proc. Natl. Acad. Sci. USA* **2014**, *111*, 1072–1077. [CrossRef] [PubMed]
142. Douglas, T.; Champagne, C.; Morizot, A.; Lapointe, J.M.; Saleh, M. The Inflammatory Caspases-1 and -11 Mediate the Pathogenesis of Dermatitis in Sharpin-Deficient Mice. *J. Immunol.* **2015**, *195*, 2365–2373. [CrossRef] [PubMed]
143. Rickard, J.A.; Anderton, H.; Etemadi, N.; Nachbur, U.; Darding, M.; Peltzer, N.; Lalaoui, N.; Lawlor, K.E.; Vanyai, H.; Hall, C.; et al. TNFR1-dependent cell death drives inflammation in Sharpin-deficient mice. *eLife* **2014**, *3*, e03464. [CrossRef] [PubMed]
144. Kumari, S.; Redouane, Y.; Lopez-Mosqueda, J.; Shiraishi, R.; Romanowska, M.; Lutzmayer, S.; Kuiper, J.; Martinez, C.; Dikic, I.; Pasparakis, M.; et al. Sharpin prevents skin inflammation by inhibiting TNFR1-induced keratinocyte apoptosis. *eLife* **2014**, *3*, e03422. [CrossRef] [PubMed]
145. HogenEsch, H.; Gijbels, M.J.; Offerman, E.; van Hooft, J.; van Bekkum, D.W.; Zurcher, C. A spontaneous mutation characterized by chronic proliferative dermatitis in C57BL mice. *Am. J. Pathol.* **1993**, *143*, 972–982.
146. Berger, S.B.; Kasparcova, V.; Hoffman, S.; Swift, B.; Dare, L.; Schaeffer, M.; Capriotti, C.; Cook, M.; Finger, J.; Hughes-Earle, A.; et al. Cutting Edge: RIP1 kinase activity is dispensable for normal development but is a key regulator of inflammation in SHARPIN-deficient mice. *J. Immunol.* **2014**, *192*, 5476–5480. [CrossRef]
147. Lukens, J.R.; Vogel, P.; Johnson, G.R.; Kelliher, M.A.; Iwakura, Y.; Lamkanfi, M.; Kanneganti, T.D. RIP1-driven autoinflammation targets IL-1alpha independently of inflammasomes and RIP3. *Nature* **2013**, *498*, 224–227. [CrossRef]
148. Gurung, P.; Fan, G.; Lukens, J.R.; Vogel, P.; Tonks, N.K.; Kanneganti, T.D. Tyrosine Kinase SYK Licenses MyD88 Adaptor Protein to Instigate IL-1alpha-Mediated Inflammatory Disease. *Immunity* **2017**, *46*, 635–648. [CrossRef]
149. Peltzer, N.; Darding, M.; Montinaro, A.; Draber, P.; Draberova, H.; Kupka, S.; Rieser, E.; Fisher, A.; Hutchinson, C.; Taraborrelli, L.; et al. LUBAC is essential for embryogenesis by preventing cell death and enabling haematopoiesis. *Nature* **2018**, *557*, 112–117. [CrossRef]

150. Mandal, P.; Feng, Y.; Lyons, J.D.; Berger, S.B.; Otani, S.; DeLaney, A.; Tharp, G.K.; Maner-Smith, K.; Burd, E.M.; Schaeffer, M.; et al. Caspase-8 Collaborates with Caspase-11 to Drive Tissue Damage and Execution of Endotoxic Shock. *Immunity* **2018**, *49*, 42–55.e6. [CrossRef]
151. Rauch, I.; Deets, K.A.; Ji, D.X.; von Moltke, J.; Tenthorey, J.L.; Lee, A.Y.; Philip, N.H.; Ayres, J.S.; Brodsky, I.E.; Gronert, K.; et al. NAIP-NLRC4 Inflammasomes Coordinate Intestinal Epithelial Cell Expulsion with Eicosanoid and IL-18 Release via Activation of Caspase-1 and -8. *Immunity* **2017**, *46*, 649–659. [CrossRef] [PubMed]
152. von Moltke, J.; Trinidad, N.J.; Moayeri, M.; Kintzer, A.F.; Wang, S.B.; van Rooijen, N.; Brown, C.R.; Krantz, B.A.; Leppla, S.H.; Gronert, K.; et al. Rapid induction of inflammatory lipid mediators by the inflammasome in vivo. *Nature* **2012**, *490*, 107–111. [CrossRef] [PubMed]
153. Maccioni, R.B.; Rojo, L.E.; Fernández, J.A.; Kuljis, R.O. The role of neuroimmunomodulation in Alzheimer's disease. *Ann. N. Y. Acad. Sci.* **2009**, *1153*, 240–246. [CrossRef] [PubMed]
154. Ofengeim, D.; Mazzitelli, S.; Ito, Y.; DeWitt, J.P.; Mifflin, L.; Zou, C.; Das, S.; Adiconis, X.; Chen, H.; Zhu, H.; et al. RIPK1 mediates a disease-associated microglial response in Alzheimer's disease. *Proc. Natl. Acad. Sci. USA* **2017**, *114*, E8788–E8797. [CrossRef]
155. Nogusa, S.; Thapa, R.J.; Dillon, C.P.; Liedmann, S.; Oguin, T.H., 3rd; Ingram, J.P.; Rodriguez, D.A.; Kosoff, R.; Sharma, S.; Sturm, O.; et al. RIPK3 activates parallel pathways of MLKL-criven necroptosis and FADD-mediated apoptosis to protect against Influenza A virus. *Cell Host Microbe* **2016**, *20*, 13–24. [CrossRef]
156. Wallace, H.L.; Wang, L.; Gardner, C.L.; Corkum, C.P.; Grant, M.D.; Hirasawa, K.; Russell, R.S. Crosstalk Between Pyroptosis and Apoptosis in Hepatitis C Virus-induced Cell Death. *Front. Immunol.* **2022**, *13*, 788138. [CrossRef]
157. Van Hauwermeiren, F.; Van Opdenbosch, N.; Van Gorp, H.; de Vasconcelos, N.; van Loo, G.; Vandenabeele, P.; Kanneganti, T.D.; Lamkanfi, M. Bacillus anthracis induces NLRP3 inflammasome activation and caspase-8-mediated apoptosis of macrophages to promote lethal anthrax. *Proc. Natl. Acad. Sci. USA* **2022**, *119*, e2116415119. [CrossRef]
158. Turner, S.; Kenshole, B.; Ruby, J. Viral modulation of the host response via crmA/SPI-2 expression. *Immunol. Cell Biol.* **1999**, *77*, 236–241. [CrossRef]
159. He, S.; Han, J. Manipulation of Host Cell Death Pathways by Herpes Simplex Virus. In *Current Topics in Microbiology and Immunology*; Springer: Berlin, Heidelberg, 2020.
160. Pauleau, A.L.; Larochette, N.; Giordanetto, F.; Scholz, S.R.; Poncet, D.; Zamzami, N.; Goldmacher, V.S.; Kroemer, G. Structure-function analysis of the interaction between Bax and the cytomegalovirus-encoded protein vMIA. *Oncogene* **2007**, *26*, 7067–7080. [CrossRef]
161. Ashida, H.; Sasakawa, C.; Suzuki, T. A unique bacterial tactic to circumvent the cell death crosstalk induced by blockade of caspase-8. *EMBO J.* **2020**, *39*, e104469. [CrossRef]

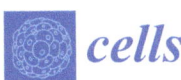

Review

Proteostasis Perturbations and Their Roles in Causing Sterile Inflammation and Autoinflammatory Diseases

Jonas Johannes Papendorf, Elke Krüger *,† and Frédéric Ebstein *,†

Institut für Medizinische Biochemie und Molekularbiologie, Universitätsmedizin Greifswald, Ferdinand-Sauerbruch-Straße, 17475 Greifswald, Germany; jonasjohannes.papendorf@med.uni-greifswald.de
* Correspondence: elke.krueger@uni-greifswald.de (E.K.); ebsteinf@uni-greifswald.de (F.E.)
† These authors contributed equally to this work.

Abstract: Proteostasis, a portmanteau of the words protein and homeostasis, refers to the ability of eukaryotic cells to maintain a stable proteome by acting on protein synthesis, quality control and/or degradation. Over the last two decades, an increasing number of disorders caused by proteostasis perturbations have been identified. Depending on their molecular etiology, such diseases may be classified into ribosomopathies, proteinopathies and proteasomopathies. Strikingly, most—if not all—of these syndromes exhibit an autoinflammatory component, implying a direct cause-and-effect relationship between proteostasis disruption and the initiation of innate immune responses. In this review, we provide a comprehensive overview of the molecular pathogenesis of these disorders and summarize current knowledge of the various mechanisms by which impaired proteostasis promotes autoinflammation. We particularly focus our discussion on the notion of how cells sense and integrate proteostasis perturbations as danger signals in the context of autoinflammatory diseases to provide insights into the complex and multiple facets of sterile inflammation.

Keywords: proteostasis; autoinflammation; ribosomopathies; proteinopathies; proteasomopathies

1. Introduction

Inflammation describes a highly conserved generally beneficial reaction—if controlled—of the body in response to a variety of danger signals [1–3]. It is triggered by the innate immune system and characterized by the rapid mobilization of specialized cells and humoral factors which combat the insult with a relatively low specificity [4–6]. Noxious signals capable of initiating innate responses are traditionally divided into exogenous and endogenous insults in order to facilitate self and non-self-discrimination [7,8]. External stimuli are typically derived from infectious agents and include a wide range of microbial products referred to as pathogen-associated molecular patterns (PAMPs) which are recognized by pathogen-recognition receptors (PRR) such as Toll-like receptors (TLR), RIG-I-like receptors (RLR), NOD-like receptors (NLR), among others [9,10]. The binding of PAMP to PRR triggers multiple intracellular signaling cascades ultimately resulting in the activation of the NF-κB and IRF3 transcription factors which in turn promote the expression of pro-inflammatory cytokines (i.e., TNFα, IL-1, IL-6) and type I and/or II interferons (IFN) [11,12]. Type I IFN is a large cytokine family consisting of 18 members with 14 IFN-α species and one single specimen each of IFN-β, IFN-κ, IFN-ω and IFN-ε which are produced by both immune and non-immune cells [13]. Following autocrine and/or paracrine binding to their receptor IFNAR1/2, type I IFN engage JAK/STAT signaling that results in the rapid transcription of a myriad of so-called IFN-stimulated genes (ISG) [14]. Prominent ISG include *PKR* and *OAS1* whose products confer the cell an antiviral state by arresting protein translation and promoting RNA degradation, respectively [14]. Internal stimuli also known as damage-associated molecular patterns (DAMPs) are widely regarded as self-molecules that accidently reach undedicated compartments following tissue injury [15,16]. Prime examples of DAMPs include extracellular and/or cytosolic DNA as well as extracellular

ATP or histones, only to name a few [17–20]. Like PAMPs, DAMPs use various PRR to elicit innate immune responses which are characterized by the prompt production of NF-κB- and IRF3-responsive genes [21,22]. As innate immunity triggered by DAMPs is pathogen-free, it is frequently categorized as sterile inflammation [23,24]. Importantly, sterile inflammation is not necessarily restricted to the unphysiological release of molecules from necrotic cells and/or damaged intracellular organelles. Disturbances in protein flux have also long been known to be immunostimulant and prominent hallmarks of a flurry of autoimmune diseases. It is indeed more than 60 years ago that extracellular protein aggregates initially called "rheumatoid factors" have been described in the plasma and synovial tissues of patients with rheumatoid arthritis (RA) [25]. It became rapidly evident that such aggregates were in fact large insoluble autoimmune complexes (IC) made up of self-reactive immunoglobulin (Ig) G [26]. It is their inefficient clearance by circulating proteases and/or phagocytes that results in their deposition in tissues and contributes to autoinflammation, notably through the stimulation of monocytes, macrophages and dendritic cells (DC) [27,28]. Herein, RA provided the first example of sterile inflammation triggered by loss of protein homeostasis. Meanwhile, over 40 autoinflammatory diseases have been reported to be associated with protein homeostasis (or more commonly referred to as "proteostasis") perturbations.

2. Proteostasis Sensors and Their Roles in Triggering Sterile Inflammation

Imbalances of protein flux are not limited to the extracellular space but can also occur within the cell as a consequence of a disequilibrium between protein synthesis at ribosomes (i.e., translation) and degradation by the ubiquitin–proteasome system (UPS) and/or autophagy [29]. Regardless of localization, it is becoming increasingly clear that proteostasis perturbations behave as danger signals and have the potential to initiate sterile inflammation. Although our current knowledge on the mechanisms perceiving and integrating these signals are not fully understood, a growing body of evidence suggests a critical role of the endoplasmic reticulum (ER) in the surveillance of intracellular proteostasis. The mechanisms monitoring proteostasis outside the cell are less clear, albeit a couple of studies point to a potential involvement of PRR in this process, as discussed below.

2.1. The Unfolded Protein Response (UPR)

As shown in Figure 1, the ER-membrane resident proteins IRE1, ATF6 and PERK belong to the mechanisms by which the cell is capable of sensing intracellular proteostasis disruption. One estimates that approximately 30–40% of the newly synthetized proteins traffic through the endoplasmic reticulum (ER) [30]. It is further understood that up to 25% of these proteins fail to achieve final conformation and that such products are recognized by the protein quality control machinery in the ER and transported back to cytosol by the ER-associated degradation (ERAD) pathway for subsequent degradation by 26S proteasomes [31]. Given that retro-translocation is driven by degradation [32–34], proteasome dysfunction ultimately results in the accumulation of misfolded proteins within the ER lumen and subsequent activation of the IRE1, ATF6 and PERK receptors. This in turn engages the so-called unfolded protein response (UPR), a compensatory reaction which mostly aims to restore proteostasis by

I.   Arresting global protein biosynthesis;
II. Upregulating specific genes coding for chaperones and ERAD components [35–37].

While transient stimulations of the UPR are physiological reactions devoid of inflammation, excessive UPR activation is considered pathological and associated with persistent innate responses [35,38]. The mechanisms by which the UPR triggers sterile inflammation are diverse, complex, poorly understood and have been already discussed elsewhere [35,39]. Of particular interest is the PERK arm of the UPR which mediates the phosphorylation of eIF2α, an event that shuts down canonical translation of 5' capped mRNA molecules and affects the steady-state level of short-lived proteins [40]. These proteins include notably IκBα whose increased turnover upon activation of the UPR facilitates the nuclear translocation of NF-κB and the subsequent production of inflammatory mediators [41,42]. As discussed later, the UPR has been proposed as a major contributor to autoinflammation in various proteinopathies [35].

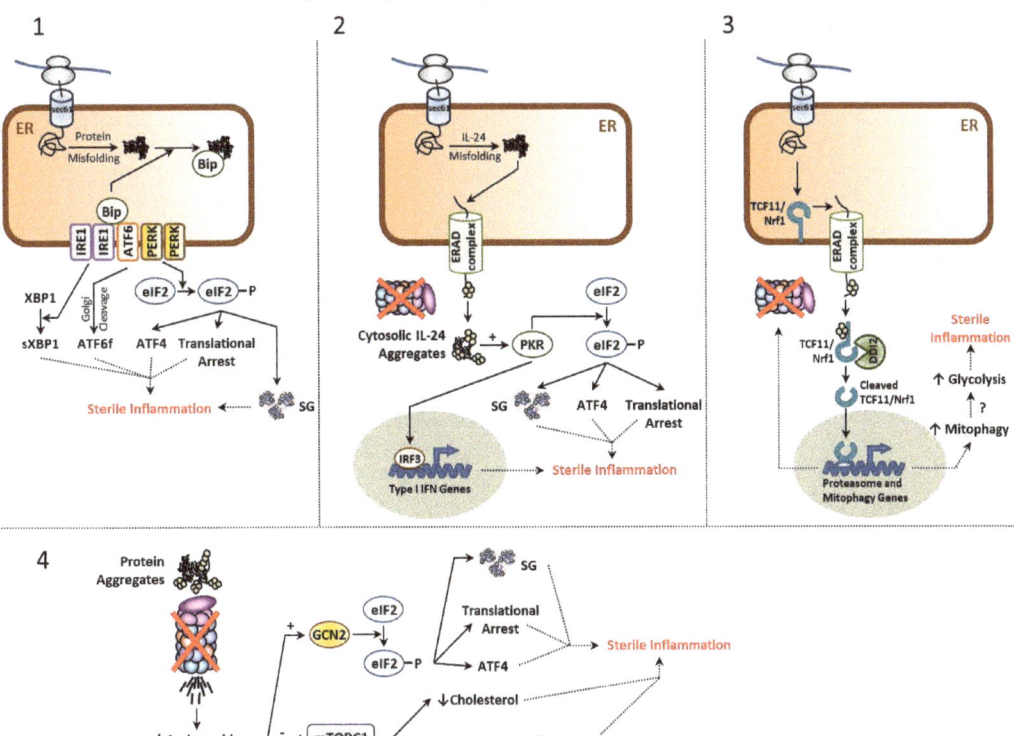

Figure 1. Most inflammatory pathways engaged following proteostasis disruption originate from the ER. Proteostasis perturbations are typically caused by proteasome dysfunction and/or excessive protein misfolding, as indicated. (**1**) Sustained misfolding of secretory proteins results in their accumulation within the ER lumen and generates ER stress, which is sensed by the IRE1, ATF6 and PERK receptors upon dissociation of the chaperone protein Bip. This, in turn, initiates the UPR that comprises the formation of sXBP1, ATF6f as well as a translational arrest, the activation of ATF4 and the formation of SGs following phosphorylation of eIF2α by PERK. Persistent activation of all UPR branches have been reported to trigger sterile inflammation by various mechanisms (for more details, see main text). (**2**) Misfolding of IL-24 typically results in its subsequent retro-translocation back to the cytosol by the ERAD machinery. In case of proteasome dysfunction, IL-24 misfolded species accumulate in the cytosol and activate PKR to trigger a type I IFN response and inflammation via eIF2α phosphorylation. (**3**) Proteome imbalance is also sensed by the short-lived ER-membrane resident protein TCF11/Nrf1 whose turnover rate decreases with increased proteasome dysfunction. This results in its proteolytic cleavage by DDI2, thereby giving rise to a transcription factor inducing the expression of proteasome genes to restore protein homeostasis and mitophagy genes that may exacerbate inflammation through persistent glycolysis, as indicated. (**4**) Proteasome defects also reduce the intracellular pool of free amino acids and result in mTORC1 downregulation. This, in turn, promotes sterile inflammation by increasing mitophagy and blocking lipid synthesis (for more details, see the main text). Amino acid depletion in the cell also activates GCN2 of the integrated stress response (ISR) which facilitates inflammation following eIF2α phosphorylation.

2.2. The Integrated Stress Response (ISR)

As proteasome-mediated protein degradation produces peptides which are further degraded into amino acids by peptidases [43], it is legitimate to assume that the intracellular pool of amino acids is regulated—at least partially—by the UPS. This hypothesis, which has been proven to be true in yeast [43], implies that proteostasis perturbations caused by impaired protein breakdown are followed by a parallel depletion of intracellular amino acids.

A major sensor of amino acid deficiency in the cell is the general control nonderepressible 2 (GCN2) kinase which undergoes activation by uncharged tRNA that accumulate upon amino acid starvation [44]. As shown in Figure 1, like PERK, GCN2 promotes the phosphorylation of eIF2α in a pathway referred to as the integrated stress response (ISR) [45] which, by definition, intersects with the UPR. As both the ISR and PERK branch of the UPR converge to eIF2α, these pathways share similar consequences regarding their proinflammatory properties in case of sustained stimulus. Another kinase of the ISR capable of phosphorylating eIF2α is protein kinase R (PKR) [46], which is primarily activated by double-stranded (ds) RNA in infected cells during viral replication [47,48]. Besides phosphorylating eIF2α, PKR also triggers a signaling cascade resulting in the nuclear translocation of the transcription factor IRF3 and subsequent transcription of type I IFN genes [49–52]. Interestingly, the PKR activation spectrum is not restricted to RNA viruses and can be expanded to a flurry of non-microbial stimuli including proteostasis disruptors such as tunicamycin, oxidative stress and heat shock [53–58]. A recent study by Davidson et al. described cytosolic IL-24 as a potent PKR activator following proteasome dysfunction [59]. In this process, misfolding of newly synthetized IL-24 within the ER lumen results in its retro-translocation back to the cytosol by ERAD where it accumulates and activates PKR to engage a type I IFN response. Supporting the notion that abnormal cytosolic accumulation of IL-24 is a danger signal alerting the immune system via PKR, cells devoid of IL-24 and/or PKR fail to exhibit a type I IFN signature in response to proteasome inhibition [59]. The work of Davidson et al. therefore unambiguously identifies the IL-24/PKR axis as a new surveillance pathway capable of initiating sterile inflammation in response to perturbed proteostasis. This notion is fully in line with the observation that PKR is found constitutively phosphorylated/activated in the CNS of patients suffering from neurodegenerative proteinopathies [60–63] and that PKR inhibition is able to delay neuroinflammation in rats [64].

2.3. The mTORC1 Signaling Complex

Apart from GCN2, major amino acid sensors include the cytosolic SESN2 and CASTOR proteins which sense leucine and arginine levels, respectively [65]. Binding of these amino acids to their respective receptors activate GATOR2, which in turn inhibits the mTORC1 complex inhibitor GATOR1 [66]. Subsequently, mTORC1 itself undergoes activation and engages several downstream signaling pathways inhibiting autophagy, while promoting protein translation, lipid biosynthesis and mitochondria biogenesis [67]. Based on the assumption that the UPS regulates amino acid homeostasis, one would expect that impaired proteostasis result in downregulation of mTORC1 signaling (Figure 1). Indeed, our recent investigation on cells isolated from patients with *PSMD12* haploinsufficiency confirmed that proteasome loss-of-function was associated with reduced activation of mTORC1 [68]. From the mTORC1 downstream pathways, lipid biosynthesis seems of particular interest regarding sterile inflammation. It was indeed recently suggested that a reduced cholesterol flux in the cell engages spontaneous type I IFN responses in a poorly understood process involving the cGAS/STING pathway [69]. Likewise, increased autophagy by reduced mTORC1 activation might be relevant with respect to sterile inflammation following proteotoxic stress. Elevated autophagy does not only imply increased lysosomal protein breakdown but also presupposes increased elimination of intracellular organelles including mitochondria, a process referred to as "mitophagy". Supporting the notion that mTORC1 is a proteostasis sensor, increased mitophagy has been observed in patients with proteasomopathies [68]. Interestingly, sustained mitophagy implies a switch of the energetic metabolism from oxidative phosphorylation to glycolysis, the latter being associated with the accumulation of PEP, succinate, citrate and itaconate all exhibiting pro-inflammatory properties (i.e., M1 phenotype) by various and sometimes poorly understood mechanisms [70]. Whether mitophagy indeed participates in the initiation of sterile inflammation in response to impaired proteostasis is not known, but the observation that glycolysis is increased in microglia and astrocytes of patients in AD [70–72] supports this notion.

2.4. Stress-Induced Granulation

A cellular feature frequently shared by many neurodegenerative proteinopathies is the formation of so-called stress granules (SGs) in the CNS [73–84]. SGs are cytoplasmic liquid-like seemingly compartmentalized structures devoid of membranes mostly containing translation factors, RNA as well as RNA-binding proteins [85–88]. Importantly, SGs are not an exclusive feature of neurodegenerative diseases, and their formation may be induced in all cell types in response to various stress reactions driven by eIF2α phosphorylation, namely following activation of the UPR and/or ISR (Figure 1) [89]. Accordingly, SGs are induced in situations in which the proteostasis network is challenged such as viral infection and proteasome inhibition and [90–92]. Interestingly, while the role of SGs in the propagation of type I IFN responses during viral infection seems to be established [93–95], their contribution to inflammation following sterile proteostasis disruption is not known. Viral SGs are thought to amplify innate immune signaling by building a platform that facilitates the recruitment of the DNA/RNA sensors cGAS, PKR and RIG-1 [96–98]. It is unclear whether viral SGs are biochemically distinct from those observed in proteinopathies. In this regard, further investigations are warranted to answer the question whether SGs due to impaired proteostasis of non-viral origin predispose the cells to generate type I IFN responses.

2.5. The TCF11/Nrf1-NGLY1-DDI2 Axis

Another proteostasis sensor is the ER membrane-resident protein TCF11/Nrf1, also referred to as nuclear factor erythroid derived 2-related factor 1 (NFE2L1) and encoded by the *NFE2L1* gene [99,100]. TCF11/Nrf1 is a highly glycosylated short-lived protein which under normal conditions is rapidly targeted to proteasome-mediated degradation by ERAD [99,100] following its de-glycosylation by the enzyme N-glycanase 1 (NGLY1) [101]. Consequently, in case of proteasome dysfunction, TCF11/Nrf1 becomes stabilized and prone to enzymatic processing by the aspartyl protease protein DDI1 homolog 2 (DDI2) at the ER membrane [102]. As shown in Figure 1, following proteolytic cleavage, processed TCF11/Nrf1 translocates into the nucleus and binds to ARE promoters to induce the transcription of 20S and 19S proteasome subunit genes and a subset of ubiquitin factors. The TCF11/Nrf1-DDI2 pathway is widely viewed as a compensatory mechanism ensuring the replacement of defective 26S complexes by newly synthetized ones. Like all proteostasis sensors, TCF11/Nrf1 seems to have the potential to engage proinflammatory programs. This assumption is based on the observation that TCF11/Nrf1 also up-regulates mitophagy genes [103]. While the safe elimination of damaged mitochondria by autophagy prevents the accidental leakage of immunostimulatory mitochondrial (mt) DNA into the cytosol, the removal of the healthy ones due to excessive mitophagy might reprogram the cells towards glycolytic processes and their inherent proinflammatory consequences. On the other hand, TCF11/Nrf1 has been shown to mitigate lipid-mediated inflammation acting as a sensor for cholesterol [104]. Altogether, these studies highlight that our current understanding of TCF11/Nrf1 in inflammation remains incomplete and warrants further investigation.

2.6. Pathogen Recognition Receptors (PRR)

Unexpectedly, works aimed to unravel the pathogenesis of neurodegenerative proteinopathies have revealed that PRR are able to sense intra- and extracellular proteostasis perturbations. Indeed, normally specialized in the recognition of PAMP and/or DAMPs, PRR are also capable of perceiving abnormal protein aggregates. For instance, extracellular α-syn oligomers and fibrils produced during the course of Parkinson disease (PD) bind to TLR4 and TLR2 expressed on microglia [105–110]. In a very similar fashion, Aβ aggregates from Alzheimer disease (AD) are captured by TLR2, 4, 6 and 9 [111–115]. In ALS, the inflammasome is activated by cytosolic TDP-43 aggregates [116–118]. These observations suggest a role for PRR beyond sensing PAMP and/or DAMP in surveilling both intra- and extracellular proteostasis disturbances. It remains however unclear whether this perception is limited to certain types of proteins and/or aggregates.

3. Causes of Proteostasis Perturbations and Associated Autoinflammatory Syndromes

Depending on the source of perturbation, proteostasis imbalances carry two possible consequences, namely

I. Protein aggregation or;
II. Protein depletion.

As illustrated in Figure 2, protein aggregation is frequently found in disorders such as proteinopathies or proteasomopathies following excessive protein misfolding or proteasome dysfunction, respectively. By contrast, intracellular protein depletion mostly occurs as a consequence of impaired translation in so-called ribosomopathies. The investigation of the molecular pathogenesis of such disorders have greatly improved our knowledge on how the innate immune respond reacts to disrupted proteostasis, as discussed below.

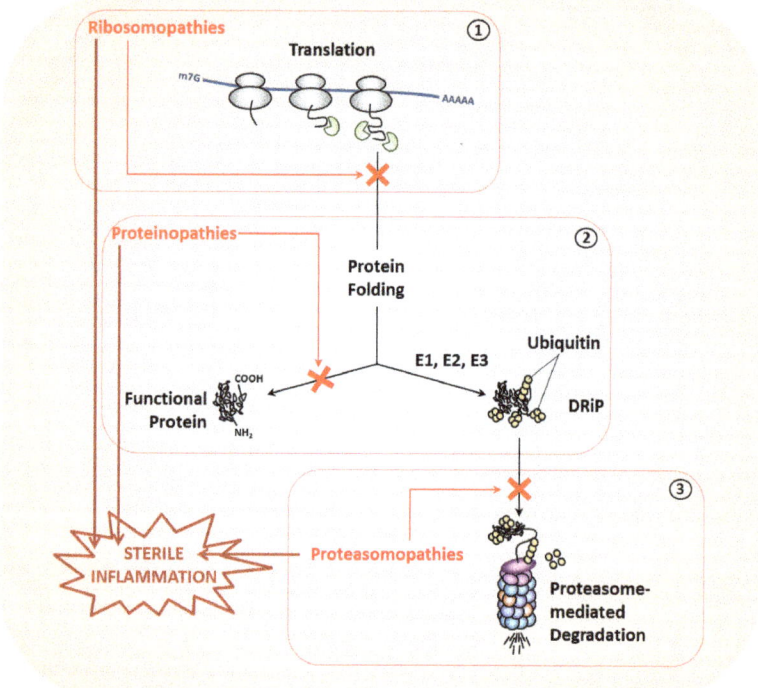

Figure 2. Proteostasis perturbations may arise at any stage of the protein life cycle and typically result in the initiation of sterile inflammation. Depicted are three pathological situations causing impaired proteostasis in which translation (**1**), protein folding (**2**) and proteasome-mediated protein degradation of defective ribosomal products (DRiPs) following their polyubiquitination by E1, E2 and E3 enzymes of the ubiquitin-conjugation pathway (**3**) are affected.

3.1. Proteostasis Perturbations Caused by Translation Deficiency

Defects in protein synthesis are typically due to loss-of-function mutations in genes encoding components of the translation machinery. Prominent vulnerable genes in this category include those coding for proteins of the 40S and 60S ribosomal subunits (RPS and RPL, respectively). Genomic alterations of the RPS and/or RPL genes generally result in ribosome assembly disruption which itself causes a wide range of disorders traditionally referred to as "ribosomopathies" [119].

At the molecular level, this group of syndromes is essentially characterized by reduced protein synthesis due to persistently depressed translation [120]. Accordingly, ribosomopathies primarily affect cells with high protein demand, particularly those of the hematopoietic lineage. Major ribosomopathies include the various forms of Diamond-Blackfan anemia (DBA), which are inherited monogenic autosomal dominant genetic disorders characterized by ineffective erythropoiesis and caused by mutations in either RPS or RPL genes [121]. Here, insufficient protein synthesis leads to protein depletion and cell death. Specifically, it is understood that the ribosomal subunits that fail to become incorporated into ribosomes initiate a so-called nucleolar stress response that results in cell cycle arrest and apoptosis [122,123]. Paradoxically, ribosomopathies also increase cancer risk overtime [124]. This seemingly inconsistency can be however easily explained by the fact that cell proliferation defects exert a strong pressure that results in the progressive selection of transformed cells that have acquired compensatory mutations in proto-oncogenes [124].

Most importantly, it was recently suggested that proteostasis disruption in DBA was associated with the generation of inflammatory gene signatures [125–127]. Autoinflammation could be confirmed in a DBA zebrafish model in which affected animals constitutively express type I IFN-stimulated genes (ISG) [128]. Further evidence for a functional cause-and-effect relationship between translation deficiency and sterile inflammation comes from the observation that mutations in RPL10 drive type I IFN responses in T cell leukemia [129]. The mechanisms by which ribosomopathies favor autoinflammation remain unclear, but it is conceivable that senescence due to prolonged cell cycle arrest might play a role in this process. Indeed, as shown in Figure 3, it was recently shown that senescence is intrinsically associated with genome instability and the subsequent leakage of DNA fragments into the cytosol which trigger type I IFN response by the cGAS/STING pathway [130,131]. Consistent with a potential role of cGAS in driving inflammatory responses upon ribosomal dysfunction, Wan et al. have shown that ribosome collision during translation results in the cytosolic accumulation of cGAS [132], thereby predisposing the cells to respond stronger to cytosolic, even background, DNA (Figure 3).

3.2. Proteostasis Perturbations Caused by Protein Misfolding

It is well established that protein biosynthesis (or mRNA translation) in eukaryotic cells is not an accurate process. Early works from Yewdell's lab estimate that approximately 30% of newly synthetized proteins fail to reach their 3D structure because of damage, premature termination and/or incorporation of wrong amino acids [133,134]. As these improperly folded proteins (or DRiPs) are non-functional and, in most cases, prone to aggregation, they are rapidly sampled and sorted out by various protein quality control (PQC) systems. One major co-translational PQC mechanism relies on the action of the molecular chaperones Hsp70 and Hsp90 that are capable of sensing hydrophobicity exposed by all misfolded nascent proteins [135]. Both Hsp70 and Hsp90 recruit E3 ubiquitin ligases such as the carboxy-terminus of the Hsc70 interacting protein (CHIP), leucine-rich repeat and sterile alpha motif-containing 1 (LRSAM1) and/or E6-associated protein (E6-AP) which themselves mediate the ubiquitination of the presented protein substrates and target them for subsequent degradation by the 26S proteasome [136,137].

Besides aging, major causes for excessive misfolding include alterations in genes coding for

(i) UPS components or;
(ii) Highly translated host (or viral) proteins.

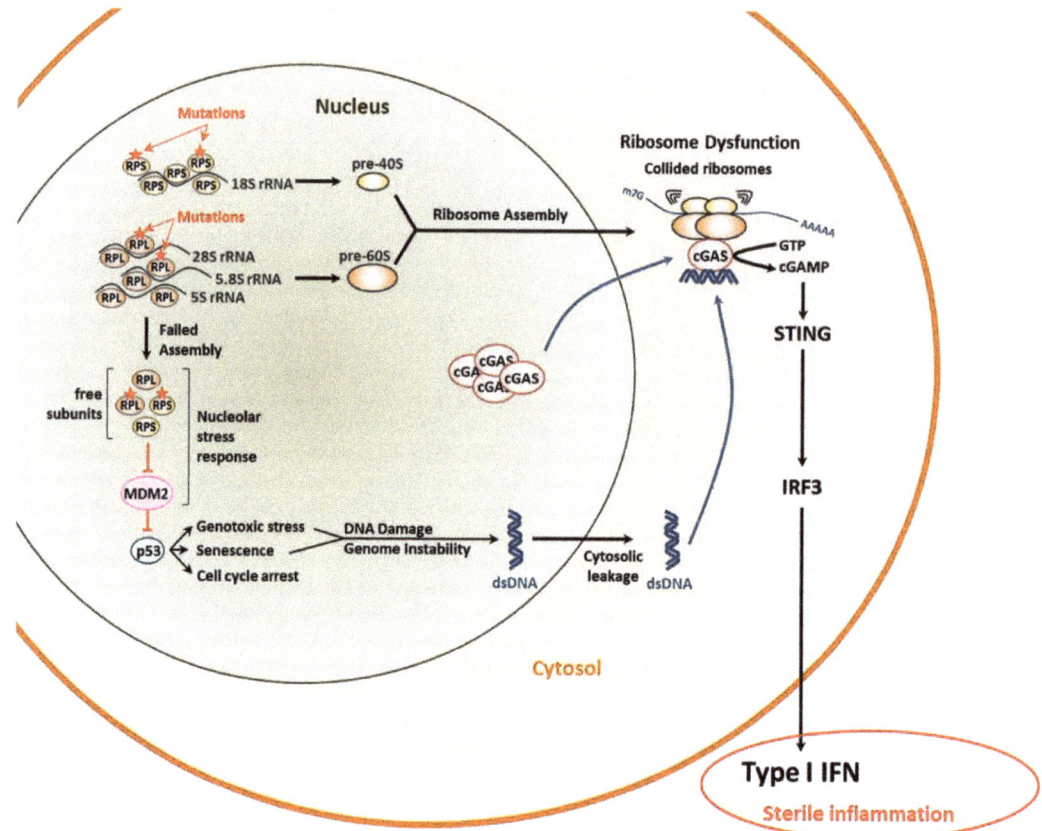

Figure 3. Molecular pathogenesis of ribosomopathies and their potential inflammatory consequences. The failure of mutant ribosomal proteins of the small 40S (RPS) and/or large 60S (RPL) ribosomal subunits to assemble into ribosomes induces the nucleolar stress response leading to p53 stabilization via persistent inactivation of the MDM2 E3 ubiquitin ligase. This, in turn, results in genome instability and subsequent leakage of double-stranded (ds)DNA into the cytosol. Cytoplasmic dsDNA is then sensed by the cyclic GMP-AMP synthase (cGAS) which promotes a type I IFN response via the STING/IRF3 signaling pathway, as indicated. The recruitment of cGAS in the cytosol is itself facilitated by defective and collided ribosomes.

These events may result in the accumulation of insoluble protein aggregates, a typical feature of a heterogenous group of disorders known as proteinopathies [138,139]. As mentioned above, proteostasis disruption in proteinopathies is not necessarily due to UPS dysfunction. Indeed, virtually every protein variant with a particularly high synthesis rate may increase protein supply and/or misfolding, thereby surpassing UPS capacity. Prime examples of protein mutants predisposed to misfolding and aggregating include the HLA-B27 allele as well as various variants of the cystic fibrosis transmembrane conductance regulator (CFTR), transthyretin (TTR), α-1 antitrypsin (AAT), amyloid protein precursor (APP), α-synuclein (SNCA), huntingtin (HTT) and transactive response RNA/DNA-binding protein (TDP-43), just to name a few. With the exception of HLA-B27, CFTR and AAT, all these proteinopathies primarily affect CNS and promote typical neurodegenerative phenotypes. The reasons for this tissue selectivity remain obscure and intriguing in view of the wide distribution of these proteins throughout the body. An undebatable issue in this field, however, is that neurodegeneration has a sterile inflammatory component—commonly referred to as neuroinflammation—predominantly triggered by glia cells (i.e., microglia, astrocytes and/or oligodendrocytes). Likewise, non-neurodegenerative proteinopathies are strongly associated with autoinflammation. These observations unambiguously point to a cause-and-effect relationship between protein aggregation and innate immunity, as discussed below.

3.2.1. Non-Neurodegenerative Proteinopathies

These disorders are essentially caused by misfolding and subsequent aggregation of protein variants outside the CNS. These typically include ankylosing spondylitis (AS), cystic fibrosis (CF), alpha-1-antitrypsin deficiency (AATD) and hereditary transthyretin amyloidosis (ATTR) which are all associated with inflammatory reactions. As a large fraction of these mutant proteins (i.e., HLA-27, CFTR and AATD in AS, CF and AATD, respectively) typically misfold within the ER lumen, persistent activation of the UPR is thought to contribute to the disease inflammatory phenotype [140–148]. Nevertheless, additional pathways may synergize with the UPR to trigger autoinflammation in these patients.

For instance, ATTR is an autosomal dominant proteinopathy with neuronal and cardiac manifestations which provides an excellent example of extracellular proteostasis perturbation. It is characterized by the extracellular deposition of transthyretin (TTR)-derived amyloid fibrils, particularly in the peripheral nervous system (PNS) [149]. The pathologic basis of ATTR are single amino acid variations in the TTR protein, among which the Val30Met and Val142Ile substitutions are the most frequent ones [150]. The TTR protein is produced by the choroid plexus and liver and found in the cerebrospinal fluid (CSF) as well as in the bloodstream where it carries thyroxin and retinol [35,151]. TTR misfolding mutations typically result in the formation of extracellular precipitates resembling β-pleated sheet structures named amyloid fibrils which cause tissue dysfunction [152]. Although patients with ATTR exhibit no evidence of systemic inflammation, they present with elevated circulating inflammatory markers [153,154]. Recent evidence suggests that activation of the innate immune system in ATTR occurs extracellularly as well with TTR aggregates capable of activating immune cells, notably neutrophils and microglia to produce proinflammatory cytokines [155,156]. The receptors involved in this process remain however ill-defined.

3.2.2. Neurodegenerative Proteinopathies

This group of proteinopathies is by far the largest and includes prominent disorders such as Alzheimer's disease (AD), Parkinson's disease (PD), Huntington's disease (HD), spinocerebellar ataxias and polyglutamine (polyQ) diseases, among others. Although these disorders are clinically and phenotypically distinct, their molecular etiology is identical and based on the uncontrolled accumulation of protein variants mostly in the CNS. As alluded to earlier, one major mechanism by which proteostasis perturbations trigger neuroinflammation in these diseases involves the release of protein aggregates into the extracellular space and their subsequent binding to PRR such as TLR and/or TREM2 on microglia [105–115]. However, recent research on the molecular pathogenesis of amyotrophic lateral sclerosis (ALS) has expanded the spectrum of the molecular pathways initiating sterile inflammation in response to proteostasis disruption.

ALS is a neurodegenerative proteinopathy characterized by a progressive loss of motor neurons [157,158]. While most cases of ALS are sporadic, a dozen of predisposition genes have been identified over the past two decades [159,160]. These include notably SOD1 and TARDBP which code for the superoxide dismutase 1 (SOD1) and transactive response DNA binding protein 43 (TDP-43), respectively [161,162]. Both proteins tend to misfold and aggregate in neurons upon specific point mutations. In particular, abnormal accumulation and/or localization of TDP-43 accounts for 90% of ALS cases [163]. TDP-43 is a ribonucleoprotein highly expressed in the CNS with functions in RNA processing [164,165] and its deposition is favored by aging, variations in the TDP-43 gene itself and/or in the C9orf72, GRN or TBK1 genes. [166–171]. Not surprisingly, ALS is associated with constitutive activation of microglia and ongoing neuroinflammation [172,173]. The mechanisms involved in the inflammatory component of ALS are diverse and seem to depend on genetic lesion. For instance, TDP-43 or its variants, as cytosolic proteins not trafficking in the ER, do not generate ER stress and/or induce the UPR [174]. By contrast, SOD1 mutant species, although devoid of signal sequence, have been shown to impair ERAD and activate the UPR [175], which itself conceivably contributes to autoinflammation (Figure 4). In addition, SOD1 aggregates are released to activate microglia via binding to TLR2, TLR4 and/or CD14 (Figure 4) [176]. The neuroinflammatory phenotype of individuals with ALS is also thought to be a direct consequence of aggregation of TDP-43 or its mutant in the mitochondria [177,178]. Indeed, a recent study showed that mislocalization of TDP-43 variants in mitochondria results in mitochondrial DNA leakage into the cytosol, subsequent activation of the cGAS/STING innate pathway and IFN signaling in ALS. (Figure 4) [118]. In addition, cytosolic TDP-43 aggregates may promote innate immune responses by activating the inflammasome (Figure 4) [116,117]. Whether these processes occur simultaneously is unclear and their respective contributions to neuroinflammation may be also difficult to assess. In any case, these works reveal that the ability of the cells to react to impaired proteostasis due to protein misfolding is broad and probably even wider than initially assumed.

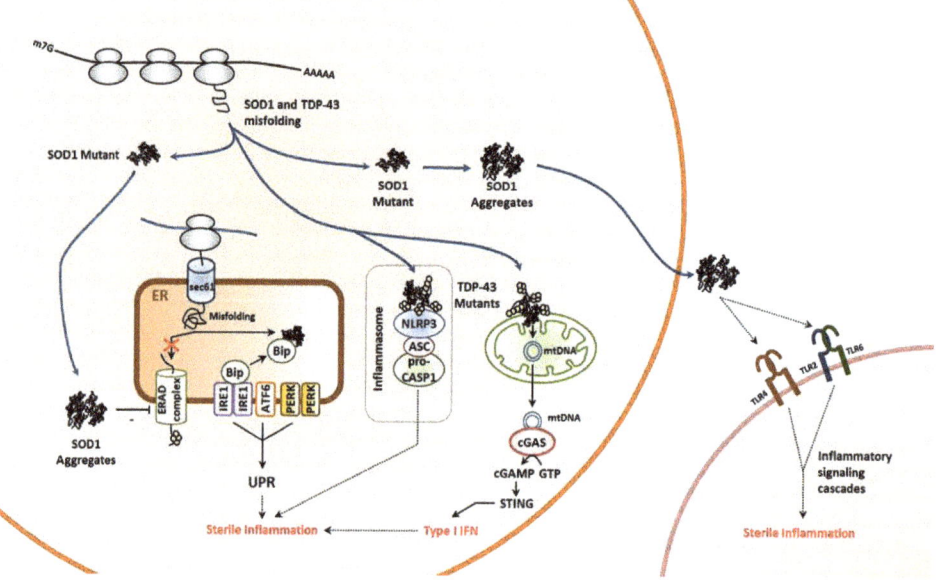

Figure 4. Neuroinflammation caused by impaired proteostasis in ALS involves multiple pathways. Pathogenic variants of superoxide dismutase 1 (SOD1) facilitate the formation of intracellular protein aggregates which themselves promote sterile inflammation by causing persistent activation of the unfolded protein response (UPR) via inhibition of the ER-associated degradation machinery (ERAD), as indicated. In addition, extracellular SOD1 protein aggregates exert their pro-inflammatory effects by binding to phagocyte pattern recognition receptors such as Toll-like receptors (TLR)-2, 4 and 6. Pathogenic mutations within the TAR DNA-binding protein 43 (TDP-43) results in protein aggregation which activates the inflammasome and triggers the release of mitochondrial (mt) DNA. The latter, in turn, initiates a type I IFN response following sensing by the cytosolic cyclic GMP-AMP (cGAS) synthase and subsequent STING activation, as indicated. NLRP3: NOD-like receptor pyrin domain-containing-3; ASC: apoptosis associated speck-like protein containing a CARD; pro-CASP1: pro-caspase 1.

3.3. Proteostasis Perturbations Caused by Impaired Protein Degradation

As alluded to earlier, the breakdown of intracellular proteins in eukaryotic cells is ensured by two major conserved machineries from yeast to humans, namely

I. The ubiquitin–proteasome system (UPS) and;
II. The autophagy–lysosomal system [179].

The UPS allows the specific elimination of ubiquitin-tagged protein by the 26S proteasome [180]. Ubiquitination is a three-step process involving three groups of enzymes (i.e., E1, E2 and E3) that catalyze the transfer of ubiquitin moieties or chains on lysine, serine, threonine or cysteine residues of target proteins (a modus operandi described in excellent reviews) [181,182]. The 26S proteasome is formed by 20S core complex and a 19S regulatory particle [183,184]. While the 20S core complex contains the three different catalytic activities that permit degradation, the 19S regulatory particle is specialized in the recognition and unfolding of ubiquitin-modified substrates [185]. Specifically, the 20S proteasome is a large complex comprised of two outer α-subunits rings (α1–7) embracing two central head-to-head oriented rings containing β-subunits (β1–7). The catalytic activity is conferred by three of the β subunits, namely β1, β2 and β5 which exhibit caspase-like, trypsin-like and chymotrypsin-like activity, respectively [186]. The 19S regulatory particle is made up of a base containing six ATPase subunits (Rpt1–6) which unfold the protein substrate and a lid carrying subunits (i.e., Rpn10, Rpn13) capable of binding ubiquitin-modified proteins [187]. Importantly, the β1, β2 and β5 standard subunits may be replaced by the so-called β1i, β2i and β5i inducible ones in newly synthetized complexes to promote a switch from constitutive proteasomes to immunoproteasomes [188,189]. It is appreciated that immunoproteasomes are more effective than their standard counterparts at degrading ubiquitin-modified proteins, making them particularly important in situations in which protein homeostasis is challenged such as during infection or oxidative stress [190–195]. Due to its unique position at the intersection of multiple pathways [196], the UPS is involved in the regulation of myriad of cellular processes, and as such any dysfunction of one of its components may carry serious consequences on cell functioning or viability.

3.3.1. The UPS and its Dysfunctions

One major cause of proteasome dysfunction is aging [197]. Although not always consistent, investigations in animals and patients suffering from sporadic aging-related neurodegenerative diseases point to a decline ability of the UPS to eliminate undesirable proteins [198–205]. Other causes of UPS impairment are loss-of-function mutations in genes encoding proteasome subunits [35]. Surprisingly, as shown in Table 1, such genomic alterations lead to two clinical distinct phenotypes, namely autoinflammation (CANDLE/PRAAS) and neurodevelopmental disorders (NDD).

3.3.2. Proteasome-Associated Autoinflammatory Syndromes (PRAAS)

From the mid-eighties, an increasing number of cases of rare autoinflammatory syndromes sharing similar clinical features such as lipodystrophy, skin lesions and recurrent fever have been reported. These conditions were referred to by a number of different names including Nakajo–Nishimura syndrome (NNS) [228–230], joint contractures, muscle atrophy and panniculitis-induced lipodystrophy (JMP) syndrome [230] and chronic atypical neutrophilic dermatitis with lipodystrophy and elevated temperatures (CANDLE) [231,232]. From 2010, it became evident that such syndromes were caused by loss-of-function mutations in genes encoding proteasome subunits and/or proteasome assembly factors and were subsequently renamed proteasome-associated autoinflammatory syndromes (PRAAS) [207,210–212,220,221,223,233] (Table 1). Two major hallmarks of PRAAS are the presence of a constitutive type I IFN gene signature in patients' blood cells and a concomitant increased accumulation of ubiquitin-modified proteins in various cell types including fibroblasts. Recent studies have identified cells of the hematopoietic lineage as decisive mediators of type I IFN in PRAAS [208,234] and in view of increased eIF2α phosphorylation in B cells isolated from PRAAS subjects [221], a possible role of the UPR has been suggested in the induction of autoinflammation in these patients [35]. This notion was supported by in vitro studies showing that blocking the IRE1 arm of the UPR prevents the upregulation of IFN-stimulated genes (ISG) in response to proteasome inhibition in microglia cells [235]. Later studies however have shown that the IL-24/PKR axis of the ISR was the key contributor to type I IFN responses in ten unrelated PRAAS subjects [59,236]. These works unambiguously identify cytosolic IL-24 and PKR as a new DAMP/PRR pair involved in proteostasis surveillance. Whether other mechanisms contribute to sterile inflammation in PRAAS, notably in cells expressing no or low levels of IL-24, is currently not known.

Table 1. Summary of the genetic characteristics and associated clinical phenotypes of the proteasome variants identified so far.

Proteasome	Gene	Variant	Genetic Model	Origin	Phenotype	Reference
20S Complex	PSMB1	p.Y103H	Homozygous, monogenic	Recessive inheritance	NDD	[206]
	PSMB4	5' UTR: c.−9G > A p.D212_V214del	Compound heterozygous, monogenic	Recessive inheritance	PRAAS	[207]
	PSMB4	p.L78Wfs * 31 c.494 + 17A > G	Compound heterozygous, monogenic	Recessive inheritance	PRAAS	[208]
	PSMB4/ PSMB8	p.Y222 * p.K105Q	Double heterozygous, digenic	Recessive inheritance	PRAAS	[207]
	PSMB8	p.G179V	Homozygous, monogenic	Recessive inheritance	PRAAS	[209]
	PSMB8	p.G201V	Homozygous, monogenic	Recessive inheritance	PRAAS	[210]
	PSMB8	p.C135 *	Homozygous, monogenic	Recessive inheritance	PRAAS	[211]
	PSMB8	p.T75M	Homozygous, monogenic	Recessive inheritance	PRAAS	[212]
	PSMB8	p.R125C p.D119N	Compound heterozygous, monogenic	Recessive inheritance	PRAAS	[213]
	PSMB8	p.Q55 * p.S118P	Compound heterozygous, monogenic	Recessive inheritance	PRAAS	[214]
	PSMB8	p.A92V p.K105Q	Compound heterozygous, monogenic	Recessive inheritance	PRAAS	[215]
	PSMB8	p.A92T	Homozygous, monogenic	Recessive inheritance	PRAAS	[216]
	PSMB8	-	Homozygous, monogenic	Recessive inheritance	PRAAS	[217]
	PSMB8/ PSMA3	p.T75M p.H111Ffs * 10	Double heterozygous, digenic	Recessive inheritance	PRAAS	[207]
	PSMB8/ PSMA3	p.T75M p.R233del	Double heterozygous, digenic	Recessive inheritance	PRAAS	[207]
	PSMB9/ PSMB4	p.G165D p.P16Sfs * 45	Double heterozygous, digenic	Recessive inheritance	PRAAS	[207]
	PSMB9	p.G156D	Heterozygous, monogenic	de novo, dominant	PRAAS	[218] [219]
	PSMB10	p.F14S	Homozygous, monogenic	Recessive inheritance	PRAAS	[220]

Table 1. Cont.

Proteasome	Gene	Variant	Genetic Model	Origin	Phenotype	Reference
Assembly Factors	POMP	p.E115Dfs * 20	Heterozygous, monogenic	de novo, dominant	PRAAS	[207]
	POMP	p.F114Lfs * 18	Heterozygous, monogenic	de novo, dominant	PRAAS	[221]
	POMP	p.I112Wfs * 3	Heterozygous, monogenic	de novo, dominant	PRAAS	[221]
	POMP	p.D109Efs * 2	Heterozygous, monogenic	de novo, dominant	PRAAS	[222]
	PSMG4	p.Y223Sfs * 2 p.N225K	Compound heterozygous, monogenic	Recessive inheritance	PRAAS	[223]
19S Complex	PSMD12	p.R123 *	Heterozygous, monogenic	de novo, dominant	NDD	
	PSMD12	p.L425 *	Heterozygous, monogenic	de novo, dominant	NDD	[224]
	PSMD12	p.R201 *	Heterozygous, monogenic	de novo, dominant	NDD	
	PSMD12	c.909−2A > G	Heterozygous, monogenic	de novo, dominant	NDD	
	PSMD12	Deletion	Heterozygous, monogenic	de novo, dominant	NDD	
	PSMD12	p.R201 *	Heterozygous, monogenic	de novo, dominant	NDD	[225]
	PSMD12	p.R182 *	Heterozygous, monogenic	de novo, dominant	NDD	
	PSMD12	p.R357fs * 3	Heterozygous, monogenic	de novo, dominant	NDD	
	PSMD12	p.T146Kfs * 3	Heterozygous, monogenic	de novo, dominant	NDD	
	PSMD12	p.E313 *	Heterozygous, monogenic	de novo, dominant	NDD	
	PSMD12	p.Q170Gfs * 40	Heterozygous, monogenic	de novo, dominant	NDD	[68]
	PSMD12	p.L149 *	Heterozygous, monogenic	de novo, dominant	NDD	
	PSMD12	p.Q106 *	Heterozygous, monogenic	de novo, dominant	NDD	
	PSMD12	p.Q345 *	Heterozygous, monogenic	de novo, dominant	NDD	
	PSMD12	c.1083 + 1G > A	Heterozygous, monogenic	de novo, dominant	NDD	
	PSMD12	p.Q416 *	Heterozygous, monogenic	de novo, dominant	NDD	
	PSMD12	p.S176Qfs * 15	Heterozygous, monogenic	de novo, dominant	NDD	
	PSMD12	c.1162−1G > A	Heterozygous, monogenic	de novo, dominant	NDD	
	PSMD12	p.S434Hfs * 2	Heterozygous, monogenic	de novo, dominant	NDD	
	PSMD12	c.795 + 1G > A	Heterozygous, monogenic	de novo, dominant	NDD	
	PSMD12	p.L50Gfs * 26	Heterozygous, monogenic	de novo, dominant	NDD	
	PSMD12	p.T146Kfs * 3	Heterozygous, monogenic	de novo, dominant	NDD	
	PSMD12	p.R182 *	Heterozygous, monogenic	de novo, dominant	NDD	
	PSMD12	p.L354Efs * 6	Heterozygous, monogenic	de novo, dominant	NDD	
	PSMD12	p.Y302 *	Heterozygous, monogenic	de novo, dominant	NDD	
	PSMD12	p.R289 *	Heterozygous, monogenic	de novo, dominant	NDD	[226]
	PSMC3	p.S376Rfs15 *	Homozygous, monogenic	Recessive inheritance	NDD	[227]

* Asterisks indicate termination codons.

3.3.3. Neurodevelopmental Disorders (NDD) Caused by Proteasome Variants

Surprisingly, the phenotypic spectrum of proteasome loss-of-function mutations is broader than initially assumed. In 2017, the identification of pathogenic variants of the *PSMD12* gene in patients showing a predominant neuronal phenotype came as a surprise [224]. Subjects with *PSMD12* mutations presented with short stature, facial dysmorphism, intellectual disability, limb anomalies and sometimes absent of speech. Later, similar manifestations were reported in patients carrying variants of the *PSMB1* and *PSMC3* genes [206,227], thereby confirming the causal relationship between proteasome loss-of-function and NDD. One particularly intriguing observation from these studies is that, in contrast to PRAAS patients, subjects with NDD were devoid of clinical signs of autoinflammation. However, recent investigation revealed that leukocytes isolated from NDD patients with *PSMD12* haploinsufficiency do exhibit a typical type I IFN gene signature [68]. The reason why the upregulation of ISG in these cells is not associated with the development of clinical autoinflammation as observed in PRAAS patients is obscure, but this phenomenon has been described in other interferonopathies [237–240]. Interestingly, it was shown that *PSMD12* haploinsufficiency was accompanied by a profound remodeling of mTORC1 and its downstream autophagy pathway. Specifically, the elimination of mitochondria by mitophagy in *PSMD12*-deficient cells was induced [68].

3.3.4. Disorders due to Deficient DUB and/or E3 Ubiquitin Ligases

A number of autoinflammatory syndromes have been described to be caused by genomic alterations in genes coding for DUB and E3 ubiquitin ligases. These include notably loss- or gain-of-function mutations in the *TNFAIP3*, *USP18* and *OTULIN*, *RNF31*, *RBCK1* genes [241–247]. However, in contrast to their proteasome counterparts, pathogenic variants from DUB and/or E3 ubiquitin ligases exert their proinflammatory effects mostly by interfering with specific PRR signaling cascades rather than by destabilizing the whole-cell proteome [248].

3.3.5. The Autophagy-Lysosomal System and Its Defects

The 2016 Nobel Prize in Physiology or Medicine went to Yoshinori Ohsumi for his discoveries of the "mechanisms of autophagy" [249,250]. Together with the UPS, autophagy is the main contributor to protein breakdown in the cell. Unlike the UPS, which is constitutive active, autophagy requires signals such as starvation, growth, etc. It relies on the formation of autophagosomes capable of sequestering intracellular material prior to delivery to lysosomes for subsequent degradation. Over the past few years, various types of autophagy have been described including micro-autophagy and macro-autophagy [251], the latter enabling the elimination of protein aggregates [252], a process frequently referred to as "aggrephagy" [253]. In this selective form of autophagy, ubiquitin-modified protein aggregates are recognized by the autophagy receptors p62, NBR1 and OPTN which themselves interact with lipidated LC3II on the inner phagophore membrane [254], thereby targeting them to autophagosomes. As such, protein homeostasis critically depends on functional autophagy under stress conditions and any and loss of autophagy has been early associated with the aggregation of abnormal proteins and neurodegeneration [255].

Another major cause of autophagy dysfunction and a fortiori protein homeostasis perturbations are loss-of-function mutations in genes encoding any one of the many components involved in this process. A particularly vulnerable gene in this regard is *SQSTM1* encoding the autophagy receptor p62 and whose pathogenic variants are associated with the onset of various metabolic, myopathic and skeletal disorders as well as neurodegenerative disease including ALS. Strikingly, syndromes caused by SQSTM1 disruption are clearly associated with signs of autoinflammation [256–258]. However, given that p62 is also directly involved in the regulation of NF-κB signaling [259,260], the precise contribution of impaired aggrephagy to inflammation in these diseases is difficult to assess. Other ALS genes potentially causing imbalanced protein homeostasis include ATG5 and

ATG7 [261,262]. Although clearly associated with protein aggregates, no inflammation was observed in these patients.

4. Conclusions and Future Directions

Altogether, these studies revealed that eukaryotic cells are equipped with various sensitive systems capable of sensing quantitative aberrations of their intra- and extracellular proteomes. Strikingly, these sensors are more or less directly connected to innate signaling pathways, and the continuous sampling of proteostasis perturbations consistently results in autoinflammation. The reason why the cell mostly responds to impaired proteostasis by the production of proinflammatory mediators is however not fully understood. One possible explanation is that inflammation might be part of autocrine program primarily aimed to help restoring proteostasis. This hypothesis is particularly based on the fact that many of the target genes (i.e., ISG) of type I IFN encode products that act on the proteostasis network at various levels. For instance, type I IFN limits the proteostatic burden by supporting a translation arrest via the induction of PKR. Conversely, by inducing immunoproteasome subunits and proteasome activators [263], type I IFN accelerates protein breakdown and as such help the cells to cope with proteotoxic stress. Given that inflammation has proliferation-promotive effects [264], it might also well be that the initiation of innate responses under these circumstances is intended to preserve integrity by generating new cellular space for the accumulating protein aggregates. Herein, when limited in time, sterile inflammation might represent a beneficial reaction rebalancing dysregulated proteostasis. However, the onset of sterile autoinflammation or neuroinflammation in patients with impaired proteostasis might signify a point of no return from which protein homeostasis cannot be rescued any longer. In this regard, a better comprehension of the mechanisms driving these processes is needed.

Author Contributions: Conceptualization: J.J.P., E.K. and F.E.; data curation: J.J.P., E.K. and F.E.; writing—original draft preparation: J.J.P. and F.E., writing—review and editing: E.K. and F.E.; funding acquisition: E.K. All authors have read and agreed to the published version of the manuscript.

Funding: This research was funded by the German Research Foundation (DFG) Research Training Group (RTG) 2719 Pro to E.K. We also acknowledge support for the Article Processing Charge from the DFG and the Open Access Publication Fund of the University of Greifswald.

Conflicts of Interest: The authors declare no conflict of interest.

References

1. A Series of Essays on Inflammation and Its Varieties. Essay, I. The Natural History of the Disease. *Med. Chir. Rev.* **1846**, *4*, 251–253.
2. Plytycz, B.; Seljelid, R. From inflammation to sickness: Historical perspective. *Arch. Immunol. Exp. (Warsz)* **2003**, *51*, 105–109. [PubMed]
3. Cavaillon, J.M. Once upon a time, inflammation. *J. Venom. Anim. Toxins Incl. Trop. Dis.* **2021**, *27*, e20200147. [CrossRef] [PubMed]
4. Diamond, G.; Legarda, D.; Ryan, L.K. The innate immune response of the respiratory epithelium. *Immunol. Rev.* **2000**, *173*, 27–38. [CrossRef]
5. Shishido, S.N.; Varahan, S.; Yuan, K.; Li, X.; Fleming, S.D. Humoral innate immune response and disease. *Clin. Immunol.* **2012**, *144*, 142–158. [CrossRef]
6. Koenderman, L.; Buurman, W.; Daha, M.R. The innate immune response. *Immunol. Lett.* **2014**, *162*, 95–102. [CrossRef]
7. Bianchi, M.E. DAMPs, PAMPs and alarmins: All we need to know about danger. *J. Leukoc. Biol.* **2007**, *81*, 1–5. [CrossRef]
8. Skoberne, M.; Beignon, A.S.; Bhardwaj, N. Danger signals: A time and space continuum. *Trends Mol. Med.* **2004**, *10*, 251–257. [CrossRef]
9. Kawai, T.; Akira, S. Toll-like receptors and their crosstalk with other innate receptors in infection and immunity. *Immunity* **2011**, *34*, 637–650. [CrossRef]
10. Sok, S.P.M.; Ori, D.; Nagoor, N.H.; Kawai, T. Sensing Self and Non-Self DNA by Innate Immune Receptors and Their Signaling Pathways. *Crit. Rev. Immunol.* **2018**, *38*, 279–301. [CrossRef]
11. Thaiss, C.A.; Levy, M.; Itav, S.; Elinav, E. Integration of Innate Immune Signaling. *Trends Immunol.* **2016**, *37*, 84–101. [CrossRef] [PubMed]
12. Kawai, T.; Akira, S. The roles of TLRs, RLRs and NLRs in pathogen recognition. *Int. Immunol.* **2009**, *21*, 317–337. [CrossRef] [PubMed]

13. Capobianchi, M.R.; Uleri, E.; Caglioti, C.; Dolei, A. Type I IFN family members: Similarity, differences and interaction. *Cytokine Growth Factor Rev.* **2015**, *26*, 103–111. [CrossRef] [PubMed]
14. Schoggins, J.W. Interferon-Stimulated Genes: What Do They All Do? *Annu Rev. Virol.* **2019**, *6*, 567–584. [CrossRef]
15. Nace, G.; Evankovich, J.; Eid, R.; Tsung, A. Dendritic cells and damage-associated molecular patterns: Endogenous danger signals linking innate and adaptive immunity. *J. Innate Immun.* **2012**, *4*, 6–15. [CrossRef]
16. Schaefer, L. Complexity of danger: The diverse nature of damage-associated molecular patterns. *J. Biol. Chem.* **2014**, *289*, 35237–35245. [CrossRef]
17. Jounai, N.; Kobiyama, K.; Takeshita, F.; Ishii, K.J. Recognition of damage-associated molecular patterns related to nucleic acids during inflammation and vaccination. *Front. Cell Infect. Microbiol.* **2012**, *2*, 168. [CrossRef]
18. Denning, N.L.; Aziz, M.; Gurien, S.D.; Wang, P. DAMPs and NETs in Sepsis. *Front. Immunol.* **2019**, *10*, 2536. [CrossRef]
19. Scaffidi, P.; Misteli, T.; Bianchi, M.E. Release of chromatin protein HMGB1 by necrotic cells triggers inflammation. *Nature* **2002**, *418*, 191–195. [CrossRef]
20. Allam, R.; Darisipudi, M.N.; Tschopp, J.; Anders, H.J. Histones trigger sterile inflammation by activating the NLRP3 inflammasome. *Eur. J. Immunol.* **2013**, *43*, 3336–3342. [CrossRef]
21. Chen, G.Y.; Nunez, G. Sterile inflammation: Sensing and reacting to damage. *Nat. Rev. Immunol.* **2010**, *10*, 826–837. [CrossRef] [PubMed]
22. Mihm, S. Danger-Associated Molecular Patterns (DAMPs): Molecular Triggers for Sterile Inflammation in the Liver. *Int. J. Mol. Sci.* **2018**, *19*, 3104. [CrossRef] [PubMed]
23. Gong, T.; Liu, L.; Jiang, W.; Zhou, R. DAMP-sensing receptors in sterile inflammation and inflammatory diseases. *Nat. Rev. Immunol.* **2020**, *20*, 95–112. [CrossRef] [PubMed]
24. Feldman, N.; Rotter-Maskowitz, A.; Okun, E. DAMPs as mediators of sterile inflammation in aging-related pathologies. *Ageing Res. Rev.* **2015**, *24*, 29–39. [CrossRef] [PubMed]
25. Franklin, E.C.; Holman, H.R.; Muller-Eberhard, H.J.; Kunkel, H.G. An unusual protein component of high molecular weight in the serum of certain patients with rheumatoid arthritis. *J. Exp. Med.* **1957**, *105*, 425–438. [CrossRef]
26. Mellors, R.C.; Heimer, R.; Corcos, J.; Korngold, L. Cellular Origin of Rheumatoid Factor. *J. Exp. Med.* **1959**, *110*, 875–886. [CrossRef]
27. Blom, A.B.; Radstake, T.R.; Holthuysen, A.E.; Sloetjes, A.W.; Pesman, G.J.; Sweep, F.G.; van de Loo, F.A.; Joosten, L.A.; Barrera, P.; van Lent, P.L.; et al. Increased expression of Fcgamma receptors II and III on macrophages of rheumatoid arthritis patients results in higher production of tumor necrosis factor alpha and matrix metalloproteinase. *Arthritis Rheum* **2003**, *48*, 1002–1014. [CrossRef] [PubMed]
28. Radstake, T.R.; Blom, A.B.; Sloetjes, A.W.; van Gorselen, E.O.; Pesman, G.J.; Engelen, L.; Torensma, R.; van den Berg, W.B.; Figdor, C.G.; van Lent, P.L.; et al. Increased FcgammaRII expression and aberrant tumour necrosis factor alpha production by mature dendritic cells from patients with active rheumatoid arthritis. *Ann. Rheum. Dis.* **2004**, *63*, 1556–1563. [CrossRef]
29. Brehm, A.; Kruger, E. Dysfunction in protein clearance by the proteasome: Impact on autoinflammatory diseases. *Semin. Immunopathol.* **2015**, *37*, 323–333. [CrossRef] [PubMed]
30. Uhlen, M.; Fagerberg, L.; Hallstrom, B.M.; Lindskog, C.; Oksvold, P.; Mardinoglu, A.; Sivertsson, A.; Kampf, C.; Sjostedt, E.; Asplund, A.; et al. Proteomics. Tissue-based map of the human proteome. *Science* **2015**, *347*, 1260419. [CrossRef]
31. Anton, L.C.; Yewdell, J.W. Translating DRiPs: MHC class I immunosurveillance of pathogens and tumors. *J. Leukoc. Biol.* **2014**, *95*, 551–562. [CrossRef] [PubMed]
32. Mancini, R.; Fagioli, C.; Fra, A.M.; Maggioni, C.; Sitia, R. Degradation of unassembled soluble Ig subunits by cytosolic proteasomes: Evidence that retrotranslocation and degradation are coupled events. *FASEB J. Off. Publ. Fed. Am. Soc. Exp. Biol.* **2000**, *14*, 769–778. [CrossRef] [PubMed]
33. Chillaron, J.; Haas, I.G. Dissociation from BiP and retrotranslocation of unassembled immunoglobulin light chains are tightly coupled to proteasome activity. *Mol. Biol. Cell* **2000**, *11*, 217–226. [CrossRef] [PubMed]
34. Mayer, T.U.; Braun, T.; Jentsch, S. Role of the proteasome in membrane extraction of a short-lived ER-transmembrane protein. *EMBO J.* **1998**, *17*, 3251–3257. [CrossRef] [PubMed]
35. Ebstein, F.; Poli Harlowe, M.C.; Studencka-Turski, M.; Kruger, E. Contribution of the Unfolded Protein Response (UPR) to the Pathogenesis of Proteasome-Associated Autoinflammatory Syndromes (PRAAS). *Front. Immunol.* **2019**, *10*, 2756. [CrossRef] [PubMed]
36. Ron, D.; Walter, P. Signal integration in the endoplasmic reticulum unfolded protein response. *Nat. Rev. Mol. Cell Biol.* **2007**, *8*, 519–529. [CrossRef]
37. Dekker, J.; Strous, G.J. Covalent oligomerization of rat gastric mucin occurs in the rough endoplasmic reticulum, is N-glycosylation-dependent, and precedes initial O-glycosylation. *J. Biol. Chem.* **1990**, *265*, 18116–18122. [CrossRef]
38. Pahl, H.L.; Baeuerle, P.A. A novel signal transduction pathway from the endoplasmic reticulum to the nucleus is mediated by transcription factor NF-kappa B. *EMBO J.* **1995**, *14*, 2580–2588. [CrossRef]
39. Grootjans, J.; Kaser, A.; Kaufman, R.J.; Blumberg, R.S. The unfolded protein response in immunity and inflammation. *Nat. Rev. Immunol.* **2016**, *16*, 469–484. [CrossRef]
40. Jaud, M.; Philippe, C.; Di Bella, D.; Tang, W.; Pyronnet, S.; Laurell, H.; Mazzolini, L.; Rouault-Pierre, K.; Touriol, C. Translational Regulations in Response to Endoplasmic Reticulum Stress in Cancers. *Cells* **2020**, *9*, 540. [CrossRef]

41. Deng, J.; Lu, P.D.; Zhang, Y.; Scheuner, D.; Kaufman, R.J.; Sonenberg, N.; Harding, H.P.; Ron, D. Translational repression mediates activation of nuclear factor kappa B by phosphorylated translation initiation factor 2. *Mol. Cell. Biol.* **2004**, *24*, 10161–10168. [CrossRef] [PubMed]
42. Kaneko, M.; Niinuma, Y.; Nomura, Y. Activation signal of nuclear factor-kappa B in response to endoplasmic reticulum stress is transduced via IRE1 and tumor necrosis factor receptor-associated factor 2. *Biol. Pharm. Bull.* **2003**, *26*, 931–935. [CrossRef] [PubMed]
43. Suraweera, A.; Munch, C.; Hanssum, A.; Bertolotti, A. Failure of amino acid homeostasis causes cell death following proteasome inhibition. *Mol. Cell* **2012**, *48*, 242–253. [CrossRef] [PubMed]
44. Dong, J.; Qiu, H.; Garcia-Barrio, M.; Anderson, J.; Hinnebusch, A.G. Uncharged tRNA activates GCN2 by displacing the protein kinase moiety from a bipartite tRNA-binding domain. *Mol. Cell* **2000**, *6*, 269–279. [CrossRef]
45. Harding, H.P.; Novoa, I.; Zhang, Y.; Zeng, H.; Wek, R.; Schapira, M.; Ron, D. Regulated translation initiation controls stress-induced gene expression in mammalian cells. *Mol. Cell* **2000**, *6*, 1099–1108. [CrossRef]
46. Dar, A.C.; Dever, T.E.; Sicheri, F. Higher-order substrate recognition of eIF2alpha by the RNA-dependent protein kinase PKR. *Cell* **2005**, *122*, 887–900. [CrossRef]
47. Clemens, M.J.; Hershey, J.W.; Hovanessian, A.C.; Jacobs, B.C.; Katze, M.G.; Kaufman, R.J.; Lengyel, P.; Samuel, C.E.; Sen, G.C.; Williams, B.R. PKR: Proposed nomenclature for the RNA-dependent protein kinase induced by interferon. *J. Interferon Res.* **1993**, *13*, 241. [CrossRef]
48. Meurs, E.; Chong, K.; Galabru, J.; Thomas, N.S.; Kerr, I.M.; Williams, B.R.; Hovanessian, A.G. Molecular cloning and characterization of the human double-stranded RNA-activated protein kinase induced by interferon. *Cell* **1990**, *62*, 379–390. [CrossRef]
49. Gilfoy, F.D.; Mason, P.W. West Nile virus-induced interferon production is mediated by the double-stranded RNA-dependent protein kinase PKR. *J. Virol.* **2007**, *81*, 11148–11158. [CrossRef]
50. Barry, G.; Breakwell, L.; Fragkoudis, R.; Attarzadeh-Yazdi, G.; Rodriguez-Andres, J.; Kohl, A.; Fazakerley, J.K. PKR acts early in infection to suppress Semliki Forest virus production and strongly enhances the type I interferon response. *J. Gen. Virol.* **2009**, *90*, 1382–1391. [CrossRef]
51. McAllister, C.S.; Toth, A.M.; Zhang, P.; Devaux, P.; Cattaneo, R.; Samuel, C.E. Mechanisms of protein kinase PKR-mediated amplification of beta interferon induction by C protein-deficient measles virus. *J. Virol.* **2010**, *84*, 380–386. [CrossRef] [PubMed]
52. Schulz, O.; Pichlmair, A.; Rehwinkel, J.; Rogers, N.C.; Scheuner, D.; Kato, H.; Takeuchi, O.; Akira, S.; Kaufman, R.J.; Reis e Sousa, C. Protein kinase R contributes to immunity against specific viruses by regulating interferon mRNA integrity. *Cell Host Microbe* **2010**, *7*, 354–361. [CrossRef] [PubMed]
53. Singh, M.; Fowlkes, V.; Handy, I.; Patel, C.V.; Patel, R.C. Essential role of PACT-mediated PKR activation in tunicamycin-induced apoptosis. *J. Mol. Biol.* **2009**, *385*, 457–468. [CrossRef] [PubMed]
54. Pyo, C.W.; Lee, S.H.; Choi, S.Y. Oxidative stress induces PKR-dependent apoptosis via IFN-gamma activation signaling in Jurkat T cells. *Biochem. Biophys. Res. Commun.* **2008**, *377*, 1001–1006. [CrossRef] [PubMed]
55. Murtha-Riel, P.; Davies, M.V.; Scherer, B.J.; Choi, S.Y.; Hershey, J.W.; Kaufman, R.J. Expression of a phosphorylation-resistant eukaryotic initiation factor 2 alpha-subunit mitigates heat shock inhibition of protein synthesis. *J. Biol. Chem.* **1993**, *268*, 12946–12951. [CrossRef]
56. Ito, T.; Yang, M.; May, W.S. RAX, a cellular activator for double-stranded RNA-dependent protein kinase during stress signaling. *J. Biol. Chem.* **1999**, *274*, 15427–15432. [CrossRef]
57. Patel, C.V.; Handy, I.; Goldsmith, T.; Patel, R.C. PACT, a stress-modulated cellular activator of interferon-induced double-stranded RNA-activated protein kinase, PKR. *J. Biol. Chem.* **2000**, *275*, 37993–37998. [CrossRef]
58. Ito, T.; Warnken, S.P.; May, W.S. Protein synthesis inhibition by flavonoids: Roles of eukaryotic initiation factor 2alpha kinases. *Biochem. Biophys. Res. Commun.* **1999**, *265*, 589–594. [CrossRef]
59. Davidson, S.; Yu, C.H.; Steiner, A.; Ebstein, F.; Baker, P.J.; Jarur-Chamy, V.; Hrovat Schaale, K.; Laohamonthonkul, P.; Kong, K.; Calleja, D.J.; et al. Protein kinase R is an innate immune sensor of proteotoxic stress via accumulation of cytoplasmic IL-24. *Sci. Immunol.* **2022**, *7*, eabi6763. [CrossRef]
60. DeTure, M.A.; Dickson, D.W. The neuropathological diagnosis of Alzheimer's disease. *Mol. Neurodegener* **2019**, *14*, 32. [CrossRef]
61. Gal-Ben-Ari, S.; Barrera, I.; Ehrlich, M.; Rosenblum, K. PKR: A Kinase to Remember. *Front. Mol. Neurosci.* **2018**, *11*, 480. [CrossRef] [PubMed]
62. Marchal, J.A.; Lopez, G.J.; Peran, M.; Comino, A.; Delgado, J.R.; Garcia-Garcia, J.A.; Conde, V.; Aranda, F.M.; Rivas, C.; Esteban, M.; et al. The impact of PKR activation: From neurodegeneration to cancer. *FASEB J. Off. Publ. Fed. Am. Soc. Exp. Biol.* **2014**, *28*, 1965–1974. [CrossRef] [PubMed]
63. Chukwurah, E.; Farabaugh, K.T.; Guan, B.J.; Ramakrishnan, P.; Hatzoglou, M. A tale of two proteins: PACT and PKR and their roles in inflammation. *FEBS J.* **2021**. [CrossRef] [PubMed]
64. Ingrand, S.; Barrier, L.; Lafay-Chebassier, C.; Fauconneau, B.; Page, G.; Hugon, J. The oxindole/imidazole derivative C16 reduces in vivo brain PKR activation. *FEBS Lett.* **2007**, *581*, 4473–4478. [CrossRef] [PubMed]
65. Goberdhan, D.C.; Wilson, C.; Harris, A.L. Amino Acid Sensing by mTORC1: Intracellular Transporters Mark the Spot. *Cell Metab.* **2016**, *23*, 580–589. [CrossRef] [PubMed]
66. Broer, S.; Broer, A. Amino acid homeostasis and signalling in mammalian cells and organisms. *Biochem. J.* **2017**, *474*, 1935–1963. [CrossRef] [PubMed]

67. Condon, K.J.; Sabatini, D.M. Nutrient regulation of mTORC1 at a glance. *J. Cell Sci.* **2019**, *132*. [CrossRef]
68. Isidor, B.; Ebstein, F.; Hurst, A.; Vincent, M.; Bader, I.; Rudy, N.L.; Cogne, B.; Mayr, J.; Brehm, A.; Bupp, C.; et al. Stankiewicz-Isidor syndrome: Expanding the clinical and molecular phenotype. *Genet. Med.* **2021**. [CrossRef]
69. York, A.G.; Williams, K.J.; Argus, J.P.; Zhou, Q.D.; Brar, G.; Vergnes, L.; Gray, E.E.; Zhen, A.; Wu, N.C.; Yamada, D.H.; et al. Limiting Cholesterol Biosynthetic Flux Spontaneously Engages Type I IFN Signaling. *Cell* **2015**, *163*, 1716–1729. [CrossRef]
70. Soto-Heredero, G.; Gomez de Las Heras, M.M.; Gabande-Rodriguez, E.; Oller, J.; Mittelbrunn, M. Glycolysis—A key player in the inflammatory response. *FEBS J.* **2020**, *287*, 3350–3369. [CrossRef]
71. Allaman, I.; Gavillet, M.; Belanger, M.; Laroche, T.; Viertl, D.; Lashuel, H.A.; Magistretti, P.J. Amyloid-beta aggregates cause alterations of astrocytic metabolic phenotype: Impact on neuronal viability. *J. Neurosci.* **2010**, *30*, 3326–3338. [CrossRef] [PubMed]
72. Ulland, T.K.; Song, W.M.; Huang, S.C.; Ulrich, J.D.; Sergushichev, A.; Beatty, W.L.; Loboda, A.A.; Zhou, Y.; Cairns, N.J.; Kambal, A.; et al. TREM2 Maintains Microglial Metabolic Fitness in Alzheimer's Disease. *Cell* **2017**, *170*, 649–663.e13. [CrossRef] [PubMed]
73. Taylor, J.P.; Brown, R.H., Jr.; Cleveland, D.W. Decoding ALS: From genes to mechanism. *Nature* **2016**, *539*, 197–206. [CrossRef] [PubMed]
74. Ramaswami, M.; Taylor, J.P.; Parker, R. Altered ribostasis: RNA-protein granules in degenerative disorders. *Cell* **2013**, *154*, 727–736. [CrossRef]
75. Li, Y.R.; King, O.D.; Shorter, J.; Gitler, A.D. Stress granules as crucibles of ALS pathogenesis. *J. Cell Biol.* **2013**, *201*, 361–372. [CrossRef]
76. Buchan, J.R.; Parker, R. Eukaryotic stress granules: The ins and outs of translation. *Mol. Cell* **2009**, *36*, 932–941. [CrossRef]
77. Ash, P.E.; Vanderweyde, T.E.; Youmans, K.L.; Apicco, D.J.; Wolozin, B. Pathological stress granules in Alzheimer's disease. *Brain Res.* **2014**, *1584*, 52–58. [CrossRef]
78. Vanderweyde, T.; Apicco, D.J.; Youmans-Kidder, K.; Ash, P.E.A.; Cook, C.; Lummertz da Rocha, E.; Jansen-West, K.; Frame, A.A.; Citro, A.; Leszyk, J.D.; et al. Interaction of tau with the RNA-Binding Protein TIA1 Regulates tau Pathophysiology and Toxicity. *Cell Rep.* **2016**, *15*, 1455–1466. [CrossRef]
79. McAleese, K.E.; Walker, L.; Erskine, D.; Thomas, A.J.; McKeith, I.G.; Attems, J. TDP-43 pathology in Alzheimer's disease, dementia with Lewy bodies and ageing. *Brain Pathol.* **2017**, *27*, 472–479. [CrossRef]
80. St-Amour, I.; Turgeon, A.; Goupil, C.; Planel, E.; Hebert, S.S. Co-occurrence of mixed proteinopathies in late-stage Huntington's disease. *Acta Neuropathol.* **2018**, *135*, 249–265. [CrossRef]
81. Coudert, L.; Nonaka, T.; Bernard, E.; Hasegawa, M.; Schaeffer, L.; Leblanc, P. Phosphorylated and aggregated TDP-43 with seeding properties are induced upon mutant Huntingtin (mHtt) polyglutamine expression in human cellular models. *Cell Mol. Life Sci* **2019**, *76*, 2615–2632. [CrossRef] [PubMed]
82. Ryan, V.H.; Fawzi, N.L. Physiological, Pathological, and Targetable Membraneless Organelles in Neurons. *Trends Neurosci.* **2019**, *42*, 693–708. [CrossRef] [PubMed]
83. Wolozin, B.; Ivanov, P. Stress granules and neurodegeneration. *Nat. Rev. Neurosci.* **2019**, *20*, 649–666. [CrossRef] [PubMed]
84. Dudman, J.; Qi, X. Stress Granule Dysregulation in Amyotrophic Lateral Sclerosis. *Front. Cell Neurosci.* **2020**, *14*, 598517. [CrossRef] [PubMed]
85. Hofmann, S.; Kedersha, N.; Anderson, P.; Ivanov, P. Molecular mechanisms of stress granule assembly and disassembly. *Biochim Biophys Acta Mol. Cell Res.* **2021**, *1868*, 118876. [CrossRef] [PubMed]
86. Yang, P.; Mathieu, C.; Kolaitis, R.M.; Zhang, P.; Messing, J.; Yurtsever, U.; Yang, Z.; Wu, J.; Li, Y.; Pan, Q.; et al. G3BP1 Is a Tunable Switch that Triggers Phase Separation to Assemble Stress Granules. *Cell* **2020**, *181*, 325–345.e28. [CrossRef]
87. Sanders, D.W.; Kedersha, N.; Lee, D.S.W.; Strom, A.R.; Drake, V.; Riback, J.A.; Bracha, D.; Eeftens, J.M.; Iwanicki, A.; Wang, A.; et al. Competing Protein-RNA Interaction Networks Control Multiphase Intracellular Organization. *Cell* **2020**, *181*, 306–324.e28. [CrossRef]
88. Guillen-Boixet, J.; Kopach, A.; Holehouse, A.S.; Wittmann, S.; Jahnel, M.; Schlussler, R.; Kim, K.; Trussina, I.; Wang, J.; Mateju, D.; et al. RNA-Induced Conformational Switching and Clustering of G3BP Drive Stress Granule Assembly by Condensation. *Cell* **2020**, *181*, 346–361.e17. [CrossRef]
89. Pakos-Zebrucka, K.; Koryga, I.; Mnich, K.; Ljujic, M.; Samali, A.; Gorman, A.M. The integrated stress response. *EMBO Rep.* **2016**, *17*, 1374–1395. [CrossRef]
90. Mazroui, R.; Di Marco, S.; Kaufman, R.J.; Gallouzi, I.E. Inhibition of the ubiquitin-proteasome system induces stress granule formation. *Mol. Biol. Cell* **2007**, *18*, 2603–2618. [CrossRef]
91. Mateju, D.; Franzmann, T.M.; Patel, A.; Kopach, A.; Boczek, E.E.; Maharana, S.; Lee, H.O.; Carra, S.; Hyman, A.A.; Alberti, S. An aberrant phase transition of stress granules triggered by misfolded protein and prevented by chaperone function. *EMBO J.* **2017**, *36*, 1669–1687. [CrossRef] [PubMed]
92. Rao, L.; Xu, Y.; Reineke, L.C.; Bhattacharya, A.; Tyryshkin, A.; Shin, J.N.; Eissa, N.T. Post-Transcriptional Regulation of Alpha One Antitrypsin by a Proteasome Inhibitor. *Int. J. Mol. Sci.* **2020**, *21*, 4318. [CrossRef] [PubMed]
93. Oh, S.W.; Onomoto, K.; Wakimoto, M.; Onoguchi, K.; Ishidate, F.; Fujiwara, T.; Yoneyama, M.; Kato, H.; Fujita, T. Leader-Containing Uncapped Viral Transcript Activates RIG-I in Antiviral Stress Granules. *PLoS Pathog.* **2016**, *12*, e1005444. [CrossRef] [PubMed]

94. Onomoto, K.; Jogi, M.; Yoo, J.S.; Narita, R.; Morimoto, S.; Takemura, A.; Sambhara, S.; Kawaguchi, A.; Osari, S.; Nagata, K.; et al. Critical role of an antiviral stress granule containing RIG-I and PKR in viral detection and innate immunity. *PLoS ONE* **2012**, *7*, e43031. [CrossRef]
95. Yoneyama, M.; Jogi, M.; Onomoto, K. Regulation of antiviral innate immune signaling by stress-induced RNA granules. *J. Biochem.* **2016**, *159*, 279–286. [CrossRef] [PubMed]
96. Hu, S.; Sun, H.; Yin, L.; Li, J.; Mei, S.; Xu, F.; Wu, C.; Liu, X.; Zhao, F.; Zhang, D.; et al. PKR-dependent cytosolic cGAS foci are necessary for intracellular DNA sensing. *Sci Signal.* **2019**, *12*. [CrossRef]
97. Liu, Z.S.; Cai, H.; Xue, W.; Wang, M.; Xia, T.; Li, W.J.; Xing, J.Q.; Zhao, M.; Huang, Y.J.; Chen, S.; et al. G3BP1 promotes DNA binding and activation of cGAS. *Nat. Immunol.* **2019**, *20*, 18–28. [CrossRef]
98. Kim, S.S.; Sze, L.; Liu, C.; Lam, K.P. The stress granule protein G3BP1 binds viral dsRNA and RIG-I to enhance interferon-beta response. *J. Biol. Chem.* **2019**, *294*, 6430–6438. [CrossRef]
99. Radhakrishnan, S.K.; Lee, C.S.; Young, P.; Beskow, A.; Chan, J.Y.; Deshaies, R.J. Transcription factor Nrf1 mediates the proteasome recovery pathway after proteasome inhibition in mammalian cells. *Mol. Cell* **2010**, *38*, 17–28. [CrossRef]
100. Steffen, J.; Seeger, M.; Koch, A.; Kruger, E. Proteasomal degradation is transcriptionally controlled by TCF11 via an ERAD-dependent feedback loop. *Mol. Cell* **2010**, *40*, 147–158. [CrossRef] [PubMed]
101. Tomlin, F.M.; Gerling-Driessen, U.I.M.; Liu, Y.C.; Flynn, R.A.; Vangala, J.R.; Lentz, C.S.; Clauder-Muenster, S.; Jakob, P.; Mueller, W.F.; Ordonez-Rueda, D.; et al. Inhibition of NGLY1 Inactivates the Transcription Factor Nrf1 and Potentiates Proteasome Inhibitor Cytotoxicity. *ACS Cent. Sci.* **2017**, *3*, 1143–1155. [CrossRef] [PubMed]
102. Koizumi, S.; Irie, T.; Hirayama, S.; Sakurai, Y.; Yashiroda, H.; Naguro, I.; Ichijo, H.; Hamazaki, J.; Murata, S. The aspartyl protease DDI2 activates Nrf1 to compensate for proteasome dysfunction. *eLife* **2016**, *5*. [CrossRef] [PubMed]
103. Yang, K.; Huang, R.; Fujihira, H.; Suzuki, T.; Yan, N. N-glycanase NGLY1 regulates mitochondrial homeostasis and inflammation through NRF1. *J. Exp. Med.* **2018**, *215*, 2600–2616. [CrossRef] [PubMed]
104. Widenmaier, S.B.; Snyder, N.A.; Nguyen, T.B.; Arduini, A.; Lee, G.Y.; Arruda, A.P.; Saksi, J.; Bartelt, A.; Hotamisligil, G.S. NRF1 Is an ER Membrane Sensor that Is Central to Cholesterol Homeostasis. *Cell* **2017**, *171*, 1094–1109.e15. [CrossRef]
105. Fellner, L.; Irschick, R.; Schanda, K.; Reindl, M.; Klimaschewski, L.; Poewe, W.; Wenning, G.K.; Stefanova, N. Toll-like receptor 4 is required for alpha-synuclein dependent activation of microglia and astroglia. *Glia* **2013**, *61*, 349–360. [CrossRef]
106. Rannikko, E.H.; Weber, S.S.; Kahle, P.J. Exogenous alpha-synuclein induces toll-like receptor 4 dependent inflammatory responses in astrocytes. *BMC Neurosci.* **2015**, *16*, 57. [CrossRef]
107. Stefanova, N.; Fellner, L.; Reindl, M.; Masliah, E.; Poewe, W.; Wenning, G.K. Toll-like receptor 4 promotes alpha-synuclein clearance and survival of nigral dopaminergic neurons. *Am. J. Pathol.* **2011**, *179*, 954–963. [CrossRef]
108. Kim, C.; Ho, D.H.; Suk, J.E.; You, S.; Michael, S.; Kang, J.; Joong Lee, S.; Masliah, E.; Hwang, D.; Lee, H.J.; et al. Neuron-released oligomeric alpha-synuclein is an endogenous agonist of TLR2 for paracrine activation of microglia. *Nat. Commun.* **2013**, *4*, 1562. [CrossRef]
109. Dzamko, N.; Gysbers, A.; Perera, G.; Bahar, A.; Shankar, A.; Gao, J.; Fu, Y.; Halliday, G.M. Toll-like receptor 2 is increased in neurons in Parkinson's disease brain and may contribute to alpha-synuclein pathology. *Acta Neuropathol.* **2017**, *133*, 303–319. [CrossRef]
110. Kim, C.; Rockenstein, E.; Spencer, B.; Kim, H.K.; Adame, A.; Trejo, M.; Stafa, K.; Lee, H.J.; Lee, S.J.; Masliah, E. Antagonizing Neuronal Toll-like Receptor 2 Prevents Synucleinopathy by Activating Autophagy. *Cell Rep.* **2015**, *13*, 771–782. [CrossRef]
111. Wang, Y.; Cella, M.; Mallinson, K.; Ulrich, J.D.; Young, K.L.; Robinette, M.L.; Gilfillan, S.; Krishnan, G.M.; Sudhakar, S.; Zinselmeyer, B.H.; et al. TREM2 lipid sensing sustains the microglial response in an Alzheimer's disease model. *Cell* **2015**, *160*, 1061–1071. [CrossRef] [PubMed]
112. Lehnardt, S.; Massillon, L.; Follett, P.; Jensen, F.E.; Ratan, R.; Rosenberg, P.A.; Volpe, J.J.; Vartanian, T. Activation of innate immunity in the CNS triggers neurodegeneration through a Toll-like receptor 4-dependent pathway. *Proc. Natl. Acad. Sci. USA* **2003**, *100*, 8514–8519. [CrossRef] [PubMed]
113. Stewart, C.R.; Stuart, L.M.; Wilkinson, K.; van Gils, J.M.; Deng, J.; Halle, A.; Rayner, K.J.; Boyer, L.; Zhong, R.; Frazier, W.A.; et al. CD36 ligands promote sterile inflammation through assembly of a Toll-like receptor 4 and 6 heterodimer. *Nat. Immunol.* **2010**, *11*, 155–161. [CrossRef] [PubMed]
114. Liu, S.; Liu, Y.; Hao, W.; Wolf, L.; Kiliaan, A.J.; Penke, B.; Rube, C.E.; Walter, J.; Heneka, M.T.; Hartmann, T.; et al. TLR2 is a primary receptor for Alzheimer's amyloid beta peptide to trigger neuroinflammatory activation. *J. Immunol.* **2012**, *188*, 1098–1107. [CrossRef]
115. Scholtzova, H.; Chianchiano, P.; Pan, J.; Sun, Y.; Goni, F.; Mehta, P.D.; Wisniewski, T. Amyloid beta and Tau Alzheimer's disease related pathology is reduced by Toll-like receptor 9 stimulation. *Acta Neuropathol. Commun.* **2014**, *2*, 101. [CrossRef]
116. Zhao, W.; Beers, D.R.; Bell, S.; Wang, J.; Wen, S.; Baloh, R.H.; Appel, S.H. TDP-43 activates microglia through NF-kappaB and NLRP3 inflammasome. *Exp. Neurol.* **2015**, *273*, 24–35. [CrossRef]
117. Kadhim, H.; Deltenre, P.; Martin, J.J.; Sebire, G. In-situ expression of Interleukin-18 and associated mediators in the human brain of sALS patients: Hypothesis for a role for immune-inflammatory mechanisms. *Med. Hypotheses* **2016**, *86*, 14–17. [CrossRef]
118. Yu, C.H.; Davidson, S.; Harapas, C.R.; Hilton, J.B.; Mlodzianoski, M.J.; Laohamonthonkul, P.; Louis, C.; Low, R.R.J.; Moecking, J.; De Nardo, D.; et al. TDP-43 Triggers Mitochondrial DNA Release via mPTP to Activate cGAS/STING in ALS. *Cell* **2020**, *183*, 636–649.e18. [CrossRef]

119. Kampen, K.R.; Sulima, S.O.; Vereecke, S.; De Keersmaecker, K. Hallmarks of ribosomopathies. *Nucleic Acids Res.* **2020**, *48*, 1013–1028. [CrossRef]
120. Berman, I.R.; Iliescu, H.; Stachura, I. Pulmonary effects of blood container materials. *Surg. Forum* **1977**, *28*, 182–184.
121. Da Costa, L.; Leblanc, T.; Mohandas, N. Diamond-Blackfan anemia. *Blood* **2020**, *136*, 1262–1273. [CrossRef] [PubMed]
122. Ellis, S.R. Nucleolar stress in Diamond Blackfan anemia pathophysiology. *Biochim. Biophys. Acta* **2014**, *1842*, 765–768. [CrossRef] [PubMed]
123. Chakraborty, A.; Uechi, T.; Kenmochi, N. Guarding the 'translation apparatus': Defective ribosome biogenesis and the p53 signaling pathway. *Wiley Interdiscip. Rev. RNA* **2011**, *2*, 507–522. [CrossRef]
124. Kang, J.; Brajanovski, N.; Chan, K.T.; Xuan, J.; Pearson, R.B.; Sanij, E. Ribosomal proteins and human diseases: Molecular mechanisms and targeted therapy. *Signal. Transduct. Target.* **2021**, *6*, 323. [CrossRef] [PubMed]
125. Kapralova, K.; Jahoda, O.; Koralkova, P.; Gursky, J.; Lanikova, L.; Pospisilova, D.; Divoky, V.; Horvathova, M. Oxidative DNA Damage, Inflammatory Signature, and Altered Erythrocytes Properties in Diamond-Blackfan Anemia. *Int. J. Mol. Sci.* **2020**, *21*, 9652. [CrossRef] [PubMed]
126. Pesciotta, E.N.; Lam, H.S.; Kossenkov, A.; Ge, J.; Showe, L.C.; Mason, P.J.; Bessler, M.; Speicher, D.W. In-Depth, Label-Free Analysis of the Erythrocyte Cytoplasmic Proteome in Diamond Blackfan Anemia Identifies a Unique Inflammatory Signature. *PLoS ONE* **2015**, *10*, e0140036. [CrossRef] [PubMed]
127. Gazda, H.T.; Kho, A.T.; Sanoudou, D.; Zaucha, J.M.; Kohane, I.S.; Sieff, C.A.; Beggs, A.H. Defective ribosomal protein gene expression alters transcription, translation, apoptosis, and oncogenic pathways in Diamond-Blackfan anemia. *Stem Cells* **2006**, *24*, 2034–2044. [CrossRef]
128. Danilova, N.; Wilkes, M.; Bibikova, E.; Youn, M.Y.; Sakamoto, K.M.; Lin, S. Innate immune system activation in zebrafish and cellular models of Diamond Blackfan Anemia. *Sci. Rep.* **2018**, *8*, 5165. [CrossRef]
129. Girardi, T.; Vereecke, S.; Sulima, S.O.; Khan, Y.; Fancello, L.; Briggs, J.W.; Schwab, C.; de Beeck, J.O.; Verbeeck, J.; Royaert, J.; et al. The T-cell leukemia-associated ribosomal RPL10 R98S mutation enhances JAK-STAT signaling. *Leukemia* **2018**, *32*, 809–819. [CrossRef]
130. Dou, Z.; Ghosh, K.; Vizioli, M.G.; Zhu, J.; Sen, P.; Wangensteen, K.J.; Simithy, J.; Lan, Y.; Lin, Y.; Zhou, Z.; et al. Cytoplasmic chromatin triggers inflammation in senescence and cancer. *Nature* **2017**, *550*, 402–406. [CrossRef]
131. Frisch, S.M.; MacFawn, I.P. Type I interferons and related pathways in cell senescence. *Aging Cell* **2020**, *19*, e13234. [CrossRef] [PubMed]
132. Wan, L.; Juszkiewicz, S.; Blears, D.; Bajpe, P.K.; Han, Z.; Faull, P.; Mitter, R.; Stewart, A.; Snijders, A.P.; Hegde, R.S.; et al. Translation stress and collided ribosomes are co-activators of cGAS. *Mol. Cell* **2021**, *81*, 2808–2822.e10. [CrossRef] [PubMed]
133. Yewdell, J.W.; Nicchitta, C.V. The DRiP hypothesis decennial: Support, controversy, refinement and extension. *Trends Immunol.* **2006**, *27*, 368–373. [CrossRef]
134. Schubert, U.; Anton, L.C.; Gibbs, J.; Norbury, C.C.; Yewdell, J.W.; Bennink, J.R. Rapid degradation of a large fraction of newly synthesized proteins by proteasomes. *Nature* **2000**, *404*, 770–774. [CrossRef] [PubMed]
135. Wegele, H.; Muller, L.; Buchner, J. Hsp70 and Hsp90—A relay team for protein folding. *Rev. Physiol. Biochem. Pharm.* **2004**, *151*, 1–44. [CrossRef]
136. Mishra, A.; Godavarthi, S.K.; Maheshwari, M.; Goswami, A.; Jana, N.R. The ubiquitin ligase E6-AP is induced and recruited to aggresomes in response to proteasome inhibition and may be involved in the ubiquitination of Hsp70-bound misfolded proteins. *J. Biol. Chem.* **2009**, *284*, 10537–10545. [CrossRef]
137. Mishra, R.; Amanullah, A.; Upadhyay, A.; Dhiman, R.; Dubey, A.R.; Singh, S.; Prasad, A.; Mishra, A. Ubiquitin ligase LRSAM1 suppresses neurodegenerative diseases linked aberrant proteins induced cell death. *Int. J. Biochem. Cell Biol.* **2020**, *120*, 105697. [CrossRef]
138. Inda, C.; Bolaender, A.; Wang, T.; Gandu, S.R.; Koren, J., 3rd. Stressing Out Hsp90 in Neurotoxic Proteinopathies. *Curr. Top. Med. Chem.* **2016**, *16*, 2829–2838. [CrossRef]
139. Olzscha, H. Posttranslational modifications and proteinopathies: How guardians of the proteome are defeated. *Biol. Chem.* **2019**, *400*, 895–915. [CrossRef]
140. Mear, J.P.; Schreiber, K.L.; Munz, C.; Zhu, X.; Stevanovic, S.; Rammensee, H.G.; Rowland-Jones, S.L.; Colbert, R.A. Misfolding of HLA-B27 as a result of its B pocket suggests a novel mechanism for its role in susceptibility to spondyloarthropathies. *J. Immunol.* **1999**, *163*, 6665–6670.
141. Dangoria, N.S.; DeLay, M.L.; Kingsbury, D.J.; Mear, J.P.; Uchanska-Ziegler, B.; Ziegler, A.; Colbert, R.A. HLA-B27 misfolding is associated with aberrant intermolecular disulfide bond formation (dimerization) in the endoplasmic reticulum. *J. Biol. Chem.* **2002**, *277*, 23459–23468. [CrossRef] [PubMed]
142. Colbert, R.A. HLA-B27 misfolding: A solution to the spondyloarthropathy conundrum? *Mol. Med. Today* **2000**, *6*, 224–230. [CrossRef]
143. Colbert, R.A.; Tran, T.M.; Layh-Schmitt, G. HLA-B27 misfolding and ankylosing spondylitis. *Mol. Immunol* **2014**, *57*, 44–51. [CrossRef] [PubMed]
144. Kerbiriou, M.; Le Drevo, M.A.; Ferec, C.; Trouve, P. Coupling cystic fibrosis to endoplasmic reticulum stress: Differential role of Grp78 and ATF6. *Biochim. Biophys. Acta* **2007**, *1772*, 1236–1249. [CrossRef]

145. Trouve, P.; Ferec, C.; Genin, E. The Interplay between the Unfolded Protein Response, Inflammation and Infection in Cystic Fibrosis. *Cells* **2021**, *10*, 2980. [CrossRef]
146. Segeritz, C.P.; Rashid, S.T.; de Brito, M.C.; Serra, M.P.; Ordonez, A.; Morell, C.M.; Kaserman, J.E.; Madrigal, P.; Hannan, N.R.F.; Gatto, L.; et al. hiPSC hepatocyte model demonstrates the role of unfolded protein response and inflammatory networks in alpha1-antitrypsin deficiency. *J. Hepatol.* **2018**, *69*, 851–860. [CrossRef]
147. Lawless, M.W.; Greene, C.M.; Mulgrew, A.; Taggart, C.C.; O'Neill, S.J.; McElvaney, N.G. Activation of endoplasmic reticulum-specific stress responses associated with the conformational disease Z alpha 1-antitrypsin deficiency. *J. Immunol.* **2004**, *172*, 5722–5726. [CrossRef]
148. Carroll, T.P.; Greene, C.M.; O'Connor, C.A.; Nolan, A.M.; O'Neill, S.J.; McElvaney, N.G. Evidence for unfolded protein response activation in monocytes from individuals with alpha-1 antitrypsin deficiency. *J. Immunol.* **2010**, *184*, 4538–4546. [CrossRef]
149. Saraiva, M.J.; Magalhaes, J.; Ferreira, N.; Almeida, M.R. Transthyretin deposition in familial amyloidotic polyneuropathy. *Curr. Med. Chem.* **2012**, *19*, 2304–2311. [CrossRef]
150. Quarta, C.C.; Buxbaum, J.N.; Shah, A.M.; Falk, R.H.; Claggett, B.; Kitzman, D.W.; Mosley, T.H.; Butler, K.R.; Boerwinkle, E.; Solomon, S.D. The amyloidogenic V122I transthyretin variant in elderly black Americans. *N. Engl. J. Med.* **2015**, *372*, 21–29. [CrossRef]
151. Kanda, Y.; Goodman, D.S.; Canfield, R.E.; Morgan, F.J. The amino acid sequence of human plasma prealbumin. *J. Biol. Chem.* **1974**, *249*, 6796–6805. [CrossRef]
152. Sousa, M.M.; Saraiva, M.J. Neurodegeneration in familial amyloid polyneuropathy: From pathology to molecular signaling. *Prog. Neurobiol.* **2003**, *71*, 385–400. [CrossRef] [PubMed]
153. Azevedo, E.P.; Guimaraes-Costa, A.B.; Bandeira-Melo, C.; Chimelli, L.; Waddington-Cruz, M.; Saraiva, E.M.; Palhano, F.L.; Foguel, D. Inflammatory profiling of patients with familial amyloid polyneuropathy. *BMC Neurol.* **2019**, *19*, 146. [CrossRef] [PubMed]
154. Sousa, M.M.; Du Yan, S.; Fernandes, R.; Guimaraes, A.; Stern, D.; Saraiva, M.J. Familial amyloid polyneuropathy: Receptor for advanced glycation end products-dependent triggering of neuronal inflammatory and apoptotic pathways. *J. Neurosci.* **2001**, *21*, 7576–7586. [CrossRef] [PubMed]
155. Azevedo, E.P.; Ledo, J.H.; Barbosa, G.; Sobrinho, M.; Diniz, L.; Fonseca, A.C.; Gomes, F.; Romao, L.; Lima, F.R.; Palhano, F.L.; et al. Activated microglia mediate synapse loss and short-term memory deficits in a mouse model of transthyretin-related oculoleptomeningeal amyloidosis. *Cell Death Dis.* **2013**, *4*, e789. [CrossRef]
156. Azevedo, E.P.; Guimaraes-Costa, A.B.; Torezani, G.S.; Braga, C.A.; Palhano, F.L.; Kelly, J.W.; Saraiva, E.M.; Foguel, D. Amyloid fibrils trigger the release of neutrophil extracellular traps (NETs), causing fibril fragmentation by NET-associated elastase. *J. Biol. Chem.* **2012**, *287*, 37206–37218. [CrossRef]
157. Williams, D.B.; Windebank, A.J. Motor neuron disease (amyotrophic lateral sclerosis). *Mayo Clin. Proc.* **1991**, *66*, 54–82. [CrossRef]
158. Rowland, L.P. Amyotrophic lateral sclerosis. *Curr. Opin. Neurol.* **1994**, *7*, 310–315. [CrossRef]
159. Chia, R.; Chio, A.; Traynor, B.J. Novel genes associated with amyotrophic lateral sclerosis: Diagnostic and clinical implications. *Lancet Neurol.* **2018**, *17*, 94–102. [CrossRef]
160. Maurel, C.; Dangoumau, A.; Marouillat, S.; Brulard, C.; Chami, A.; Hergesheimer, R.; Corcia, P.; Blasco, H.; Andres, C.R.; Vourc'h, P. Causative Genes in Amyotrophic Lateral Sclerosis and Protein Degradation Pathways: A Link to Neurodegeneration. *Mol. Neurobiol.* **2018**, *55*, 6480–6499. [CrossRef]
161. Rosen, D.R.; Siddique, T.; Patterson, D.; Figlewicz, D.A.; Sapp, P.; Hentati, A.; Donaldson, D.; Goto, J.; O'Regan, J.P.; Deng, H.X.; et al. Mutations in Cu/Zn superoxide dismutase gene are associated with familial amyotrophic lateral sclerosis. *Nature* **1993**, *362*, 59–62. [CrossRef] [PubMed]
162. Kabashi, E.; Valdmanis, P.N.; Dion, P.; Spiegelman, D.; McConkey, B.J.; Vande Velde, C.; Bouchard, J.P.; Lacomblez, L.; Pochigaeva, K.; Salachas, F.; et al. TARDBP mutations in individuals with sporadic and familial amyotrophic lateral sclerosis. *Nat. Genet.* **2008**, *40*, 572–574. [CrossRef] [PubMed]
163. Ling, S.C.; Polymenidou, M.; Cleveland, D.W. Converging mechanisms in ALS and FTD: Disrupted RNA and protein homeostasis. *Neuron* **2013**, *79*, 416–438. [CrossRef] [PubMed]
164. Buratti, E.; Baralle, F.E. Multiple roles of TDP-43 in gene expression, splicing regulation, and human disease. *Front. Biosci.* **2008**, *13*, 867–878. [CrossRef] [PubMed]
165. Buratti, E.; Baralle, F.E. TDP-43: Gumming up neurons through protein-protein and protein-RNA interactions. *Trends Biochem. Sci.* **2012**, *37*, 237–247. [CrossRef] [PubMed]
166. DeJesus-Hernandez, M.; Mackenzie, I.R.; Boeve, B.F.; Boxer, A.L.; Baker, M.; Rutherford, N.J.; Nicholson, A.M.; Finch, N.A.; Flynn, H.; Adamson, J.; et al. Expanded GGGGCC hexanucleotide repeat in noncoding region of C9ORF72 causes chromosome 9p-linked FTD and ALS. *Neuron* **2011**, *72*, 245–256. [CrossRef]
167. Renton, A.E.; Majounie, E.; Waite, A.; Simon-Sanchez, J.; Rollinson, S.; Gibbs, J.R.; Schymick, J.C.; Laaksovirta, H.; van Swieten, J.C.; Myllykangas, L.; et al. A hexanucleotide repeat expansion in C9ORF72 is the cause of chromosome 9p21-linked ALS-FTD. *Neuron* **2011**, *72*, 257–268. [CrossRef]
168. Cook, C.N.; Wu, Y.; Odeh, H.M.; Gendron, T.F.; Jansen-West, K.; Del Rosso, G.; Yue, M.; Jiang, P.; Gomes, E.; Tong, J.; et al. C9orf72 poly(GR) aggregation induces TDP-43 proteinopathy. *Sci Transl Med.* **2020**, *12*. [CrossRef]

169. Neumann, M.; Sampathu, D.M.; Kwong, L.K.; Truax, A.C.; Micsenyi, M.C.; Chou, T.T.; Bruce, J.; Schuck, T.; Grossman, M.; Clark, C.M.; et al. Ubiquitinated TDP-43 in frontotemporal lobar degeneration and amyotrophic lateral sclerosis. *Science* **2006**, *314*, 130–133. [CrossRef]
170. Cirulli, E.T.; Lasseigne, B.N.; Petrovski, S.; Sapp, P.C.; Dion, P.A.; Leblond, C.S.; Couthouis, J.; Lu, Y.F.; Wang, Q.; Krueger, B.J.; et al. Exome sequencing in amyotrophic lateral sclerosis identifies risk genes and pathways. *Science* **2015**, *347*, 1436–1441. [CrossRef]
171. Freischmidt, A.; Wieland, T.; Richter, B.; Ruf, W.; Schaeffer, V.; Muller, K.; Marroquin, N.; Nordin, F.; Hubers, A.; Weydt, P.; et al. Haploinsufficiency of TBK1 causes familial ALS and fronto-temporal dementia. *Nat. Neurosci.* **2015**, *18*, 631–636. [CrossRef] [PubMed]
172. Geloso, M.C.; Corvino, V.; Marchese, E.; Serrano, A.; Michetti, F.; D'Ambrosi, N. The Dual Role of Microglia in ALS: Mechanisms and Therapeutic Approaches. *Front. Aging Neurosci.* **2017**, *9*, 242. [CrossRef] [PubMed]
173. Henkel, J.S.; Beers, D.R.; Zhao, W.; Appel, S.H. Microglia in ALS: The good, the bad, and the resting. *J. Neuroimmune Pharm.* **2009**, *4*, 389–398. [CrossRef] [PubMed]
174. Shahheydari, H.; Ragagnin, A.; Walker, A.K.; Toth, R.P.; Vidal, M.; Jagaraj, C.J.; Perri, E.R.; Konopka, A.; Sultana, J.M.; Atkin, J.D. Protein Quality Control and the Amyotrophic Lateral Sclerosis/Frontotemporal Dementia Continuum. *Front. Mol. Neurosci.* **2017**, *10*, 119. [CrossRef] [PubMed]
175. Nishitoh, H.; Kadowaki, H.; Nagai, A.; Maruyama, T.; Yokota, T.; Fukutomi, H.; Noguchi, T.; Matsuzawa, A.; Takeda, K.; Ichijo, H. ALS-linked mutant SOD1 induces ER stress- and ASK1-dependent motor neuron death by targeting Derlin-1. *Genes Dev.* **2008**, *22*, 1451–1464. [CrossRef] [PubMed]
176. Zhao, W.; Beers, D.R.; Henkel, J.S.; Zhang, W.; Urushitani, M.; Julien, J.P.; Appel, S.H. Extracellular mutant SOD1 induces microglial-mediated motoneuron injury. *Glia* **2010**, *58*, 231–243. [CrossRef] [PubMed]
177. Magrane, J.; Cortez, C.; Gan, W.B.; Manfredi, G. Abnormal mitochondrial transport and morphology are common pathological denominators in SOD1 and TDP43 ALS mouse models. *Hum. Mol. Genet.* **2014**, *23*, 1413–1424. [CrossRef]
178. Wang, W.; Li, L.; Lin, W.L.; Dickson, D.W.; Petrucelli, L.; Zhang, T.; Wang, X. The ALS disease-associated mutant TDP-43 impairs mitochondrial dynamics and function in motor neurons. *Hum. Mol. Genet.* **2013**, *22*, 4706–4719. [CrossRef]
179. Varshavsky, A. The Ubiquitin System, Autophagy, and Regulated Protein Degradation. *Annu Rev. Biochem.* **2017**, *86*, 123–128. [CrossRef]
180. Cetin, G.; Klafack, S.; Studencka-Turski, M.; Kruger, E.; Ebstein, F. The Ubiquitin-Proteasome System in Immune Cells. *Biomolecules* **2021**, *11*, 60. [CrossRef]
181. Pickart, C.M.; Fushman, D. Polyubiquitin chains: Polymeric protein signals. *Curr. Opin. Chem. Biol.* **2004**, *8*, 610–616. [CrossRef] [PubMed]
182. Pickart, C.M.; Eddins, M.J. Ubiquitin: Structures, functions, mechanisms. *Biochim. Biophys. Acta* **2004**, *1695*, 55–72. [CrossRef] [PubMed]
183. Tanaka, K.; Mizushima, T.; Saeki, Y. The proteasome: Molecular machinery and pathophysiological roles. *Biol. Chem.* **2012**, *393*, 217–234. [CrossRef] [PubMed]
184. Tanaka, K. The proteasome: Overview of structure and functions. *Proc. Jpn. Acad. Ser. B Phys. Biol. Sci.* **2009**, *85*, 12–36. [CrossRef] [PubMed]
185. Bard, J.A.M.; Goodall, E.A.; Greene, E.R.; Jonsson, E.; Dong, K.C.; Martin, A. Structure and Function of the 26S Proteasome. *Annu. Rev. Biochem.* **2018**, *87*, 697–724. [CrossRef] [PubMed]
186. Dahlmann, B. Proteasomes. *Essays Biochem.* **2005**, *41*, 31–48. [CrossRef]
187. Greene, E.R.; Dong, K.C.; Martin, A. Understanding the 26S proteasome molecular machine from a structural and conformational dynamics perspective. *Curr. Opin. Struct. Biol.* **2020**, *61*, 33–41. [CrossRef]
188. Ebstein, F.; Kloetzel, P.M.; Kruger, E.; Seifert, U. Emerging roles of immunoproteasomes beyond MHC class I antigen processing. *Cell Mol. Life Sci.* **2012**, *69*, 2543–2558. [CrossRef]
189. Tubio-Santamaria, N.; Ebstein, F.; Heidel, F.H.; Kruger, E. Immunoproteasome Function in Normal and Malignant Hematopoiesis. *Cells* **2021**, *10*, 1577. [CrossRef]
190. Seifert, U.; Bialy, L.P.; Ebstein, F.; Bech-Otschir, D.; Voigt, A.; Schroter, F.; Prozorovski, T.; Lange, N.; Steffen, J.; Rieger, M.; et al. Immunoproteasomes preserve protein homeostasis upon interferon-induced oxidative stress. *Cell* **2010**, *142*, 613–624. [CrossRef] [PubMed]
191. Ebstein, F.; Voigt, A.; Lange, N.; Warnatsch, A.; Schroter, F.; Prozorovski, T.; Kuckelkorn, U.; Aktas, O.; Seifert, U.; Kloetzel, P.M.; et al. Immunoproteasomes are important for proteostasis in immune responses. *Cell* **2013**, *152*, 935–937. [CrossRef] [PubMed]
192. Yun, Y.S.; Kim, K.H.; Tschida, B.; Sachs, Z.; Noble-Orcutt, K.E.; Moriarity, B.S.; Ai, T.; Ding, R.; Williams, J.; Chen, L.; et al. mTORC1 Coordinates Protein Synthesis and Immunoproteasome Formation via PRAS40 to Prevent Accumulation of Protein Stress. *Mol. Cell* **2016**, *61*, 625–639. [CrossRef] [PubMed]
193. Niewerth, D.; Kaspers, G.J.; Assaraf, Y.G.; van Meerloo, J.; Kirk, C.J.; Anderl, J.; Blank, J.L.; van de Ven, P.M.; Zweegman, S.; Jansen, G.; et al. Interferon-gamma-induced upregulation of immunoproteasome subunit assembly overcomes bortezomib resistance in human hematological cell lines. *J. Hematol. Oncol.* **2014**, *7*, 7. [CrossRef]
194. Opitz, E.; Koch, A.; Klingel, K.; Schmidt, F.; Prokop, S.; Rahnefeld, A.; Sauter, M.; Heppner, F.L.; Volker, U.; Kandolf, R.; et al. Impairment of immunoproteasome function by beta5i/LMP7 subunit deficiency results in severe enterovirus myocarditis. *PLoS Pathog.* **2011**, *7*, e1002233. [CrossRef] [PubMed]

195. Kruger, E.; Kloetzel, P.M. Immunoproteasomes at the interface of innate and adaptive immune responses: Two faces of one enzyme. *Curr. Opin. Immunol.* **2012**, *24*, 77–83. [CrossRef] [PubMed]
196. Goetzke, C.C.; Ebstein, F.; Kallinich, T. Role of Proteasomes in Inflammation. *J. Clin. Med.* **2021**, *10*, 1783. [CrossRef] [PubMed]
197. Chondrogianni, N.; Gonos, E.S. Proteasome function determines cellular homeostasis and the rate of aging. *Adv. Exp. Med. Biol.* **2010**, *694*, 38–46. [CrossRef]
198. Keller, J.N.; Huang, F.F.; Markesbery, W.R. Decreased levels of proteasome activity and proteasome expression in aging spinal cord. *Neuroscience* **2000**, *98*, 149–156. [CrossRef]
199. Tydlacka, S.; Wang, C.E.; Wang, X.; Li, S.; Li, X.J. Differential activities of the ubiquitin-proteasome system in neurons versus glia may account for the preferential accumulation of misfolded proteins in neurons. *J. Neurosci.* **2008**, *28*, 13285–13295. [CrossRef]
200. Giannini, C.; Kloss, A.; Gohlke, S.; Mishto, M.; Nicholson, T.P.; Sheppard, P.W.; Kloetzel, P.M.; Dahlmann, B. Poly-Ub-substrate-degradative activity of 26S proteasome is not impaired in the aging rat brain. *PLoS ONE* **2013**, *8*, e64042. [CrossRef]
201. Keller, J.N.; Hanni, K.B.; Markesbery, W.R. Impaired proteasome function in Alzheimer's disease. *J. Neurochem.* **2000**, *75*, 436–439. [CrossRef] [PubMed]
202. Lopez Salon, M.; Morelli, L.; Castano, E.M.; Soto, E.F.; Pasquini, J.M. Defective ubiquitination of cerebral proteins in Alzheimer's disease. *J. Neurosci. Res.* **2000**, *62*, 302–310. [CrossRef]
203. Jenner, P.; Olanow, C.W. Understanding cell death in Parkinson's disease. *Ann. Neurol.* **1998**, *44*, 72–84. [CrossRef] [PubMed]
204. McNaught, K.S.; Jenner, P. Proteasomal function is impaired in substantia nigra in Parkinson's disease. *Neurosci. Lett.* **2001**, *297*, 191–194. [CrossRef]
205. McNaught, K.S.; Belizaire, R.; Isacson, O.; Jenner, P.; Olanow, C.W. Altered proteasomal function in sporadic Parkinson's disease. *Exp. Neurol.* **2003**, *179*, 38–46. [CrossRef] [PubMed]
206. Ansar, M.; Ebstein, F.; Ozkoc, H.; Paracha, S.A.; Iwaszkiewicz, J.; Gesemann, M.; Zoete, V.; Ranza, E.; Santoni, F.A.; Sarwar, M.T.; et al. Biallelic variants in PSMB1 encoding the proteasome subunit beta6 cause impairment of proteasome function, microcephaly, intellectual disability, developmental delay and short stature. *Hum. Mol. Genet.* **2020**, *29*, 1132–1143. [CrossRef]
207. Brehm, A.; Liu, Y.; Sheikh, A.; Marrero, B.; Omoyinmi, E.; Zhou, Q.; Montealegre, G.; Biancotto, A.; Reinhardt, A.; Almeida de Jesus, A.; et al. Additive loss-of-function proteasome subunit mutations in CANDLE/PRAAS patients promote type I IFN production. *J. Clin. Investig.* **2015**, *125*, 4196–4211. [CrossRef]
208. Verhoeven, D.; Schonenberg-Meinema, D.; Ebstein, F.; Papendorf, J.J.; Baars, P.A.; van Leeuwen, E.M.M.; Jansen, M.H.; Lankester, A.C.; van der Burg, M.; Florquin, S.; et al. Hematopoietic stem cell transplantation in a patient with proteasome-associated auto-inflammatory syndrome (PRAAS). *J. Allergy Clin. Immunol.* **2021**. [CrossRef]
209. Kitamura, A.; Maekawa, Y.; Uehara, H.; Izumi, K.; Kawachi, I.; Nishizawa, M.; Toyoshima, Y.; Takahashi, H.; Standley, D.M.; Tanaka, K.; et al. A mutation in the immunoproteasome subunit PSMB8 causes autoinflammation and lipodystrophy in humans. *J. Clin. Investig.* **2011**, *121*, 4150–4160. [CrossRef]
210. Arima, K.; Kinoshita, A.; Mishima, H.; Kanazawa, N.; Kaneko, T.; Mizushima, T.; Ichinose, K.; Nakamura, H.; Tsujino, A.; Kawakami, A.; et al. Proteasome assembly defect due to a proteasome subunit beta type 8 (PSMB8) mutation causes the autoinflammatory disorder, Nakajo-Nishimura syndrome. *Proc. Natl Acad Sci USA* **2011**, *108*, 14914–14919. [CrossRef]
211. Liu, Y.; Ramot, Y.; Torrelo, A.; Paller, A.S.; Si, N.; Babay, S.; Kim, P.W.; Sheikh, A.; Lee, C.C.; Chen, Y.; et al. Mutations in proteasome subunit beta type 8 cause chronic atypical neutrophilic dermatosis with lipodystrophy and elevated temperature with evidence of genetic and phenotypic heterogeneity. *Arthritis Rheum.* **2012**, *64*, 895–907. [CrossRef] [PubMed]
212. Agarwal, A.K.; Xing, C.; DeMartino, G.N.; Mizrachi, D.; Hernandez, M.D.; Sousa, A.B.; Martinez de Villarreal, L.; dos Santos, H.G.; Garg, A. PSMB8 encoding the beta5i proteasome subunit is mutated in joint contractures, muscle atrophy, microcytic anemia, and panniculitis-induced lipodystrophy syndrome. *Am. J. Hum. Genet.* **2010**, *87*, 866–872. [CrossRef] [PubMed]
213. Jia, T.; Zheng, Y.; Feng, C.; Yang, T.; Geng, S. A Chinese case of Nakajo-Nishimura syndrome with novel compound heterozygous mutations of the PSMB8 gene. *BMC Med. Genet.* **2020**, *21*, 126. [CrossRef]
214. Patel, P.N.; Hunt, R.; Pettigrew, Z.J.; Shirley, J.B.; Vogel, T.P.; de Guzman, M.M. Successful treatment of chronic atypical neutrophilic dermatosis with lipodystrophy and elevated temperature (CANDLE) syndrome with tofacitinib. *Pediatr. Derm.* **2021**, *38*, 528–529. [CrossRef] [PubMed]
215. Boyadzhiev, M.; Marinov, L.; Boyadzhiev, V.; Iotova, V.; Aksentijevich, I.; Hambleton, S. Disease course and treatment effects of a JAK inhibitor in a patient with CANDLE syndrome. *Pediatr. Rheumatol. Online J.* **2019**, *17*, 19. [CrossRef] [PubMed]
216. Yamazaki-Nakashimada, M.A.; Santos-Chavez, E.E.; de Jesus, A.A.; Rivas-Larrauri, F.; Guzman-Martinez, M.N.; Goldbach-Mansky, R.; Espinosa-Padilla, S.; Saez-de-Ocariz, M.D.; Orozco-Covarrubias, L.; Blancas-Galicia, L. Systemic Autoimmunity in a Patient With CANDLE Syndrome. *J. Investig. Allergol. Clin. Immunol.* **2019**, *29*, 75–76. [CrossRef]
217. Cardis, M.A.; Montealegre Sanchez, G.A.; Goldbach-Mansky, R.; Richard Lee, C.C.; Cowen, E.W. Recurrent fevers, progressive lipodystrophy, and annular plaques in a child. *J. Am. Acad. Dermatol.* **2019**, *80*, 291–295. [CrossRef]
218. Kataoka, S.; Kawashima, N.; Okuno, Y.; Muramatsu, H.; Miwata, S.; Narita, K.; Hamada, M.; Murakami, N.; Taniguchi, R.; Ichikawa, D.; et al. Successful treatment of a novel type I interferonopathy due to a de novo PSMB9 gene mutation with a Janus kinase inhibitor. *J. Allergy Clin. Immunol.* **2021**. [CrossRef]
219. Kanazawa, N.; Hemmi, H.; Kinjo, N.; Ohnishi, H.; Hamazaki, J.; Mishima, H.; Kinoshita, A.; Mizushima, T.; Hamada, S.; Hamada, K.; et al. Heterozygous missense variant of the proteasome subunit beta-type 9 causes neonatal-onset autoinflammation and immunodeficiency. *Nat. Commun.* **2021**, *12*, 6819. [CrossRef]

220. Sarrabay, G.; Mechin, D.; Salhi, A.; Boursier, G.; Rittore, C.; Crow, Y.; Rice, G.; Tran, T.A.; Cezar, R.; Duffy, D.; et al. PSMB10, the last immunoproteasome gene missing for PRAAS. *J. Allergy Clin. Immunol.* **2019**. [CrossRef]
221. Poli, M.C.; Ebstein, F.; Nicholas, S.K.; de Guzman, M.M.; Forbes, L.R.; Chinn, I.K.; Mace, E.M.; Vogel, T.P.; Carisey, A.F.; Benavides, F.; et al. Heterozygous Truncating Variants in POMP Escape Nonsense-Mediated Decay and Cause a Unique Immune Dysregulatory Syndrome. *Am. J. Hum. Genet.* **2018**, *102*, 1126–1142. [CrossRef] [PubMed]
222. Meinhardt, A.; Ramos, P.C.; Dohmen, R.J.; Lucas, N.; Lee-Kirsch, M.A.; Becker, B.; de Laffolie, J.; Cunha, T.; Niehues, T.; Salzer, U.; et al. Curative Treatment of POMP-Related Autoinflammation and Immune Dysregulation (PRAID) by Hematopoietic Stem Cell Transplantation. *J. Clin. Immunol.* **2021**, *41*, 1664–1667. [CrossRef] [PubMed]
223. de Jesus, A.A.; Brehm, A.; VanTries, R.; Pillet, P.; Parentelli, A.S.; Montealegre Sanchez, G.A.; Deng, Z.; Paut, I.K.; Goldbach-Mansky, R.; Kruger, E. Novel proteasome assembly chaperone mutations in PSMG2/PAC2 cause the autoinflammatory interferonopathy CANDLE/PRAAS4. *J. Allergy Clin. Immunol.* **2019**, *143*, 1939–1943.e8. [CrossRef] [PubMed]
224. Kury, S.; Besnard, T.; Ebstein, F.; Khan, T.N.; Gambin, T.; Douglas, J.; Bacino, C.A.; Craigen, W.J.; Sanders, S.J.; Lehmann, A.; et al. De Novo Disruption of the Proteasome Regulatory Subunit PSMD12 Causes a Syndromic Neurodevelopmental Disorder. *Am. J. Hum. Genet.* **2017**, *100*, 352–363. [CrossRef] [PubMed]
225. Khalil, R.; Kenny, C.; Hill, R.S.; Mochida, G.H.; Nasir, R.; Partlow, J.N.; Barry, B.J.; Al-Saffar, M.; Egan, C.; Stevens, C.R.; et al. PSMD12 haploinsufficiency in a neurodevelopmental disorder with autistic features. *Am. J. Med. Genet. B Neuropsychiatr. Genet.* **2018**, *177*, 736–745. [CrossRef]
226. Yan, K.; Zhang, J.; Lee, P.Y.; Tao, P.; Wang, J.; Wang, S.; Zhou, Q.; Dong, M. Haploinsufficiency of PSMD12 causes proteasome dysfunction and subclinical autoinflammation. *Arthritis Rheumatol.* **2022**. [CrossRef]
227. Kroll-Hermi, A.; Ebstein, F.; Stoetzel, C.; Geoffroy, V.; Schaefer, E.; Scheidecker, S.; Bar, S.; Takamiya, M.; Kawakami, K.; Zieba, B.A.; et al. Proteasome subunit PSMC3 variants cause neurosensory syndrome combining deafness and cataract due to proteotoxic stress. *EMBO Mol. Med.* **2020**, *12*, e11861. [CrossRef]
228. Kitano, Y.; Matsunaga, E.; Morimoto, T.; Okada, N.; Sano, S. A syndrome with nodular erythema, elongated and thickened fingers, and emaciation. *Arch. Derm.* **1985**, *121*, 1053–1056. [CrossRef]
229. Tanaka, M.; Miyatani, N.; Yamada, S.; Miyashita, K.; Toyoshima, I.; Sakuma, K.; Tanaka, K.; Yuasa, T.; Miyatake, T.; Tsubaki, T. Hereditary lipo-muscular atrophy with joint contracture, skin eruptions and hyper-gamma-globulinemia: A new syndrome. *Intern. Med.* **1993**, *32*, 42–45. [CrossRef]
230. Kasagi, S.; Kawano, S.; Nakazawa, T.; Sugino, H.; Koshiba, M.; Ichinose, K.; Ida, H.; Eguchi, K.; Kumagai, S. A case of periodic-fever-syndrome-like disorder with lipodystrophy, myositis, and autoimmune abnormalities. *Mod. Rheumatol.* **2008**, *18*, 203–207. [CrossRef]
231. Torrelo, A.; Patel, S.; Colmenero, I.; Gurbindo, D.; Lendinez, F.; Hernandez, A.; Lopez-Robledillo, J.C.; Dadban, A.; Requena, L.; Paller, A.S. Chronic atypical neutrophilic dermatosis with lipodystrophy and elevated temperature (CANDLE) syndrome. *J. Am. Acad. Dermatol.* **2010**, *62*, 489–495. [CrossRef] [PubMed]
232. Ramot, Y.; Czarnowicki, T.; Maly, A.; Navon-Elkan, P.; Zlotogorski, A. Chronic atypical neutrophilic dermatosis with lipodystrophy and elevated temperature syndrome: A case report. *Pediatr. Derm.* **2011**, *28*, 538–541. [CrossRef] [PubMed]
233. Kimura, H.; Usui, F.; Karasawa, T.; Kawashima, A.; Shirasuna, K.; Inoue, Y.; Komada, T.; Kobayashi, M.; Mizushina, Y.; Kasahara, T.; et al. Immunoproteasome subunit LMP7 Deficiency Improves Obesity and Metabolic Disorders. *Sci. Rep.* **2015**, *5*, 15883. [CrossRef]
234. Martinez, C.A.; Ebstein, F.; Nicholas, S.K.; De Guzman, M.; Forbes, L.R.; Delmonte, O.M.; Bosticardo, M.; Castagnoli, R.; Krance, R.; Notarangelo, L.D.; et al. HSCT corrects primary immunodeficiency and immune dysregulation in patients with POMP-related auto-inflammatory disease. *Blood* **2021**. [CrossRef]
235. Studencka-Turski, M.; Cetin, G.; Junker, H.; Ebstein, F.; Kruger, E. Molecular Insight Into the IRE1alpha-Mediated Type I Interferon Response Induced by Proteasome Impairment in Myeloid Cells of the Brain. *Front. Immunol.* **2019**, *10*, 2900. [CrossRef] [PubMed]
236. Minton, K. Sensing proteotoxic stress. *Nat. Rev. Immunol.* **2022**. [CrossRef] [PubMed]
237. Crow, Y.J.; Manel, N. Aicardi-Goutieres syndrome and the type I interferonopathies. *Nat. Rev. Immunol.* **2015**, *15*, 429–440. [CrossRef]
238. Sullivan, K.D.; Evans, D.; Pandey, A.; Hraha, T.H.; Smith, K.P.; Markham, N.; Rachubinski, A.L.; Wolter-Warmerdam, K.; Hickey, F.; Espinosa, J.M.; et al. Trisomy 21 causes changes in the circulating proteome indicative of chronic autoinflammation. *Sci. Rep.* **2017**, *7*, 14818. [CrossRef]
239. Sullivan, K.D.; Lewis, H.C.; Hill, A.A.; Pandey, A.; Jackson, L.P.; Cabral, J.M.; Smith, K.P.; Liggett, L.A.; Gomez, E.B.; Galbraith, M.D.; et al. Trisomy 21 consistently activates the interferon response. *eLife* **2016**, *5*. [CrossRef]
240. Waugh, K.A.; Araya, P.; Pandey, A.; Jordan, K.R.; Smith, K.P.; Granrath, R.E.; Khanal, S.; Butcher, E.T.; Estrada, B.E.; Rachubinski, A.L.; et al. Mass Cytometry Reveals Global Immune Remodeling with Multi-lineage Hypersensitivity to Type I Interferon in Down Syndrome. *Cell Rep.* **2019**, *29*, 1893–1908.e4. [CrossRef]
241. Zhou, Q.; Wang, H.; Schwartz, D.M.; Stoffels, M.; Park, Y.H.; Zhang, Y.; Yang, D.; Demirkaya, E.; Takeuchi, M.; Tsai, W.L.; et al. Loss-of-function mutations in TNFAIP3 leading to A20 haploinsufficiency cause an early-onset autoinflammatory disease. *Nat. Genet.* **2016**, *48*, 67–73. [CrossRef] [PubMed]

242. Damgaard, R.B.; Walker, J.A.; Marco-Casanova, P.; Morgan, N.V.; Titheradge, H.L.; Elliott, P.R.; McHale, D.; Maher, E.R.; McKenzie, A.N.J.; Komander, D. The Deubiquitinase OTULIN Is an Essential Negative Regulator of Inflammation and Autoimmunity. *Cell* **2016**, *166*, 1215–1230. [CrossRef] [PubMed]
243. Damgaard, R.B.; Elliott, P.R.; Swatek, K.N.; Maher, E.R.; Stepensky, P.; Elpeleg, O.; Komander, D.; Berkun, Y. OTULIN deficiency in ORAS causes cell type-specific LUBAC degradation, dysregulated TNF signalling and cell death. *EMBO Mol. Med.* **2019**, *11*. [CrossRef] [PubMed]
244. Meuwissen, M.E.; Schot, R.; Buta, S.; Oudesluijs, G.; Tinschert, S.; Speer, S.D.; Li, Z.; van Unen, L.; Heijsman, D.; Goldmann, T.; et al. Human USP18 deficiency underlies type 1 interferonopathy leading to severe pseudo-TORCH syndrome. *J. Exp. Med.* **2016**, *213*, 1163–1174. [CrossRef] [PubMed]
245. Boisson, B.; Laplantine, E.; Dobbs, K.; Cobat, A.; Tarantino, N.; Hazen, M.; Lidov, H.G.; Hopkins, G.; Du, L.; Belkadi, A.; et al. Human HOIP and LUBAC deficiency underlies autoinflammation, immunodeficiency, amylopectinosis, and lymphangiectasia. *J. Exp. Med.* **2015**, *212*, 939–951. [CrossRef]
246. Boisson, B.; Laplantine, E.; Prando, C.; Giliani, S.; Israelsson, E.; Xu, Z.; Abhyankar, A.; Israel, L.; Trevejo-Nunez, G.; Bogunovic, D.; et al. Immunodeficiency, autoinflammation and amylopectinosis in humans with inherited HOIL-1 and LUBAC deficiency. *Nat. Immunol.* **2012**, *13*, 1178–1186. [CrossRef] [PubMed]
247. Oda, H.; Beck, D.B.; Kuehn, H.S.; Sampaio Moura, N.; Hoffmann, P.; Ibarra, M.; Stoddard, J.; Tsai, W.L.; Gutierrez-Cruz, G.; Gadina, M.; et al. Second Case of HOIP Deficiency Expands Clinical Features and Defines Inflammatory Transcriptome Regulated by LUBAC. *Front. Immunol.* **2019**, *10*, 479. [CrossRef]
248. Di Donato, G.; d'Angelo, D.M.; Breda, L.; Chiarelli, F. Monogenic Autoinflammatory Diseases: State of the Art and Future Perspectives. *Int. J. Mol. Sci.* **2021**, *22*, 6360. [CrossRef]
249. Zimmermann, A.; Kainz, K.; Andryushkova, A.; Hofer, S.; Madeo, F.; Carmona-Gutierrez, D. Autophagy: One more Nobel Prize for yeast. *Microb. Cell* **2016**, *3*, 579–581. [CrossRef]
250. Tooze, S.A.; Dikic, I. Autophagy Captures the Nobel Prize. *Cell* **2016**, *167*, 1433–1435. [CrossRef]
251. Galluzzi, L.; Baehrecke, E.H.; Ballabio, A.; Boya, P.; Bravo-San Pedro, J.M.; Cecconi, F.; Choi, A.M.; Chu, C.T.; Codogno, P.; Colombo, M.I.; et al. Molecular definitions of autophagy and related processes. *EMBO J.* **2017**, *36*, 1811–1836. [CrossRef] [PubMed]
252. Kitada, M.; Koya, D. Autophagy in metabolic disease and ageing. *Nat. Rev. Endocrinol.* **2021**, *17*, 647–661. [CrossRef] [PubMed]
253. Tan, S.; Wong, E. Kinetics of Protein Aggregates Disposal by Aggrephagy. *Methods Enzym.* **2017**, *588*, 245–281. [CrossRef]
254. Gatica, D.; Lahiri, V.; Klionsky, D.J. Cargo recognition and degradation by selective autophagy. *Nat. Cell Biol.* **2018**, *20*, 233–242. [CrossRef] [PubMed]
255. Hara, T.; Nakamura, K.; Matsui, M.; Yamamoto, A.; Nakahara, Y.; Suzuki-Migishima, R.; Yokoyama, M.; Mishima, K.; Saito, I.; Okano, H.; et al. Suppression of basal autophagy in neural cells causes neurodegenerative disease in mice. *Nature* **2006**, *441*, 885–889. [CrossRef]
256. Haack, T.B.; Ignatius, E.; Calvo-Garrido, J.; Iuso, A.; Isohanni, P.; Maffezzini, C.; Lonnqvist, T.; Suomalainen, A.; Gorza, M.; Kremer, L.S.; et al. Absence of the Autophagy Adaptor SQSTM1/p62 Causes Childhood-Onset Neurodegeneration with Ataxia, Dystonia, and Gaze Palsy. *Am. J. Hum. Genet.* **2016**, *99*, 735–743. [CrossRef]
257. Roodman, G.D.; Kurihara, N.; Ohsaki, Y.; Kukita, A.; Hosking, D.; Demulder, A.; Smith, J.F.; Singer, F.R. Interleukin 6. A potential autocrine/paracrine factor in Paget's disease of bone. *J. Clin. Investig.* **1992**, *89*, 46–52. [CrossRef]
258. Poloni, M.; Facchetti, D.; Mai, R.; Micheli, A.; Agnoletti, L.; Francolini, G.; Mora, G.; Camana, C.; Mazzini, L.; Bachetti, T. Circulating levels of tumour necrosis factor-alpha and its soluble receptors are increased in the blood of patients with amyotrophic lateral sclerosis. *Neurosci. Lett.* **2000**, *287*, 211–214. [CrossRef]
259. Wooten, M.W.; Geetha, T.; Seibenhener, M.L.; Babu, J.R.; Diaz-Meco, M.T.; Moscat, J. The p62 scaffold regulates nerve growth factor-induced NF-kappaB activation by influencing TRAF6 polyubiquitination. *J. Biol. Chem.* **2005**, *280*, 35625–35629. [CrossRef]
260. Rea, S.L.; Walsh, J.P.; Layfield, R.; Ratajczak, T.; Xu, J. New insights into the role of sequestosome 1/p62 mutant proteins in the pathogenesis of Paget's disease of bone. *Endocr. Rev.* **2013**, *34*, 501–524. [CrossRef]
261. Kim, M.; Sandford, E.; Gatica, D.; Qiu, Y.; Liu, X.; Zheng, Y.; Schulman, B.A.; Xu, J.; Semple, I.; Ro, S.H.; et al. Mutation in ATG5 reduces autophagy and leads to ataxia with developmental delay. *eLife* **2016**, *5*. [CrossRef] [PubMed]
262. Collier, J.J.; Guissart, C.; Olahova, M.; Sasorith, S.; Piron-Prunier, F.; Suomi, F.; Zhang, D.; Martinez-Lopez, N.; Leboucq, N.; Bahr, A.; et al. Developmental Consequences of Defective ATG7-Mediated Autophagy in Humans. *N. Engl. J. Med.* **2021**, *384*, 2406–2417. [CrossRef] [PubMed]
263. Shin, E.C.; Seifert, U.; Urban, S.; Truong, K.T.; Feinstone, S.M.; Rice, C.M.; Kloetzel, P.M.; Rehermann, B. Proteasome activator and antigen-processing aminopeptidases are regulated by virus-induced type I interferon in the hepatitis C virus-infected liver. *J. Interferon Cytokine Res.* **2007**, *27*, 985–990. [CrossRef] [PubMed]
264. Bousoik, E.; Montazeri Aliabadi, H. "Do We Know Jack" About JAK? A Closer Look at JAK/STAT Signaling Pathway. *Front. Oncol.* **2018**, *8*, 287. [CrossRef] [PubMed]

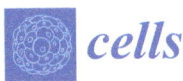

Article

Effect of Thrombin on the Metabolism and Function of Murine Macrophages

Ürün Ukan [1], Fredy Delgado Lagos [1], Sebastian Kempf [1], Stefan Günther [2], Mauro Siragusa [1], Beate Fisslthaler [1] and Ingrid Fleming [1,3,4,*]

[1] Institute for Vascular Signalling, Centre for Molecular Medicine, Goethe University, 60596 Frankfurt am Main, Germany; ukan@vrc.uni-frankfurt.de (Ü.U.); lagos@vrc.uni-frankfurt.de (F.D.L.); kempf@vrc.uni-frankfurt.de (S.K.); siragusa@vrc.uni-frankfurt.de (M.S.); fisslthaler@vrc.uni-frankfurt.de (B.F.)
[2] Bioinformatics and Deep Sequencing Platform, Max Planck Institute for Heart and Lung Research, 61231 Bad Nauheim, Germany; stefan.guenther@mpi-bn.mpg.de
[3] German Center of Cardiovascular Research (DZHK), Partner Site RheinMain, 60596 Frankfurt am Main, Germany
[4] CardioPulmonary Institute, Goethe University, 60596 Frankfurt am Main, Germany
* Correspondence: fleming@em.uni-frankfurt.de

Abstract: Macrophages are plastic and heterogeneous immune cells that adapt pro- or anti-inflammatory phenotypes upon exposure to different stimuli. Even though there has been evidence supporting a crosstalk between coagulation and innate immunity, the way in which protein components of the hemostasis pathway influence macrophages remains unclear. We investigated the effect of thrombin on macrophage polarization. On the basis of gene expression and cytokine secretion, our results suggest that polarization with thrombin induces an anti-inflammatory, M2-like phenotype. In functional studies, thrombin polarization promoted oxLDL phagocytosis by macrophages, and conditioned medium from the same cells increased endothelial cell proliferation. There were, however, clear differences between the classical M2a polarization and the effects of thrombin on gene expression. Finally, the deletion and inactivation of secreted modular Ca^{2+}-binding protein 1 (SMOC1) attenuated phagocytosis by thrombin-stimulated macrophages, a phenomenon revered by the addition of recombinant SMOC1. Manipulation of SMOC1 levels also had a pronounced impact on the expression of TGF-β-signaling-related genes. Taken together, our results show that thrombin induces an anti-inflammatory macrophage phenotype with similarities as well as differences to the classical alternatively activated M2 polarization states, highlighting the importance of tissue levels of SMOC1 in modifying thrombin-induced macrophage polarization.

Keywords: SMOC1; macrophage polarization; thrombin

1. Introduction

The coagulation cascade and the innate immune system are activated in response to insult or injury and act to stop blood loss; eradicate invading pathogens; and, later on, to re-establish homeostasis. Despite evidence of collaboration between the two pathways, humoral connections between blood constituents and inflammatory macrophages are not well understood. One potential molecular mediator of such communication is the serine protease thrombin [1]. Best known for its actions on fibrinogen and platelets, thrombin exerts its effects via the activation of G-protein-coupled receptors belonging to the protease activated receptor (PAR) family [2]. Four different PARs are expressed by different cell types, and thrombin interacts with PAR1, 3, and 4 to initiate downstream actions [3]. The best studied are probably the PAR1- and PAR4-mediated effects on platelet aggregation [4], but thrombin plays an important nonhemostatic role in the disruption of endothelial cell barrier function [5] and endothelial cell activation, leading to monocyte adhesion [6,7] and even cancer [8,9].

PARs are also expressed by monocytes where their activation has been linked with atherosclerosis [10,11], but the consequences of thrombin on macrophage responses are unclear. Indeed, in mice, thrombin has been reported to activate PAR2 to promote macrophage polarization into a classically activated or M1-like phenotype to induce inflammatory responses [12,13] and to sensitize macrophages to M1 polarization induced by interferon-γ (IFN-γ) [14]. However, thrombin has also been reported to induce alternative or M2 macrophage polarization with impaired plasticity [15,16]. There are a number of proteins known to inhibit thrombin activity, but recently, a matricellular protein, i.e., secreted modular Ca^{2+}-binding protein (SMOC 1), was reported to bind to and activate thrombin to promote platelet activation [17]. The aim of the present study was, therefore, to revisit the topic of thrombin-induced macrophage polarization and to determine how SMOC1 affects thrombin-induced macrophage polarization.

2. Materials and Methods

2.1. Animals

Wild-type (C57BL/6) mice were from Charles River (Sulzfeld, Germany), SMOC1 (B6D2-Smoc1 < Tn(sb-lacZ,GFP)PV384Jtak > /JtakRbrc) mice ($SMOC1^{+/-}$) were from the RIKEN BioResource Center (Tsukuba, Japan), and mTnG (B6.129(Cg)-Gt(ROSA)26Sortm4 (ACTB-tdTomato,-EGFP)Luo/) mice were kindly provided by Ralf Adams (Münster). All animals were housed in conditions that conform to the Guide for the Care and Use of Laboratory Animals published by the U.S. National Institutes of Health (NIH publication no. 85-23). Both the University Animal Care Committee and the Federal Authority for Animal Research at the Regierungspräsidium Darmstadt (Hessen, Germany) approved the study protocol (V54-19c, 2.04.2020). For the isolation of bone marrow, mice were sacrificed using 4% isoflurane in air and cervical dislocation.

2.2. Monocyte Isolation and Culture

Murine monocytes: Monocytes were isolated from the bone marrow of 8–10-week-old mice and cultured in RPMI 1640 medium (Invitrogen, Karlsruhe, Germany, Baden-Wurtemberg) supplemented with M-CSF (15 ng/mL; Peprotech, Hamburg, Germany) and GM-CSF (15 ng/mL; Peprotech, Hamburg, Germany) for 7 days to generate macrophages.

2.3. Macrophage Polarization

Macrophages were polarized to classical activated M1 macrophages by treating with LPS (human: 100 ng/mL, murine: 10 ng/mL; Sigma-Aldrich, Munich, Germany) and IFN-γ (human: 20 ng/mL, murine: 1 ng/mL; Peprotech, Hamburg, Germany) for 12 h and to alternative M2a macrophages by treating with IL-4 (20 ng/mL; Peprotech, Hamburg, Germany) for 24 h. Pro-resolving M2c macrophages were repolarized from M1 macrophages by the addition of TGF-β1 (10 ng/mL; Peprotech, Hamburg) for 48 h. Thrombin-induced macrophage polarization was achieved by incubating macrophages with thrombin (0.1 or 1 U/mL; Haemochrom Diagnostica Essen, Germany) for up to 48 h.

2.4. Immunoblotting

Bone-marrow-derived macrophages were lysed in ice-cold Triton X-100 lysis buffer (20 mmol/L Tris/HCl (pH 7.5), 1% Triton X-100, 25 mmol/L β-glycerolphosphate, 150 mmol/L NaCl, 10 mmol/L Na pyrophosphate, 20 mmol/L NaF) containing 2 mmol/L Na orthovanadate, 10 mmol/L okadaic acid, and a protease inhibitor mix (2 µg/mL antipain, 2 µg/mL aprotinin, 2 µg/mL chymostatin, 2 µg/mL leupeptin, 2 µg/mL pepstatin, 2 µg trypsin inhibitor, and 40 µg/mL phenylmethysulfonylfluoride). Samples were then separated by SDS-PAGE and subjected to Western blotting. Detection was performed by enhanced chemiluminescence using a commercially available kit (Amersham, Freiburg, Germany) as described [18].

2.5. RT-qPCR

Total RNA was extracted and purified from wild-type and SMOC1+/− macrophages using Tri Reagent (ThermoFisher Scientific, Karlsruhe, Germany) according to the manufacturer's instructions. RNA was eluted in nuclease-free water, and RNA concentration was spectrophotometrically determined at 260 nm using a NanoDrop ND-1000 (ThermoFischer Scientific, Karlsruhe, Germany). For the generation of complementary DNA (cDNA), total RNA (250 ng) was reverse-transcribed using SuperScript IV (ThermoFischer Scientific, Karlsruhe, Germany) and random hexamer primers (Promega, Madison, WI, USA) according to the manufacturer's protocol. qPCR was performed using SYBR green master mix (Biozym, Hessisch Oldendorf, Germany) and appropriate primers (Table 1) in a MIC-RUN quantitative PCR system (Bio Molecular Systems, Upper Coomera, Australia). Relative RNA levels were determined using a serial dilution of a positive control. The data are shown relative to the mean of the housekeeping genes, elongation factor (EF) 2 and 18S RNA.

Table 1. PCR primers used.

Gene	Forward	Reverse
NOS	GTGGTGACAAGCACATTTGG	GTTCGTCCCCTTCTCCTGTT
TNF-α	GGCCTTCCTACCTTCAGACC	CCGGCCTTCCAAATAAATAC
FIZZ-1	CCCTTCTCATCTGCATCTCC	CAGTAGCAGTCATCCCAGCA
CD206	TGGATGGATGGGAGCAAAGT	GCTGCTGTTATGTCTCTGGC
MMP9	GAAGGCAAACCCTGTGTGTT	AGAGTACTGCTTGCCCAGGA
CD36	AAACCCAGATGACGTGGCAA	AAGATGGCTCCATTGGGCTG
EF2	GACATCACCAAGGGTGTGCAG	GCGGTCAGCACACTGGCATA
18S	CTTTGGTCGCTCGCTCCTC	CTGACCGGGTTGGTTTTGAT

2.6. Phagocytosis Assays

Murine bone-marrow-derived monocytes were seeded onto 96-well plates and differentiated into macrophages by treating with MCSF and GMCSF for 7 days. After differentiation was complete, macrophages were polarized as described above, or treated with thrombin for up to 48 h. Thereafter, either dil-oxLDL (1:200; Thermofisher, Darmstadt, Germany) or pHrodo Green zymosan bioparticles (1 mg/mL, Thermofisher, Darmstadt, Germany) was added, and phagocytosis was monitored over 24 h using an automated live cell imaging system (IncuCyte; Sartorius, Göttingen Germany).

2.7. FACS Analysis

Detection of the pro-inflammatory cytokine, and chemokine secretion was performed according to the instructions of manufacturer (BioLegend, LEGENDplex Mouse Proinflammatory Chemokine Panel). In brief, macrophage supernatant was collected in 1.5 mL tubes, snap froze with liquid nitrogen, and kept in −80 °C until measurement. Samples and standards provided by the kit were transferred onto a 96-well filter plate, then incubated with equal amounts of assay buffer, and in beads for 2 h at room temperature on a shaker. Wells were washed with wash buffer twice, followed by an incubation with the detection antibody for an hour again on a shaker. At the end of incubation, SA-PE was added into the wells, and the plate was left to incubate for 30 min on a shaker; then, wells were again washed with wash buffer twice, and samples were re-suspended with wash buffer for immediate FACS analysis.

2.8. RNA Sequencing

Total RNA was isolated from macrophages by using an RNeasy Micro kit (Qiagen, Hilden, Germany) on the basis of the manufacturer's instructions. The RNA concentrations were determined by using NanoDrop ND-1000 (TFS, Waltham, MA, USA; λ 600 nm). Total RNA (1 μg) was used as input for the SMARTer Stranded Total RNA Sample Prep Kit—HI Mammalian (Takara Bio, Kusatsu shi, Japan).

Trimmomatic version 0.39 was employed to trim reads after a quality drop below a mean of Q20 in a window of 20 nucleotides and keeping only filtered reads longer than 15 nucleotides [19]. Reads were aligned versus Ensembl mouse genome version mm10 (Ensembl release 101) with STAR 2.7.10a [20]. Aligned reads were filtered to remove duplicates with Picard 2.25.5 (Picard: A set of tools (in Java) for working with next-generation sequencing data in the BAM format), multi-mapping, ribosomal, or mitochondrial reads. Gene counts were established with featureCounts 2.0.2 by aggregating reads overlapping exons on the correct strand, excluding those overlapping multiple genes [21]. The raw count matrix was normalized with DESeq2 version 1.30.1 [22]. Contrasts were created with DESeq2 on the basis of the raw count matrix. Genes were classified as significantly differentially expressed at average count > 5, multiple testing adjusted p-value < 0.05, and $-0.585 < \log2FC > 0.585$. The Ensemble annotation was enriched with UniProt data [23].

2.9. Metabolomics

Metabolites for targeted metabolomics were extracted by scraping the cells on ice, with ice-cold extraction buffer, containing methanol, formic acid (0.1%), TCEP (1 mmol/L), and sodium ascorbate (1 mmol/L). After centrifugation and removal of protein, the sample extract was divided into equal fractions for amino acid and TCA cycle analysis.

2.9.1. Amino Acid Analyses

Samples were spiked with an internal standard mix and dried (Concentrator plus; Eppendorf, Hamburg, Germany) at 45 °C. The dried samples were reconstituted in 20 μL HCl (20 mmol/L) and derivatized according to the AccQ-Tag derivatization kit protocol (Waters GmbH, Eschborn, Germany) by adding 70 μL borate buffer and 20 μL ACQ-Tag reagent and incubating at 55 °C for 10 min. For data acquisition, an Agilent 1290 Infinity II ultra-performance liquid chromatography (UPLC) system coupled to a QTrap 5500 LC–MS/MS system from ABSciex (Darmstadt, Germany) was used in positive ion mode. Metabolite separation of derivatized amino acids was achieved with a flow rate of 300 μL/min at 35 °C on an Extend C18-column (150 × 2.1 mm, 1.8 μm; Agilent). Raw data extraction and peak identification was performed using the SCIEX OS (2.2) software.

2.9.2. TCA Cycle

An internal standard mix was added to the corresponding fraction, and samples were freeze-dried (Alpha 3–4 LSCbasic; Christ, Osterode am Harz, Germany). Dried samples were reconstituted in formic acid (0.5%) and introduced to an Agilent 1290 Infinity UPLC platform coupled to an Agilent 6495 Triple quadrupole LC/MS system (Santa Clara, CA, USA) used in negative ion mode. Metabolites were separated on an ACQUITY UPLC HSS T3 column (150 × 2.1 mm, 1.8 μm; Waters) at a flow rate of 300 μL/min at 40 °C. Raw data extraction and peak identification were performed using the MassHunter Quantitative Analysis software.

Data analysis was performed after normalization to the protein content. For the unsupervised principal component analysis, MetboAnalyst 5.0 (www.metaboanalyst.ca (accessed on 22 March 2022)) was used.

2.10. Immunofluorescence

After polarizations were completed, macrophages were treated with diloxLDL 1:200 (Thermo Fischer Scientific) for 15 min, then fixed with 4% Rotifix, and blocked with 3% horse serum for an hour. At the end of incubation macrophages were incubated with primary antibodies overnight at +4 °C on a shaker, then washed 3 times with 1X PBS. After the washing was completed, macrophages were incubated with secondary antibodies for an hour on a shaker and washed again 3 times with phosphate-buffered saline. Finally, macrophages were incubated with Hoechst (1:1000), and images were taken with a confocal microscope (LSM-780; Zeiss, Jena, Germany) with ZEN Software (Zeiss).

2.11. Endothelial Cell Proliferation

Murine pulmonary endothelial cells were isolated from mTnG mice as described previously [18] and used at passage 5 following repurification with CD31-antibody-coated magnetic beads. Thereafter, cells (10^4 cells/96-well) were seeded in DMEM/F12 containing glucose/L (5 mmol/L), 20% FCS, endothelial cell growth supplement with heparin, and penicillin and streptomycin (each 50 ug/mL). After complete adherence (4 to 6 h), the medium was exchanged to 50% MLEC basal medium (2% FCS but without ECGS-H) and 50% macrophage-conditioned medium. Pictures for phase contrast and GFP-emitted fluorescence were taken every 4 h with an InCucyteS3 (Sartorius, Göttingen, Germany) to monitor cell division and plate coverage. Green nuclei were normalized to the number of nuclei at 4 h.

2.12. Statistical Analyses

Data are expressed as mean ± SEM. One-way ANOVA was used for comparison of three or more groups with one variable, and two-way ANOVA was used for comparison of variance between multiple groups and two variables. ANOVA was followed by Bonferroni's or Tukey's multiple comparison tests. Values of $p < 0.05$ were considered statistically significant.

3. Results

3.1. Effects of Thrombin on Macrophage Gene Expression

Murine bone-marrow-derived macrophages were maintained in culture or treated with LPS and IFN-γ to generate classically activated M1 macrophages, with IL-4 to generate alternatively activated M2a macrophages, or with LPS and IFN-γ followed by TGF-β to result in pro-resolving M2c macrophages. The expression of routinely used polarization markers was then assessed and compared with the effects of incubating macrophages with thrombin (1 U/mL) for up to 48 h. Different time points of thrombin stimulation were assessed as the M1 response usually peaks at or before 12 h, while the pro-resolving polarization takes up to 48 h.

Thrombin–treated macrophages did not express classical M1 markers such as tumor necrosis factor-α (TNF-α), inducible nitric oxide synthase (iNOS), or the M2 marker gene found in inflammatory zone-1 (Fizz-1) (Figure 1A). Thrombin did, however, increase the expression of MRC-1, MMP9, and CD36, with slightly higher expression detected after 48 rather than 24 h. The lack of effect on iNOS was confirmed at the protein level, as was the inability to induce the phosphorylation of STAT6 (Figure 1B), which tends to be elevated in M2a-polarized macrophages [24]. Different cytokines are secreted by macrophages in different polarization states [25]. For example, CCL5 (RANTES) and CCL2 (monocyte chemoattractant protein-1) were produced by M1- and M2c-polarized macrophages, but high levels of CCL22 (macrophage-derived chemokine) were only generated by M2c macrophages. This contrasted with previous reports of it being elevated in M2a-polarized cells [26]. Thrombin did not elicit the expression of CCL2 or CCL5 but did increase CCL22 levels (Figure 1C). These observations indicate that thrombin elicits changes in macrophage gene expression that are consistent with a state intermediate between M2a and M2c.

3.2. Metabolic Characterization of Thrombin-Polarized Macrophages

Monitoring metabolism provides a more accurate indication of functional similarities than the analysis of specific marker genes. Therefore, TCA cycle pathway metabolites as well as amino acids were quantified in M0-, M1-, M2a-, M2c-, and thrombin-polarized murine macrophages. Principal component analysis revealed metabolic signatures that were clearly distinct in M0-, M1-, M2a-, and M2c-polarized cells (Figure 2A). Thrombin-treated macrophages were most similar to M2a-polarized cells after 24 h and most similar to the M0 state after 48 h. Metabolites of the TCA cycle were largely comparable in M2a- and thrombin-polarized macrophages (Figure 2B). An analysis of amino acid levels, however, revealed clear differences between the M2a- and thrombin-polarized groups

(Figure 3A,B). While levels of citruilline, allantoin, and tryptophan were comparable in M2a- and thrombin-polarized macrophages (Figure 3C), levels of arginine, lysine, alanine, anthranilic acid, ethanolamine, and itaconate were clearly different. These metabolic data confirmed the results on the expression studies, i.e., that thrombin does not induce an M1-like activation of macrophages but rather reprograms them to a state with some similarities to M2 states.

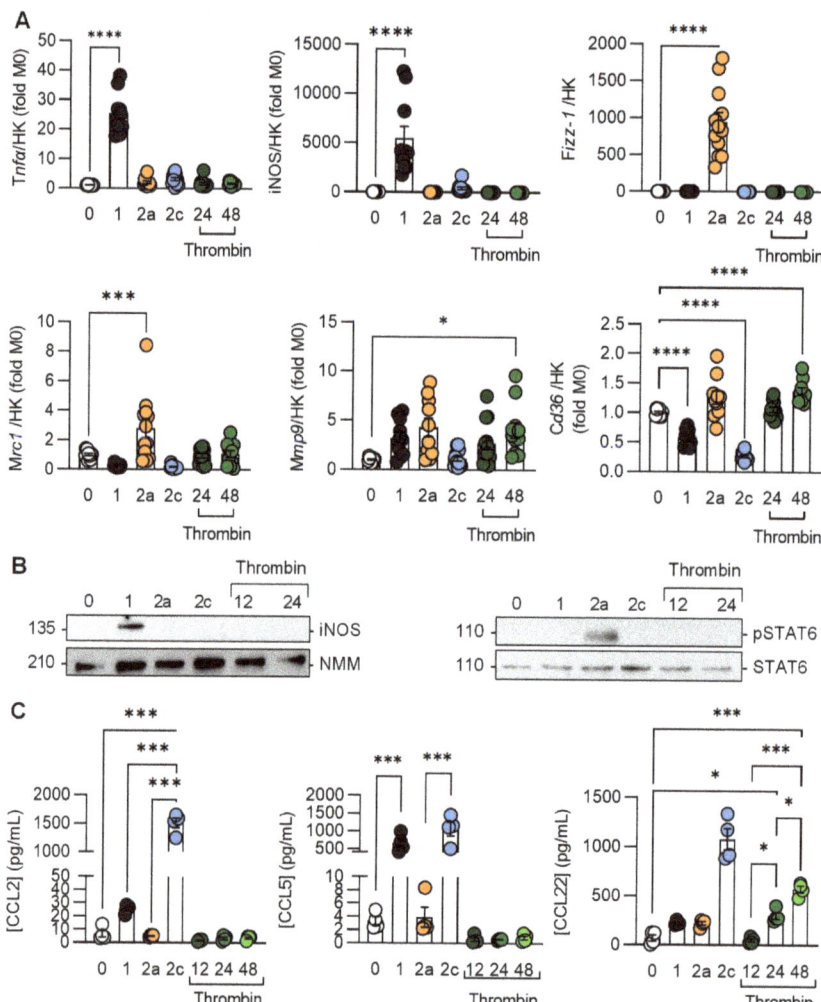

Figure 1. Effects of thrombin in murine macrophage chemokines. Murine bone-marrow-monocyte-derived macrophages were treated with either solvent (MØ) or with the combination of LPS (10 ng/mL) and INF-γ (1 ng/mL) for M1 polarization; IL-4 (20 ng/mL) for M2a polarization; and thrombin (1 U/mL) for 12, 24, and 48 h for Mth polarization. M1 macrophages were treated with TGF-β1 (10 ng/mL) for 48 h for M2c polarization. (**A**) mRNA expression of macrophage phenotype markers with qPCR; n = 6 mice. HK = housekeeping genes. (**B**) Representative blots showing the expression of iNOS and the phosphorylation of STAT6 (pSTAT6) in differently polarized macrophages; n = 4 mice. NMM = non muscle myosin. (**C**) Cytokine levels in the macrophage supernatant; n = 4 mice. All experiments were performed at least twice. (**A,C**) One-way ANOVA followed by Tukey's multiple comparison test. * $p < 0.05$, *** $p < 0.001$, **** $p < 0.0001$.

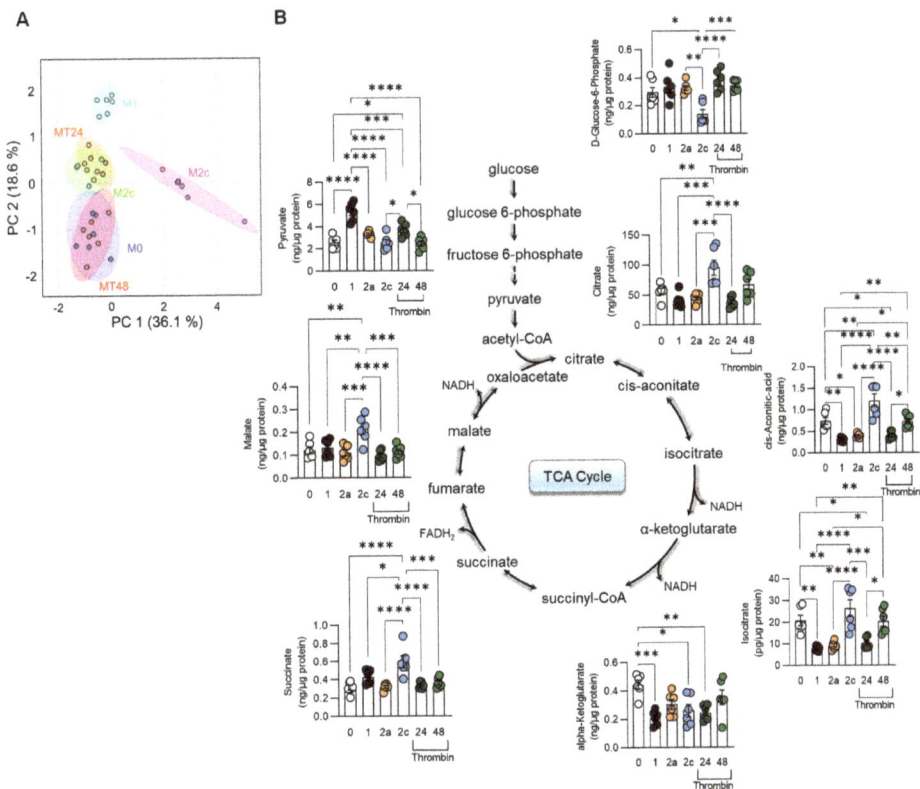

Figure 2. Effects of thrombin on macrophage TCA cycle metabolites. (**A**) Principal component (PC) analysis of TCA and glycolysis-related metabolites of the different macrophage polarization states versus cells treated with thrombin for 24 (MT24) or 48 h (MT48). (**B**) Polarization-dependent changes in specific glycolytic pathway and TCA cycle metabolites; n = 6 mice (one-way ANOVA and Tukey's multiple comparison test). * $p < 0.05$, ** $p < 0.01$, *** $p < 0.001$, **** $p < 0.0001$.

3.3. Functional Characterization of Thrombin-Polarized Macrophages

Alternatively activated or M2 macrophages are regarded as a continuum of functionally and phenotypically related cells, with a critical role in type II inflammation and in the resolution and tissue repair phases [27]. These cells can be subdivided into M2a and M2b, corresponding to type-II-activated macrophages obtained by triggering Fcγ receptors in the presence of a Toll receptor stimulus, and M2c, which includes deactivation programs elicited by agents such as transforming growth factor β (TGF-β) [27]. There is even an M2d phenotype that results from adenosine-dependent "switching" of M1 [28].

One characteristic of M2 macrophages is their ability to clear apoptotic cell debris, as well as to take up different lipids by phagocytosis [29]. We, therefore, compared the phagocytosis of oxidized low-density lipoprotein (ox-LDL) by polarized murine macrophages and observed the expected low uptake by M1-polarized cells (Figure 4A). There was, however, a clear increase in phagocytosis following M2a and M2c polarization that was even surpassed by the effects seen in cells pretreated with thrombin for 48 h. A similar phenomenon was observed using pHrodo-labelled zymosan (Figure 4B,C). M2-polarized macrophages also release exosomes and a number of soluble factors to promote angiogenesis. Therefore, conditioned medium from polarized macrophages was collected and added to subconfluent pulmonary endothelial cells from mice expressing GFP in their nuclei. Conditioned medium from thrombin-treated macrophages clearly increased endothelial cell proliferation (Figure 4D) and was equally as effective as medium from M1- and M2a-polarized macrophages, which is consistent with the well-described effects of cytokines on angiogenesis [30].

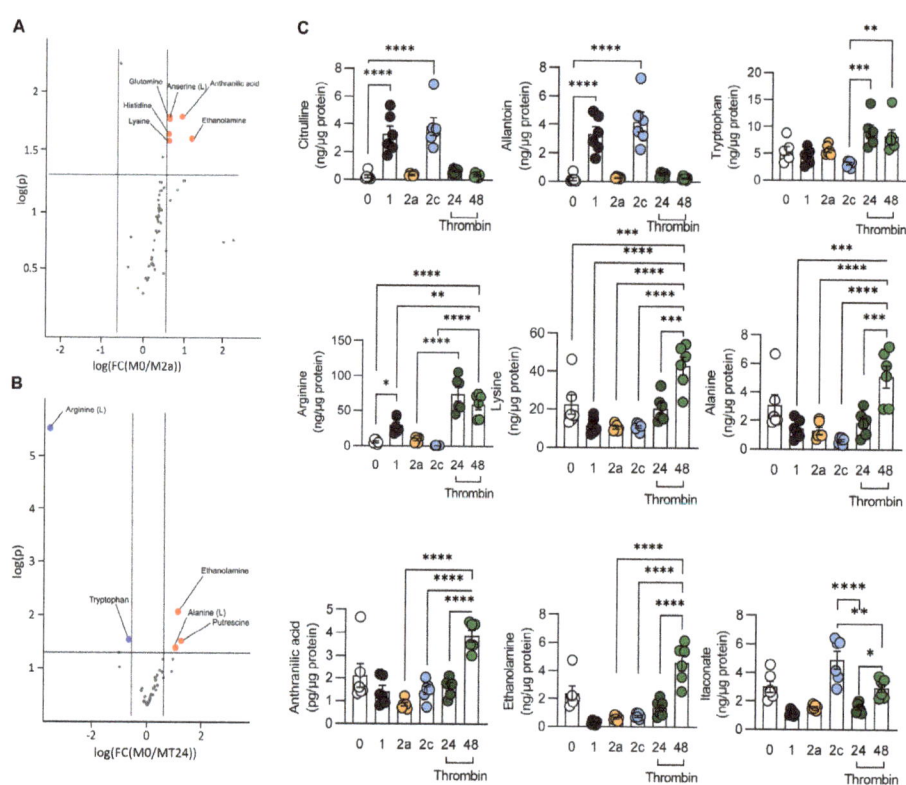

Figure 3. Effects of thrombin on macrophage amino acid metabolism. (**A**) Volcano plot comparing amino acid levels in M0 versus M2a macrophages. (**B**) Volcano plot comparing amino acid levels in M0 macrophages compared to macrophages treated with thrombin for 24 h (MT24). (**C**) Levels of selected amino acids in M0-, M1-, M2a-, and M2c-polarized macrophages versus macrophages treated with thrombin for up to 48 h; n = 6 mice (one-way ANOVA and Tukey's multiple comparison test). * $p < 0.05$, ** $p < 0.01$, *** $p < 0.001$, **** $p < 0.0001$.

3.4. Transcriptional Characterization of Thrombin-Polarized Macrophages

In order to gain insight into the impact of thrombin stimulation on alterations in macrophage gene expression, we performed RNA sequencing. While our metabolic data showed similar clustering between naïve, anti-inflammatory, and thrombin-polarized macrophages, the gene profile of thrombin-stimulated macrophages was clearly distinct from that of M0 macrophages (Figure 5A). For example, thrombin-polarized macrophages expressed higher levels of genes related to the TGF-β pathway, e.g., Id1, Id3, Smad6, and Smad9 than M0 cells. The expression of more inflammatory genes, e.g., Ifi213, Ifi44, Ifi206, Irf7, Tnfsf8, and Ccl5 was, on the other hand, lower, following stimulation with thrombin. There were also distinct differences between the expression profiles of M2a and thrombin-polarized cells, e.g., the classical M2a marker genes Il4i1, Arg1, Jak2, and Klf4 were significantly lower following thrombin stimulation (Figure 5B). GO term analysis revealed that while M2a macrophages favored pathways related to the cell cycle, thrombin-polarized macrophages expressed genes linked to responses to viruses and interferons as well as phagocytosis and engulfment (Figure S1).

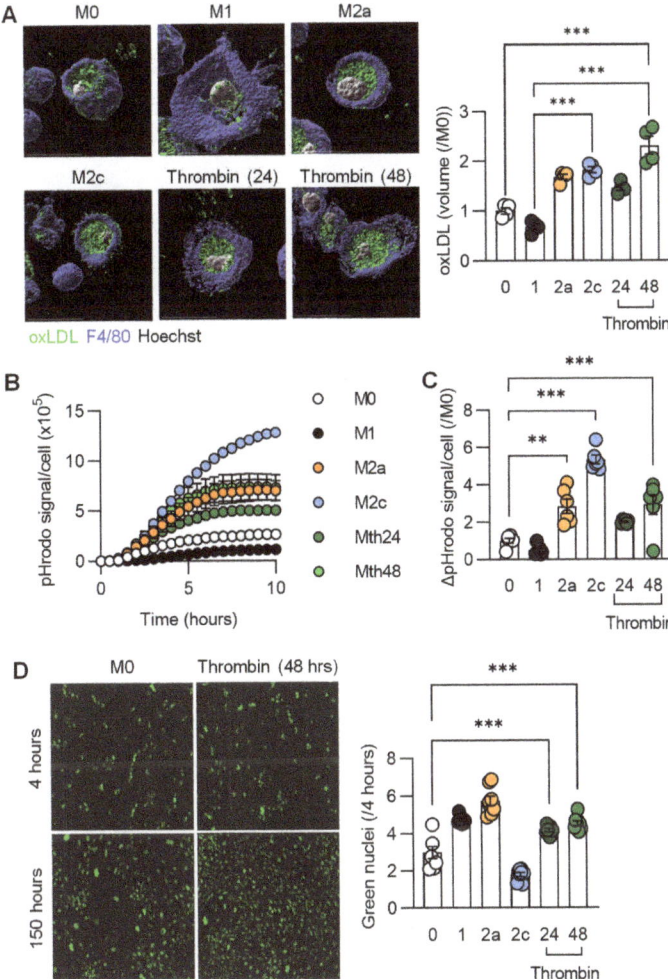

Figure 4. Consequences of thrombin polarization on macrophage function. Murine bone-marrow-monocyte-derived macrophages (M0) were either treated with solvent; polarized to the M1, M2a, or M2c phenotypes; or incubated with thrombin for up to 48 h. (**A**) Volume of dil-labeled oxLDL taken up over 15 min; n = 4 mice per group. (**B**) Time course of the phagocytosis of pHrodo-labaled particles over 10 h; n = 6 mice. (**C**) Quantification of phagocytic cells per field after 5 h; n = 6 mice. (**D**) Endothelial cell proliferation assay upon treatment with thrombin-polarized macrophage supernatants; n = 4 independent cell batches/mice. All experiments were performed at least twice. (**A,C,D**) One-way ANOVA and Bonferroni's multiple comparisons test. ** $p < 0.01$, *** $p < 0.001$.

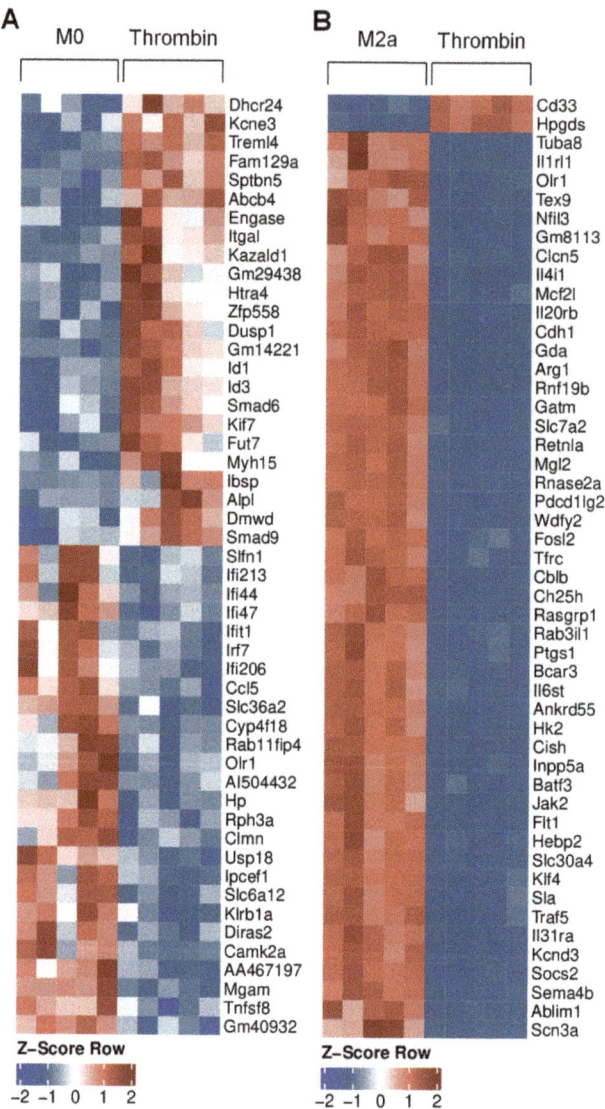

Figure 5. Thrombin-induced changes in macrophage gene expression. Murine bone-marrow-monocyte-derived macrophages (M0) were either treated with solvent, polarized to the M2a phenotype, or incubated with thrombin (0.1 U/mL, 24 h). (**A**) Top 50 differentially regulated genes between M0 and thrombin-treated macrophages; n = 5 mice. (**B**) Top 50 differentially regulated genes between M2a and thrombin-treated macrophages; n = 5 mice per group.

3.5. Impact of SMOC1 on Thrombin Polarized Macrophages

SMOC1 was recently identified as a platelet-derived thrombin activator, and antibodies directed against the protein attenuated the thrombin-induced aggregation of murine and human platelets [17]. Given the close association between platelets and macrophages, we determined the impact of SMOC1 on macrophage gene expression and function. When gene expression was compared in macrophages treated with thrombin in the absence and presence of SMOC1 antibodies, we observed the differential regulation of several of the genes reported above. In particular, the expression of transcripts involved in TGF-β signaling (*Id1*, *Id3*, *Smad6*, *Smad9*) were all downregulated by the antibody, while members of the interferon signaling pathway increased (Figure 6A).

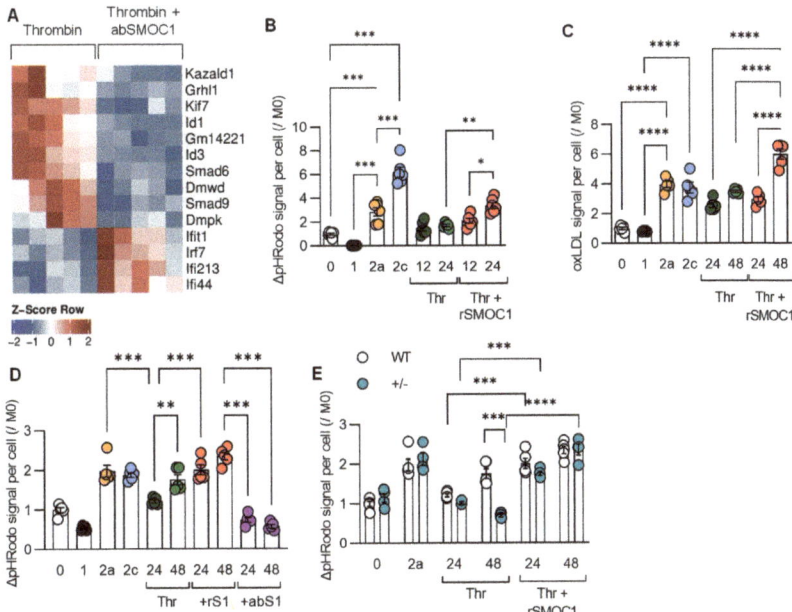

Figure 6. Modulation of thrombin-induced macrophage polarization by SMOC1. (**A**) Differentially regulated genes in murine bone-marrow-monocyte-derived macrophages treated with thrombin (0.1 U/mL, 24 h) in the absence and presence of an antibody directed against SMOC1 (1 µg/µL); n = 5 mice. (**B**) Phagocytosis of pHrodo zymosan in M0-, M1-, M2a-, and M2c-polarized macrophages compared to thrombin stimulation (Thr; 1 U/mL, up to 24 h) in the absence and presence of recombinant SMOC1 (rSMOC1; 0.5 µg/mL). n = 3 mice with all experiments preformed in duplicate. (**C**) Uptake of dil-oxLDL under the same conditions as in (B); n = 5 mice. (**D**) Phagocytosis of pHrodo zymosan in M0-, M1-, M2a-, and M2c-polarized macrophages compared to stimulation by thrombin (0.1 U/mL, up to 24 h) in the absence and presence of recombinant SMOC1 (rS1; 0.5 µg/mL) or an antibody directed against SMOC1 (abS1; 1 µg/µL); n = 5 mice. (**E**) Phagocytosis of pHrodo zymosan in M0- and M2a-polarized macrophages from wild-type (WT) and SMOC1+/− mice (+/−) compared to stimulation by thrombin (0.1 U/mL, up to 24 h) in the absence and presence of recombinant SMOC1 (rSMOC1; 0.5 µg/mL); n = 5 mice. Experiments (B–D) were performed at least twice. One-way ANOVA and Bonferroni's multiple comparisons test (B–D), and two-way ANOVA and Bonferroni's multiple comparisons test (E). * $p < 0.05$, ** $p < 0.01$, *** $p < 0.001$, **** $p < 0.0001$.

To determine the effect of SMOC1 on macrophage function, we focused on the phagocytosis of zymosan and ox-LDL. As was the case previously, the phagocytosis was highest in M2a- and M2c-polarized macrophages, but thrombin also stimulated phagocytosis (Figure 6B,C). Importantly, the addition of recombinant SMOC1 to macrophages amplified responses to thrombin, particularly to a low concentration of thrombin (0.1 U/mL), while an antibody directed against SMOC1 attenuated responses (Figure 6D). SMOC1−/− mice die shortly after birth [31,32], but the phagocytosis of zymosan induced by thrombin was attenuated in macrophages from SMOC1+/− mice and was rescued by the addition of recombinant SMOC1 (Figure 6E). Thus, the presence of SMOC1 has pronounced effects on the polarization of macrophages by thrombin.

4. Discussion

The results or our study indicate that thrombin elicits effects on macrophages that are distinct from the phenotype induced by classical activation protocols. Rather, thrombin stimulation resulted in macrophages adopting a pro-resolving phenotype characterized by the secretion of CCL22, a cytokine most akin to M2 and tumor-associated macrophages that impacted expression of genes of the TGF-β pathway. The manipulation of SMOC1 levels had a pronounced impact on the expression of TGF-β signaling-related genes as well as on macrophage function, highlighting the fact that tissue levels of SMOC1 can clearly modify thrombin-induced macrophage polarization.

The phenotypic characterization of macrophages is highly complicated, and there are many more distinct genetic fingerprints and metabolic states than are reflected in a basic M0/M1/M2 classification [33,34]. There is even still controversy about the cellular markers for each of the reported phenotypes and how in vitro polarization studies can be compared with the in vivo situation [35]. Such discrepancies in markers or the timing of the experiments may account for the previous reports that thrombin stimulation results in the M1-like [12–14] as well as M2-like polarization of macrophages [15]. In the current study, we characterized macrophages by virtue of classical polarization marker levels as well as by their ability to phagocytose extracellular material and to promote endothelial cell proliferation. The expression of genes regularly used to identify polarization subtypes indicated that thrombin induced an M2a-like polarization. For example, we observed comparable levels of CD36, which is a scavenger receptor for oxLDL uptake [36], and MMP9, which is also highly expressed by M2-type macrophages [37], in M2a- and thrombin-treated macrophages. However, levels of Fizz-1 were clearly induced by M2a polarization but unaffected by thrombin.

Changes in macrophage polarization are linked with changes in cell metabolism, not only that these alterations affect energy metabolism and biosynthesis but also influence immune function of the resulting macrophage phenotype. For example, pro-inflammatory macrophages display enhanced glycolysis and impaired TCA cycle function to meet with their metabolic needs and regulate the production of reactive oxygen species and inflammasome formation (for a review, see reference [38]). Conversely, alternatively activated M2 macrophages rely on oxidative phosphorylation and the TCA cycle to promote tissue remodeling and the reestablishment of homeostasis. Changes in arginine and citrulline levels generally reflect alterations in the activity of iNOS and arginase. Thus, the decreased citrulline and increased arginine levels in thrombin-polarized macrophages contrasts clearly with the M1 phenotype and has more similarity with M2a-polarized cells. However, there were some clear differences between M2a and thrombin-treated macrophages, and our finding that ethanolamine was higher in thrombin-polarized than in classical M2a-polarized macrophages may reflect their increased ability to phagocytose ox-LDL. Indeed, ethanolamine is the most frequent head group present in mammalian plasmalogens [39], and membrane ethanolamine plasmalogen deficiency has been reported to result in a decreased phagocytosis capacity [40]. There were also differences in itaconate, which is generated by diverting aconitate away from the TCA cycle during inflammatory macrophage activation and has been reported to link cell metabolism with stress and immune responses [41]. We found that itaconate levels were higher in more transitional phenotypes, i.e., repolarized M2c macrophages as well as thrombin-stimulated macrophages. Functionally, we focused on the ability of macrophages to phagocytose ox-LDL and zymosan, as well as the effects of the macrophage supernatant on endothelial cell growth, two classical functions of M2-polarized macrophages. In all of these assays, the function of M2a and thrombin-treated macrophages were similar, but there was a tendency for thrombin-treated macrophages to take up ox-LDL more efficiently.

RNA sequencing, however, clearly revealed distinctions between the M0 and M2a phenotypes and that induced by thrombin, including altered TGF-β signaling. Indeed, the expression of *Id1* and *Id3*, which partner with TGF-β to regulate cell proliferation and survival [42], were increased in thrombin-stimulated versus naïve M0 macrophages, as were *Smad6* and *Smad9*, which are inhibitors of the TGF-β [43] and BMP [44] pathways, respectively. In agreement with the phenotypic and metabolic data, thrombin decreased the expression of bona fide pro-inflammatory genes, several of them related to IFN-γ (*Ifi213*, *Ifi44*, *Ifi206*, *Irf7*), TNF-α (*Tnfsf8*), and chemokine (*Ccl5*) pathways. Moreover, several genes that drive polarization towards M2a such as *Arg* [45], *Il4i1* [46], *Klf4* [47], *Jak2* [48], and *Socs2* [49] were clearly attenuated by thrombin stimulation.

In addition to our focus on clarifying the effects of thrombin on macrophage polarization, we set out to determine the impact of SMOC1 on thrombin-induced responses. SMOC1 is a matricellular protein that is generally localized to the basement membrane of different tissues [50–53]. Little is known about its role in physiology or pathophysiology, but it has been associated with both Waardenburg anophthalmia syndrome [31,32] and Alzheimer's disease [54–56]. More recently, SMOC1 was identified as a glucose-responsive hepatokine important for glycemic control in mice [57], a phenomenon that could not be confirmed in a human population [58]. Rather, circulating levels of SMOC1 were found to increase in subjects with type 2 diabetes in parallel with platelet hyperactivity to thrombin [17]. To date, nothing is known about effects of SMOC1 in macrophages, but SMOC1 expression is at least partly regulated by miR-223 [59], and decreased levels of miR-223 in monocytes/macrophages have been linked with atherosclerosis and macrophage activation [60–62], as well as the transition between inflammation and cancer [63,64]. Given that SMOC1 expression is regulated by miR-223 [59], which when secreted can potentiate the actions of thrombin [17], it was tempting to suggest that the combination of thrombin and SMOC1 could affect innate immune responses. We found that SMOC1 did, indeed, increase phagocytosis by thrombin-treated macrophages, and that effects were attenuated in SMOC1+/− mice as well as by antibodies directed against SMOC1 and rescued by the addition of recombinant SMOC1 protein. All of these observations indicate that the macrophage expression of SMOC1 has a major impact on thrombin-induced macrophage polarization. At the level of gene expression, antibodies directed against SMOC1 reversed the thrombin-induced changes in a subset of genes, particularly those relating to TGF-β signaling and inflammatory interferon signaling. The overall effect was that the inactivation of SMOC1 in macrophages curbed the anti-inflammatory effects of thrombin.

Taken together, we have shown that thrombin stimulation polarizes macrophages to a distinct phenotype that initially seemed to be closest to the alternatively activated M2a phenotype. At first sight, this observation was unexpected, given the pro-inflammatory role attributed to thrombin in atherosclerosis [65] and reports that negative regulators of thrombin have athero-protective effects. For example, heparin cofactor II can protect elderly persons against carotid atherosclerotic lesions and hirudin; another thrombin inhibitor has been shown to decrease restenosis after angiography (for a review, see reference [66]). However, an M2a-like polarization of macrophages has previously been linked to a pro-fibrotic state, which could impact on wound healing [16]. Moreover, there is a well-established link between thrombosis and cancer [8], where thrombin-induced PAR1 signaling has been suggested to promote the immunosuppressive microenvironment that protects the tumor against host antitumor immune responsiveness [67]. There are also links between thrombin and epithelial–mesenchymal transition in several cancer cells, which is a key process implicated in cancer invasion and metastasis [68,69]. SMOC1 levels are elevated in some forms of cancer [70–72], and given that the cleavage of osteopontin by thrombin initiates its tumor promoting activity [73], it will be interesting to determine whether or not the interaction between SMOC1 and thrombin underlies some of this tumor-promoting ability.

Supplementary Materials: The following supporting information can be downloaded at: https://www.mdpi.com/article/10.3390/cells11101718/s1, Figure S1: Thrombin induced changes in macrophage gene expression.

Author Contributions: Conceptualization Ü.U., F.D.L., M.S., B.F. and I.F.; methodology Ü.U., F.D.L., S.K., S.G. and B.F.; data analysis, Ü.U., F.D.L., S.K., S.G., M.S., B.F. and I.F.; writing—review and editing, Ü.U. and I.F.; project administration and funding acquisition, I.F. All authors have read and agreed to the published version of the manuscript.

Funding: This work was supported by the Deutsche Forschungsgemeinschaft (GRK 2336 TP05 Project ID 321115009, SFB 834/3 A5 Project ID: 75732319, Cardio-Pulmonary Institute, EXC 2026, Project ID: 390649896).

Institutional Review Board Statement: The animal study protocol was approved by the Institutional Review Board at the Medical Faculty of the Goethe University in Frankfurt and the Federal Authority for Animal Research at the Regierungspräsidium Darmstadt (Hessen, Germany). Approved study protocol V54-19c, 2.04.2020.

Informed Consent Statement: Not applicable.

Data Availability Statement: All of the data supporting the reported results can be found in the manuscript and its supplementary files.

Acknowledgments: The authors are indebted to Katharina Herbig, Mechtild Piepenbrock, and Xiaoming Li for expert technical assistance.

Conflicts of Interest: The authors declare no conflict of interest.

References

1. Popović, M.; Smiljanić, K.; Dobutović, B.; Syrovets, T.; Simmet, T.; Isenović, E.R. Thrombin and vascular inflammation. *Mol. Cell. Biochem.* **2012**, *359*, 301–313. [CrossRef] [PubMed]
2. Hirano, K. The roles of proteinase-activated receptors in the vascular physiology and pathophysiology. *Arter. Thromb. Vasc. Biol.* **2007**, *27*, 27–36. [CrossRef] [PubMed]
3. Posma, J.J.N.; Posthuma, J.J.; Spronk, H.M.H. Coagulation and non-coagulation effects of thrombin. *J. Thromb. Haemost.* **2016**, *14*, 1908–1916. [CrossRef] [PubMed]
4. de Candia, E.; Hall, S.W.; Rutella, S.; Landolfi, R.; Andrews, R.K.; de Cristofaro, R. Binding of thrombin to glycoprotein Ib accelerates the hydrolysis of Par-1 on intact platelets. *J. Biol. Chem.* **2001**, *276*, 4692–4698. [CrossRef] [PubMed]
5. Bogatcheva, N.V.; Garcia, J.G.N.; Verin, A.D. Molecular mechanisms of thrombin-induced endothelial cell permeability. *Biochemistry* **2002**, *67*, 75–84. [CrossRef] [PubMed]
6. Kyselova, A.; Elgheznawy, A.; Wittig, I.; Heidler, J.; Mann, A.W.; Ruf, W.; Fleming, I.; Randriamboavonjy, V. Platelet-derived calpain cleaves the endothelial protease-activated receptor 1 to induce vascular inflammation in diabetes. *Basic. Res. Cardiol.* **2020**, *115*, 75. [CrossRef]
7. Szaba, F.M.; Smiley, S.T. Roles for thrombin and fibrin(ogen) in cytokine/chemokine production and macrophage adhesion in vivo. *Blood* **2002**, *99*, 1053–1059. [CrossRef]
8. Cantrell, R.; Palumbo, J.S. The thrombin–inflammation axis in cancer progression. *Thromb. Res.* **2020**, *191*, S117–S122. [CrossRef]
9. Snyder, K.M.; Kessler, C.M. The pivotal role of thrombin in cancer biology and tumorigenesis. *Semin. Thromb. Hemost.* **2008**, *34*, 734–741. [CrossRef]
10. Hara, T.; Phuong, P.T.; Fukuda, D.; Yamaguchi, K.; Murata, C.; Nishimoto, S.; Yagi, S.; Kusunose, K.; Yamada, H.; Soeki, T.; et al. Protease-activated receptor-2 plays a critical role in vascular inflammation and atherosclerosis in apolipoprotein E-deficient mice. *Circulation* **2018**, *138*, 1706–1719. [CrossRef]
11. Jones, S.M.; Mann, A.; Conrad, K.; Saum, K.; Hall, D.E.; McKinney, L.M.; Robbins, N.; Thompson, J.; Peairs, A.D.; Camerer, E.; et al. PAR2 (protease-activated receptor 2) deficiency attenuates atherosclerosis in mice. *Arter. Thromb. Vasc. Biol.* **2018**, *38*, 1271–1282. [CrossRef] [PubMed]
12. López-Zambrano, M.; Rodriguez-Montesinos, J.; Crespo-Avilan, G.E.; Muñoz-Vega, M.; Preissner, K.T. Thrombin promotes macrophage polarization into M1-like phenotype to induce inflammatory Responses. *Thromb. Haemost.* **2020**, *120*, 658–670. [CrossRef]
13. Chen, L.; Gao, B.; Zhang, Y.; Lu, H.; Li, X.; Pan, L.; Yin, X.; Zhi, X. PAR2 promotes M1 macrophage polarization and inflammation via FOXO1 pathway. *J. Cell. Biochem.* **2019**, *120*, 9799–9809. [CrossRef] [PubMed]
14. Wilkinson, H.; Leonard, H.; Chen, D.; Lawrence, T.; Robson, M.; Goossens, P.; McVey, J.H.; Dorling, A. PAR-1 signaling on macrophages is required for effective in vivo delayed-type hypersensitivity responses. *iScience* **2021**, *24*, 101981. [CrossRef] [PubMed]
15. García-González, G.; Sánchez-González, A.; Hernández-Bello, R.; González, G.M.; Franco-Molina, M.A.; Coronado-Cerda, E.E.; Palma-Nicolás, J.P. Triggering of protease-activated receptors (PARs) induces alternative M2 macrophage polarization with impaired plasticity. *Mol. Immunol.* **2019**, *114*, 278–288. [CrossRef]

16. White, M.J.V.; Gomer, R.H. Trypsin, tryptase, and thrombin polarize macrophages towards a pro-fibrotic M2a phenotype. *PLoS ONE* **2015**, *10*, e0138748. [CrossRef]
17. Delgado Lagos, F.; Elgheznawy, A.; Kyselova, A.; Meyer Zu Heringdorf, D.; Ratiu, C.; Randriamboavonjy, V.; Mann, A.W.; Fisslthaler, B.; Siragusa, M.; Fleming, I. Secreted modular calcium-binding protein 1 binds and activates thrombin to account for platelet hyperreactivity in diabetes. *Blood* **2021**, *137*, 1641–1651. [CrossRef]
18. Fleming, I.; Fisslthaler, B.; Dixit, M.; Busse, R. Role of PECAM-1 in the shear-stress-induced activation of Akt and the endothelial nitric oxide synthase (eNOS) in endothelial cells. *J. Cell Sci.* **2005**, *118*, 4103–4111. [CrossRef]
19. Bolger, A.M.; Lohse, M.; Usadel, B. Trimmomatic: A flexible trimmer for Illumina sequence data. *Bioinformatics* **2014**, *30*, 2114–2120. [CrossRef]
20. Dobin, A.; Davis, C.A.; Schlesinger, F.; Drenkow, J.; Zaleski, C.; Jha, S.; Batut, P.; Chaisson, M.; Gingeras, T.R. STAR: Ultrafast universal RNA-seq aligner. *Bioinformatics* **2013**, *29*, 15–21. [CrossRef]
21. Liao, Y.; Smyth, G.K.; Shi, W. featureCounts: An efficient general purpose program for assigning sequence reads to genomic features. *Bioinformatics* **2014**, *30*, 923–930. [CrossRef] [PubMed]
22. Love, M.I.; Huber, W.; Anders, S. Moderated estimation of fold change and dispersion for RNA-seq data with DESeq2. *Genome Biol.* **2014**, *15*, 550. [CrossRef] [PubMed]
23. UniProt Consortium. Activities at the Universal Protein Resource (UniProt). *Nucleic Acids Res.* **2014**, *42*, D191–D198. [CrossRef] [PubMed]
24. Yu, T.; Gan, S.; Zhu, Q.; Dai, D.; Li, N.; Wang, H.; Chen, X.; Hou, D.; Wang, Y.; Pan, Q.; et al. Modulation of M2 macrophage polarization by the crosstalk between Stat6 and Trim24. *Nat. Commun.* **2019**, *10*, 4353. [CrossRef] [PubMed]
25. Mantovani, A.; Sica, A.; Sozzani, S.; Allavena, P.; Vecchi, A.; Locati, M. The chemokine system in diverse forms of macrophage activation and polarization. *Trends. Immunol.* **2004**, *25*, 677–686. [CrossRef]
26. Yao, Y.; Xu, X.-H.; Jin, L. Macrophage polarization in physiological and pathological pregnancy. *Front. Immunol.* **2019**, *10*, 792. [CrossRef]
27. Martinez, F.O.; Sica, A.; Mantovani, A.; Locati, M. Macrophage activation and polarization. *Front. Biosci.* **2008**, *13*, 453–461. [CrossRef]
28. Ferrante, C.J.; Pinhal-Enfield, G.; Elson, G.; Cronstein, B.N.; Hasko, G.; Outram, S.; Leibovich, S.J. The adenosine-dependent angiogenic switch of macrophages to an M2-like phenotype is independent of interleukin-4 receptor alpha (IL-4Rα) signaling. *Inflammation* **2013**, *36*, 921–931. [CrossRef]
29. Boada-Romero, E.; Martinez, J.; Heckmann, B.L.; Green, D.R. The clearance of dead cells by efferocytosis. *Nat. Rev. Mol. Cell Biol.* **2020**, *21*, 398–414. [CrossRef]
30. Zippel, N.; Malik, R.A.; Frömel, T.; Popp, R.; Bess, E.; Strilic, B.; Wettschureck, N.; Fleming, I.; Fisslthaler, B. Transforming growth factor-β-activated kinase 1 regulates angiogenesis via AMP-activated protein kinase-α1 and redox balance in endothelial cells. *Arterioscler. Thromb. Vasc. Biol.* **2013**, *33*, 2792–2799. [CrossRef]
31. Abouzeid, H.; Boisset, G.; Favez, T.; Youssef, M.; Marzouk, I.; Shakankiry, N.; Bayoumi, N.; Descombes, P.; Agosti, C.; Munier, F.L.; et al. Mutations in the SPARC-related modular calcium-binding protein 1 gene, SMOC1, cause Waardenburg anophthalmia syndrome. *Am. J. Hum. Genet.* **2011**, *88*, 92–98. [CrossRef] [PubMed]
32. Okada, I.; Hamanoue, H.; Terada, K.; Tohma, T.; Megarbane, A.; Chouery, E.; Abou-Ghoch, J.; Jalkh, N.; Cogulu, O.; Ozkinay, F.; et al. SMOC1 is essential for ocular and limb development in humans and mice. *Am. J. Hum. Genet.* **2011**, *88*, 30–41. [CrossRef] [PubMed]
33. Sica, A.; Mantovani, A. Macrophage plasticity and polarization: In vivo veritas. *J. Clin. Investig.* **2012**, *122*, 787–795. [CrossRef] [PubMed]
34. Wang, L.-X.; Zhang, S.-X.; Wu, H.-J.; Rong, X.-L.; Guo, J. M2b macrophage polarization and its roles in diseases. *J. Leukoc. Biol.* **2019**, *106*, 345–358. [CrossRef]
35. Orecchioni, M.; Ghosheh, Y.; Pramod, A.B.; Ley, K. Macrophage polarization: Different gene signatures in M1(LPS+) vs. classically and M2(LPS-) vs. alternatively activated macrophages. *Front. Immunol.* **2019**, *10*, 1084. [CrossRef]
36. Collot-Teixeira, S.; Martin, J.; McDermott-Roe, C.; Poston, R.; McGregor, J.L. CD36 and macrophages in atherosclerosis. *Cardiovasc. Res.* **2007**, *75*, 468–477. [CrossRef]
37. Tian, K.; Du, G.; Wang, X.; Wu, X.; Li, L.; Liu, W.; Wu, R. MMP-9 secreted by M2-type macrophages promotes Wilms' tumour metastasis through the PI3K/AKT pathway. *Mol. Biol. Rep.* **2022**, 1–12. [CrossRef]
38. Saha, S.; Shalova, I.N.; Biswas, S.K. Metabolic regulation of macrophage phenotype and function. *Immunol. Rev.* **2017**, *280*, 102–111. [CrossRef]
39. Yamashita, A.; Hayashi, Y.; Nemoto-Sasaki, Y.; Ito, M.; Oka, S.; Tanikawa, T.; Waku, K.; Sugiura, T. Acyltransferases and transacylases that determine the fatty acid composition of glycerolipids and the metabolism of bioactive lipid mediators in mammalian cells and model organisms. *Prog. Lipid. Res.* **2014**, *53*, 18–81. [CrossRef]
40. Rubio, J.M.; Astudillo, A.M.; Casas, J.; Balboa, M.A.; Balsinde, J. Regulation of phagocytosis in macrophages by membrane ethanolamine plasmalogens. *Front. Immunol.* **2018**, *9*, 1723. [CrossRef]
41. O'Neill, L.A.J.; Artyomov, M.N. Itaconate: The poster child of metabolic reprogramming in macrophage function. *Nat. Rev. Immunol.* **2019**, *19*, 273–281. [CrossRef] [PubMed]

42. Zhang, Y.; Alexander, P.B.; Wang, X.-F. TGF-β family signaling in the control of cell proliferation and survival. *Cold Spring Harb. Perspect. Biol.* **2017**, *9*, a022145. [CrossRef] [PubMed]
43. Imamura, T.; Takase, M.; Nishihara, A.; Oeda, E.; Hanai, J.; Kawabata, M.; Miyazono, K. Smad6 inhibits signalling by the TGF-beta superfamily. *Nature* **1997**, *389*, 622–626. [CrossRef] [PubMed]
44. Tsukamoto, S.; Mizuta, T.; Fujimoto, M.; Ohte, S.; Osawa, K.; Miyamoto, A.; Yoneyama, K.; Murata, E.; Machiya, A.; Jimi, E.; et al. Smad9 is a new type of transcriptional regulator in bone morphogenetic protein signaling. *Sci. Rep.* **2014**, *4*, 7596. [CrossRef] [PubMed]
45. Yang, Z.; Ming, X.-F. Functions of arginase isoforms in macrophage inflammatory responses: Impact on cardiovascular diseases and metabolic disorders. *Front. Immunol.* **2014**, *5*, 533. [CrossRef]
46. Yue, Y.; Huang, W.; Liang, J.; Guo, J.; Ji, J.; Yao, Y.; Zheng, M.; Cai, Z.; Lu, L.; Wang, J. IL4I1 is a novel regulator of M2 macrophage polarization that can inhibit T cell activation via L-tryptophan and arginine depletion and IL-10 production. *PLoS ONE* **2015**, *10*, e0142979. [CrossRef]
47. Liao, X.; Sharma, N.; Kapadia, F.; Zhou, G.; Lu, Y.; Hong, H.; Paruchuri, K.; Mahabeleshwar, G.H.; Dalmas, E.; Venteclef, N.; et al. Krüppel-like factor 4 regulates macrophage polarization. *J. Clin. Investig.* **2011**, *121*, 2736–2749. [CrossRef]
48. Chen, H.; Li, M.; Sanchez, E.; Soof, C.M.; Bujarski, S.; Ng, N.; Cao, J.; Hekmati, T.; Zahab, B.; Nosrati, J.D.; et al. JAK1/2 pathway inhibition suppresses M2 polarization and overcomes resistance of myeloma to lenalidomide by reducing TRIB1, MUC1, CD44, CXCL12, and CXCR4 expression. *Br. J. Haematol.* **2020**, *188*, 283–294. [CrossRef]
49. Wilson, H.M. SOCS proteins in macrophage polarization and function. *Front. Immunol.* **2014**, *5*, 357. [CrossRef]
50. Gersdorff, N.; Muller, M.; Schall, A.; Miosge, N. Secreted modular calcium-binding protein-1 localization during mouse embryogenesis. *Histochem. Cell. Biol.* **2006**, *126*, 705–712. [CrossRef]
51. Vannahme, C.; Smyth, N.; Miosge, N.; Gosling, S.; Frie, C.; Paulsson, M.; Maurer, P.; Hartmann, U. Characterization of SMOC-1, a novel modular calcium-binding protein in basement membranes. *J. Biol. Chem.* **2002**, *277*, 37977–37986. [CrossRef] [PubMed]
52. Bradshaw, A.D. Diverse biological functions of the SPARC family of proteins. *Int. J. Biochem. Cell Biol.* **2012**, *44*, 480–488. [CrossRef] [PubMed]
53. Choi, Y.A.; Lim, J.; Kim, K.M.; Acharya, B.; Cho, J.Y.; Bae, Y.C.; Shin, H.I.; Kim, S.Y.; Park, E.K. Secretome analysis of human BMSCs and identification of SMOC1 as an important ECM protein in osteoblast differentiation. *J. Proteome. Res.* **2010**, *9*, 2946–2956. [CrossRef] [PubMed]
54. Zhou, M.; Haque, R.U.; Dammer, E.B.; Duong, D.M.; Ping, L.; Johnson, E.C.B.; Lah, J.J.; Levey, A.I.; Seyfried, N.T. Targeted mass spectrometry to quantify brain-derived cerebrospinal fluid biomarkers in Alzheimer's disease. *Clin. Proteom.* **2020**, *17*, 19. [CrossRef] [PubMed]
55. Sathe, G.; Albert, M.; Darrow, J.; Saito, A.; Troncoso, J.; Pandey, A.; Moghekar, A. Quantitative proteomic analysis of the frontal cortex in Alzheimer's disease. *J. Neurochem.* **2020**, *156*, 988–1002. [CrossRef]
56. Bai, B.; Wang, X.; Li, Y.; Chen, P.-C.; Yu, K.; Dey, K.K.; Yarbro, J.M.; Han, X.; Lutz, B.M.; Rao, S.; et al. Deep multilayer brain proteomics identifies molecular networks in Alzheimer's disease progression. *Neuron* **2020**, *105*, 975–991. [CrossRef]
57. Montgomery, M.K.; Bayliss, J.; Devereux, C.; Bezawork-Geleta, A.; Roberts, D.; Huang, C.; Schittenhelm, R.B.; Ryan, A.; Townley, S.L.; Selth, L.A.; et al. SMOC1 is a glucose-responsive hepatokine and therapeutic target for glycemic control. *Sci. Transl. Med.* **2020**, *12*, eaaz8048. [CrossRef]
58. Ghodsian, N.; Gagnon, E.; Bourgault, J.; Gobeil, É.; Manikpurage, H.D.; Perrot, N.; Girard, A.; Mitchell, P.L.; Arsenault, B.J. Blood levels of the SMOC1 hepatokine are not causally linked with type 2 diabetes: A bidirectional mendelian randomization study. *Nutrients* **2021**, *13*, 4208. [CrossRef]
59. Awwad, K.; Hu, J.; Shi, L.; Mangels, N.; Abdel Malik, R.; Zippel, N.; Fisslthaler, B.; Eble, J.A.; Pfeilschifter, J.; Popp, R.; et al. Role of secreted modular calcium binding protein 1 (SMOC1) in transforming growth factor β signaling and angiogenesis. *Cardiovasc. Res.* **2015**, *106*, 284–294. [CrossRef]
60. You, D.; Qiao, Q.; Ono, K.; Wei, M.; Tan, W.; Wang, C.; Liu, Y.; Liu, G.; Zheng, M. miR-223-3p inhibits the progression of atherosclerosis via down-regulating the activation of MEK1/ERK1/2 in macrophages. *Aging* **2022**, *14*, 1865–1878. [CrossRef]
61. Wang, J.; Bai, X.; Song, Q.; Fan, F.; Hu, Z.; Cheng, G.; Zhang, Y. miR-223 inhibits lipid deposition and inflammation by suppressing Toll-like receptor 4 signaling in macrophages. *Int. J. Mol. Sci.* **2015**, *16*, 24965–24982. [CrossRef] [PubMed]
62. Long, F.-Q.; Kou, C.-X.; Li, K.; Wu, J.; Wang, Q.-Q. MiR-223-3p inhibits rTp17-induced inflammasome activation and pyroptosis by targeting NLRP3. *J. Cell Mol. Med.* **2020**, *24*, 14405–14414. [CrossRef] [PubMed]
63. Favero, A.; Segatto, I.; Perin, T.; Belletti, B. The many facets of miR-223 in cancer: Oncosuppressor, oncogenic driver, therapeutic target, and biomarker of response. *Wiley Interdiscip Rev. RNA* **2021**, *12*, e1659. [CrossRef] [PubMed]
64. Jeffries, J.; Zhou, W.; Hsu, A.Y.; Deng, Q. miRNA-223 at the crossroads of inflammation and cancer. *Cancer Lett.* **2019**, *451*, 136–141. [CrossRef] [PubMed]
65. Jaberi, N.; Soleimani, A.; Pashirzad, M.; Abdeahad, H.; Mohammadi, F.; Khoshakhlagh, M.; Khazaei, M.; Ferns, G.A.; Avan, A.; Hassanian, S.M. Role of thrombin in the pathogenesis of atherosclerosis. *J. Cell Biochem.* **2019**, *120*, 4757–4765. [CrossRef]
66. Gray, E.; Hogwood, J.; Mulloy, B. The anticoagulant and antithrombotic mechanisms of heparin. *Handb. Exp. Pharm.* **2012**, *207*, 43–61. [CrossRef]

67. Schweickert, P.G.; Yang, Y.; White, E.E.; Cresswell, G.M.; Elzey, B.D.; Ratliff, T.L.; Arumugam, P.; Antoniak, S.; Mackman, N.; Flick, M.J.; et al. Thrombin-PAR1 signaling in pancreatic cancer promotes an immunosuppressive microenvironment. *J. Thromb. Haemost.* **2021**, *19*, 161–172. [CrossRef]
68. Zhong, Y.-C.; Zhang, T.; Di, W.; Li, W.-P. Thrombin promotes epithelial ovarian cancer cell invasion by inducing epithelial-mesenchymal transition. *J. Gynecol. Oncol.* **2013**, *24*, 265–272. [CrossRef]
69. Otsuki, T.; Fujimoto, D.; Hirono, Y.; Goi, T.; Yamaguchi, A. Thrombin conducts epithelial-mesenchymal transition via protease-activated receptor-1 in human gastric cancer. *Int. J. Oncol.* **2014**, *45*, 2287–2294. [CrossRef]
70. Brellier, F.; Ruggiero, S.; Zwolanek, D.; Martina, E.; Hess, D.; Brown-Luedi, M.; Hartmann, U.; Koch, M.; Merlo, A.; Lino, M.; et al. SMOC1 is a tenascin-C interacting protein over-expressed in brain tumors. *Matrix Biol.* **2011**, *30*, 225–233. [CrossRef]
71. Gong, X.; Liu, L.; Xiong, J.; Li, X.; Xu, J.; Xiao, Y.; Li, J.; Luo, X.; Mao, D.; Liu, L. Construction of a prognostic gene signature associated with immune infiltration in glioma: A comprehensive analysis based on the CGGA. *J. Oncol.* **2021**, *2021*, 6620159. [CrossRef] [PubMed]
72. Walline, H.M.; Komarck, C.M.; McHugh, J.B.; Bellile, E.L.; Brenner, J.C.; Prince, M.E.; McKean, E.L.; Chepeha, D.B.; Wolf, G.T.; Worden, F.P.; et al. Genomic integration of high risk HPV alters gene expression in oropharyngeal squamous cell carcinoma. *Mol. Cancer Res.* **2016**, *14*, 941–952. [CrossRef] [PubMed]
73. Peraramelli, S.; Zhou, Q.; Zhou, Q.; Wanko, B.; Zhao, L.; Nishimura, T.; Leung, T.H.; Mizuno, S.; Ito, M.; Myles, T.; et al. Thrombin cleavage of osteopontin initiates osteopontin's tumor-promoting activity. *J. Thromb. Haemost.* **2022**, *20*, 1256–1270. [CrossRef] [PubMed]

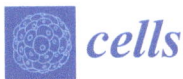

Article

The Cellular Innate Immune Response of the Invasive Pest Insect *Drosophila suzukii* against *Pseudomonas entomophila* Involves the Release of Extracellular Traps

Tessa Carrau [1,†], Susanne Thümecke [2,†], Liliana M. R. Silva [3,*], David Perez-Bravo [4], Ulrich Gärtner [5], Anja Taubert [3], Carlos Hermosilla [3], Andreas Vilcinskas [1,2] and Kwang-Zin Lee [1,*]

1. Department Pests and Vector Insect Control, Fraunhofer Institute for Molecular Biology and Applied Ecology, Ohlebergsweg 12, D-35394 Giessen, Germany; tessa.carrau@gmail.com (T.C.); andreas.vilcinskas@ime.fraunhofer.de (A.V.)
2. Institute for Insect Biotechnology, Justus Liebig University, Heinrich Buff Ring 26-32, D-35392 Giessen, Germany; susanne.thuemecke@uni-rostock.de
3. Institute of Parasitology, Justus Liebig University, Schubert Strasse 81, D-35392 Giessen, Germany; anja.taubert@vetmed.uni-giessen.de (A.T.); carlos.r.hermosilla@vetmed.uni-giessen.de (C.H.)
4. Department of Internal Medicine (Pulmonology), University of Giessen and Marburg Lung Center (UGMLC), Member of the German Center for Lung Research (DZL), Aulweg 123, D-35394 Giessen, Germany; david.perez.bravo89@gmail.com
5. Institute of Anatomy and Cell Biology, Justus Liebig University, Aulweg 123, D-35392 Giessen, Germany; ulrich.gaertner@anatomie.med.uni-giessen.de
* Correspondence: liliana.silva@vetmed.uni-giessen.de (L.M.R.S.); kwang-zin.lee@ime.fraunhofer.de (K.-Z.L.)
† These authors contributed equally to this study.

Abstract: *Drosophila suzukii* is a neobiotic invasive pest that causes extensive damage to fruit crops worldwide. The biological control of this species has been unsuccessful thus far, in part because of its robust cellular innate immune system, including the activity of professional phagocytes known as hemocytes and plasmatocytes. The in vitro cultivation of primary hemocytes isolated from *D. suzukii* third-instar larvae is a valuable tool for the investigation of hemocyte-derived effector mechanisms against pathogens such as wasp parasitoid larvae, bacteria, fungi and viruses. Here, we describe the morphological characteristics of *D. suzukii* hemocytes and evaluate early innate immune responses, including extracellular traps released against the entomopathogen *Pseudomonas entomophila* and lipopolysaccharides. We show for the first time that *D. suzukii* plasmatocytes cast extracellular traps to combat *P. entomophila*, along with other cell-mediated reactions, such as phagocytosis and the formation of filopodia.

Keywords: cell culture; *Drosophila suzukii*; hemocytes; plasmatocytes; extracellular traps

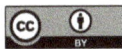

1. Introduction

Drosophila suzukii Matsumura (Diptera: Drosophilidae), also known as the spotted wing *Drosophila*, is a neobiotic invasive pest native to Asia that has spread all over the world and now infests a broad range of fruit crops [1–4]. Female flies are equipped with a serrated ovipositor that can penetrate intact fruit skins [5]. Eggs are laid inside intact fruits, protecting the developing larvae from topical pesticides [6,7]. The high reproduction rate and rapid life cycle of *D. suzukii* pose a serious economic threat to fruit and wine production. A natural innate resistance to pathogenic stressors appears to reflect the high hemocyte count of infected individuals and efficient hemocyte recruitment to infection sites [8–10]. Hemocytes mediate diverse innate defense mechanisms, such as phagocytosis, degranulation, nodulation and encapsulation, as part of the arthropod innate immune system [11,12].

Hematopoiesis in *Drosophila* species produces two hemocyte populations, one originating from the head mesoderm during early embryogenesis and the other arising later from the mesodermal lymph glands [12]. Differentiation of the embryonic hemocytes into lamellocytes, crystal cells and plasmatocytes occurs during the final stage of embryogenesis. The lamellocytes are an independent hemocyte lineage maintained in low numbers, but the population expands significantly in response to parasitoid wasp invasion [13]. These large flat cells encapsulate invading organisms that are too large to be phagocytosed [14]. Crystal cells are involved in the melanization of pathogens and also produce free radicals, such as reactive oxygen species (ROS) [14]. Plasmatocytes are small, spherical cells capable of phagocytosis. They originate in the procephalic mesoderm and migrate to colonize the entire embryo, making up the majority of all hemocytes in vivo [14–20]. Plasmatocytes act as macrophages by recognizing and eliminating microorganisms and apoptotic cells [19–21].

Hemocytes have been studied extensively in the model organism *Drosophila melanogaster* [13]. However, much less is known about these cells in *D. suzukii*. Similarities to mammalian leukocytes, such as neutrophils, suggest a conserved set of functions (and consequences of dysfunction) [20–23]. In vertebrates, polymorphonuclear neutrophils (PMNs) are the first leukocytes to arrive at an infection site, where they facilitate the removal of pathogens not only by phagocytosis, ROS production and degranulation, but also by NETosis, the release of neutrophil extracellular traps (NETs) [23]. These extracellular webs are composed mainly of DNA decorated with nuclear histones (H1A, H2A/H2B, H3 and H4) and various antimicrobial molecules [24–26]. The release of extracellular traps is not limited to PMNs, but also occurs as a highly conserved mechanism in other vertebrate nucleated immune cells (e.g., monocytes, macrophages, eosinophils and mast cells), as well as their invertebrate counterparts [27–32]. In insects, for example, extracellular traps are produced by hemocytes in the larvae of the greater wax moth (*Galleria mellonella*) [32].

The systemic and oral infection of *Drosophila* by the entomopathogenic bacteria *Pseudomonas entomophila* has been shown to be a well-suited model system for the analysis of the insects' humoral and cellular immune response mechanisms [33]. Assuming the bacterial infection would similarly activate defense responses in *D. suzukii* hemolymph, we investigated the ability of different hemocytes to cast extracellular traps following exposure to live *P. entomophila* cells or lipopolysaccharides (LPSs). We found that the coculture of *P. entomophila* with *D. suzukii* plasmatocytes not only triggered the extrusion of extracellular traps, but also resulted in firm bacterial entrapment. Primary cultures of *D. suzukii* plasmatocytes therefore provide a useful in vitro model for the analysis of insect innate immunity, particularly the formation of extracellular traps.

2. Materials and Methods

2.1. Preparation of Drosophila suzukii Fly Stocks

Flies were maintained at 26 °C and 60% humidity with a 12 h photoperiod. They were reared on a soybean and cornmeal medium comprising 10.8% (w/v) soybean and cornmeal mix, 0.8% (w/v) agar, 8% (w/v) malt, 2.2% (w/v) molasses, 1% (w/v) nipagin and 0.625% propionic acid. To avoid contamination, the food was cooked using a MediaClave 10 media sterilizer (WVR International). Before the experiments, the stock was tested for pathogens as previously described [34], including a panel of viruses that commonly infect *D. suzukii* [35].

2.2. Hemocyte Collection and Identification

Third-instar larvae (L3) were washed up to 10 times in distilled water to remove debris. Then, larvae were immobilized and dissected as described by Tracy et al. [36]. The latter protocol was followed for hemocyte isolation with slight modifications: hemocytes were isolated directly in Nunc Lab-Tek II chamber slides (Thermo Fisher Scientific, Schwerte, Germany) containing Grace's insect medium (Thermo Fisher Scientific, Schwerte, Germany) supplemented with 0.1% (w/v) phenylthiourea (Merck, Darmstadt, Germany) and 10% fetal bovine serum (Merck, Darmstadt, Germany). Up to 100 larvae per well/condition were required to recover 5000 hemocytes. The hemocytes were allowed to attach to the surface of the chamber for at least 30 min and were then washed several times with sterile PBS to prevent cross-contamination [36]. For morphological characterization, isolated hemocytes were fixed in 4% paraformaldehyde (PFA) for 5 min at room temperature and stained with 1% toluidine blue (Merck, Darmstadt, Germany), and at least 100 hemocytes per sample were counted under a Leica DM4 B microscope (Leica Microsystems, Wetzlar, Germany).

2.3. Cell Viability Assay

Hemocytes (n = 100) were resuspended in imaging medium, which is Grace's insect medium containing Hoechst (diluted 1:1000) to label DNA and SYTOX Green (diluted 1:2000), to label dead cells. For 3D holotomography, hemocytes in imaging medium were seeded into 35 mm low-rimmed tissue culture µ-dishes (Ibidi®, Gewerbehof, Germany) and allowed to settle for 10–15 min. Images were acquired using a 3D Cell Explorer-fluo microscope (Nanolive®, Tolochenaz, Switzerland) equipped with 60× magnification (λ = 520 nm, sample exposure 0.2 mW/mm^2) and a depth of field of 30 µm and an Ibidi® top-stage chamber (Ibidi®, Gewerbehof, Germany) to keep the temperature stable (RT). At the end of the experiment, images were analyzed using Steve® software v.2.6 (Nanolive®, Tolochenaz, Switzerland) to obtain refractive index (RI)-based z-stacks [37]. Further, 3D rendering and digital staining were performed based on RI values and thereafter illustrated. Additionally, each channel was exported separately using Steve® software v.2.6 (Nanolive®, Tolochenaz, Switzerland) and managed with Image J Fiji v1.7 (NIH, Bethesda, MD, USA) as described elsewhere [38,39].

2.4. Immunofluorescence Staining

Plasmatocytes were identified using an anti-NimC1 antibody mix (diluted 1:30) containing antibodies P1a and P1b [40]. Lamellocytes were identified using the L1 anti-Atilla antibody mix (diluted 1:300) containing antibodies L1a, L1b and L1c [40]. The NimC1 and L1 antibodies were kindly provided by István Andó (Biological Research Centre, Szeged, Hungary). Crystal cells were identified using antibody HC12F6 (diluted 1:30) kindly provided by Martin Speckmann and Tina Trenczek (Justus Liebig University, Giessen, Germany). Nuclear histones within hemocyte-derived extracellular traps were detected using the global anti-histone antibody MAB3422 (Merck, Darmstadt, Germany) recognizing H1, H2A/H2B, H3 and H4 (diluted 1:1000).

Samples were washed in sterile PBS, fixed with 4% PFA for 5 min and blocked for 5 min in sterile PBS containing 2% bovine serum albumin (Merck, Darmstadt, Germany) and 0.1% Triton X-100 (Merck, Darmstadt, Germany). After incubation with the primary antibodies described above at room temperature for 1 h, binding was detected with a goat anti-mouse Alexa Fluor 555 secondary antibody (Thermo Fisher Scientific, Schwerte, Germany, diluted 1:500) at RT for 1 h. The samples were then washed in PBS and mounted in Fluoromount-G anti-fading medium (Thermo Fisher Scientific, Schwerte, Germany) for analysis by confocal microscopy on an LSM 710 instrument (Zeiss, Oberkochen, Germany) with 63× magnification and a numerical aperture of 1.2 µm. Each experiment was repeated three times (using 100 larvae per condition; obtaining $n \approx 5000$ hemocytes). Imaging processing was performed in Image J Fiji v1.7 using merged channels plugins and restricting to minor adjustment of brightness and contrast.

2.5. Detection of Plasmatocyte Phagocytosis and Extracellular Traps

Phagocytosis by activated hemocytes was induced in vitro by exposure to a *P. entomophila* strain (OD 600 nm = 0.1) expressing green fluorescent protein (GFP), kindly provided by Bruno Lemaitre (École Polytechnique Fédérale de Lausanne, France) [41]. Different ODs were previously tested for the scope of this experiment; however, this led to an excess of background. To this end, OD 600 nm = 0.1 was shown to trigger the desired immune responses without interfering with the imaging background. The formation of filopodia was induced by adding 500 mg/mL LPS (Merck, Darmstadt, Germany) [42]. Bacteria or LPS were added to Grace's insect medium containing 0.001% Hoechst and were incubated at room temperature for 1 h. The medium was then removed and hemocyte monolayers were gently washed with PBS before fixing with 4% PFA for 10 min. Plasmatocyte immunostaining was carried out as described above. Actin was stained using Texas Red-X phalloidin (Thermo Fisher Scientific, diluted 1:500) at room temperature for 90 min. For the visualization of extracellular DNA filaments, cells were stained with DAPI for 5 min. Bacteria were identified by visualizing GFP expression. Each experiment was repeated three times (using 100 larvae per condition; obtaining $n \approx 5000$ hemocytes) and a representative image was chosen. Imaging processing was performed in Image J Fiji v1.7 using merged channels plugins and restricting to minor adjustment of brightness and contrast.

2.6. Scanning Electron Microscopy (SEM)

Plasmatocytes from *D. suzukii* were co-cultivated with GFP$^+$ *P. entomophila* (OD 600 nm = 0.1) for 1 h on 10 mm coverslips (Thermo Fisher Scientific, Schwerte, Germany) pre-coated with 0.01% poly-L-lysine (Merck, Darmstadt, Germany) for 15 min at RT. The cells were then fixed in 2.5% glutaraldehyde (Merck, Darmstadt, Germany), post-fixed in 1% osmium tetroxide (Merck, Darmstadt, Germany) and washed in distilled water before dehydration and critical point drying with CO_2. Finally, the cells were gold coated by sputtering and viewed on a Philips XL30 scanning electron microscope (Institute of Anatomy and Cell Biology, Justus Liebig University, Giessen, Germany). Each experiment was repeated three times (using 100 larvae per condition; obtaining $n \approx 5000$ hemocytes) and a representative image was chosen.

3. Results

3.1. Characterization of D. suzukii Larval Hemocytes

Hemocytes isolated from *D. suzukii* L3 larvae ranged in diameter from 10 to 50 μm. The isolated cells were classified by their morphology after toluidine blue staining (Figure 1A–C) followed by staining with hemocyte-specific antibodies (Figure 1D–F). Round granular cells, presenting an average diameter of 9.69 ± 2.96 μm and ranging from 5.14 to 14.70 μm ($n = 100$) (Figure 1A), that were stained by the NimC1/P1 antibody (Figure 1D), were identified as plasmatocytes. The crystal cells were similar in size (average diameter of 9.66 ± 2.07 μm, ranging from 5.82 μm to 13.41 μm; $n = 100$) to the plasmatocytes, but were stained darkly with toluidine blue due to the presence of crystals in the cytoplasm (Figure 1B). They were also stained by the C1-specific antibody, which reacts with prophenoloxidase 2 (PPO2) in *Drosophila* spp. [32] (Figure 1E). The lamellocytes ranged in morphology from oval to elongated forms (average diameter of 28.24 ± 9.66 μm, ranging from 17.89 μm to 47.89 μm; $n = 100$) with a dark nucleus (Figure 1C), but they could be identified by staining with the L1 Atilla-specific antibody (Figure 1F). The most abundant cells (Figure 1G) were plasmatocytes (89.9%), followed by crystal cells (7.5%) and lamellocytes (2.6%).

3.2. Viability of Freshly Isolated D. suzukii Larval Plasmatocytes

The viability of plasmatocytes from *D. suzukii* L3 larvae was assessed by 3D holotomography [38]. Freshly isolated cells were incubated in an imaging medium at room temperature until more than 90% of the cells were dead. At the beginning of the incubation period, plasmatocytes were generally rounded (Figure 2, RI), with a central nucleus stained with Hoechst (Figure 2, DNA). Visible granules surrounding the nucleus registered higher RI values than the rest of the cell contents (Figure 2, zoomed images). After 2 h of isolation, circa 50% of the cells remained viable (Figure 2, absence of SYTOX Green staining) but 90% of the cells were stained with SYTOX Green after 4 h (Figure 2, survival rate), indicating cell death, even though the cells maintained their shapes. Accordingly, all subsequent experiments were limited to 2 h post-isolation to ensure that most of the freshly isolated plasmatocytes were viable.

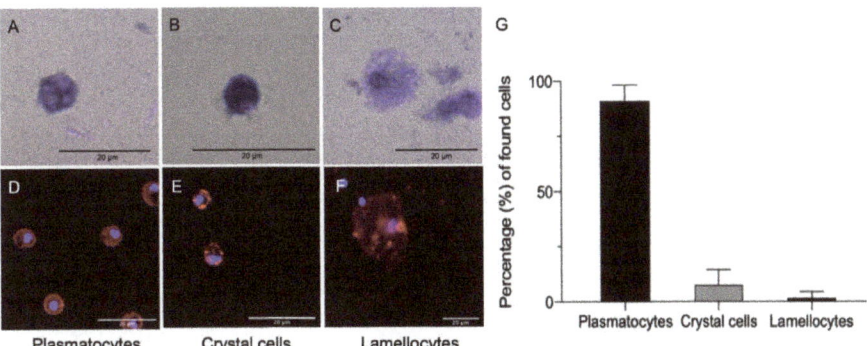

Figure 1. Characterization of hemocytes from *Drosophila suzukii* L3 larvae. Cells isolated from the hemolymph of *D. suzukii* L3 larvae were fixed with 4% paraformaldehyde for 5 min at room temperature and stained with 1% toluidine blue (**A–C**) followed by immunofluorescence staining (**D–F**). Plasmatocytes (**A**), identified by staining with the anti-NimC1 antibody (**D**), were rounded cells with central nuclei. Crystal cells (**B**), identified by staining with antibody HC12F6 (**E**), were rounded cells containing crystals that were stained densely with toluidine blue. Lamellocytes (**C**), identified by staining with the L1 anti-Atilla antibody (**F**), were oval or elongated cells. Nuclei were counterstained with DAPI (**D–F**, blue). Cell population analysis (**G**) revealed plasmatocytes to be the most abundant cells (89.9%), followed by crystal cells (7.5%) and lamellocytes (2.6%). Scale bar = 20 µm.

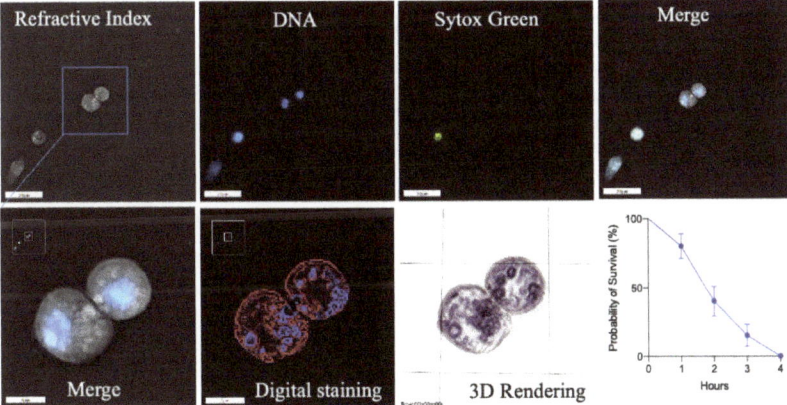

Figure 2. Plasmatocyte viability assay and characterization by 3D holotomography. Plasmatocytes were mostly rounded cells (RI) with a central nucleus (DNA) and perinuclear granules (zoomed images on bottom row). SYTOX Green staining, which is specific for dead cells, showed that circa half of the cells remained viable for at least 2 h but that 90% were dead after 4 h. Scale bar = 5 µm.

3.3. Response of D. suzukii L3 Plasmatocytes to P. entomophila

The exposure of *D. suzukii* plasmatocytes to a GFP$^+$ *P. entomophila* strain triggered the formation of extracellular trap structures with a range of phenotypes (Figure 3), as described for other species elsewhere [42–44]. Electron microscopy confirmed that *D. suzukii* plasmatocytes react against *P. entomophila*, not only by casting extracellular traps, but also by forming filopodia (Figure 3).

The plasmatocytes were able to cast short spread extracellular traps (sprETs) that captured the cocultured bacteria (Figure 3A, green arrows). Some filigree filaments (Figure 3A,B, blue arrows) were also attached to bacterial cells, but not to hemocytes. These were probably extracellular DNA filaments derived from sprETs that were damaged by the evasion attempts of bacteria or by experimental handling. We also observed the presence of so-called aggregated extracellular traps (*agg*ETs) in response to GFP⁺ *P. entomophila* (Figure 3B,C). These formed large meshes of extracellular fibers containing many immune cells releasing individual extracellular traps (Figure 3C, green arrows) and were able to trap several bacteria at once (Figure 3B, white arrows).

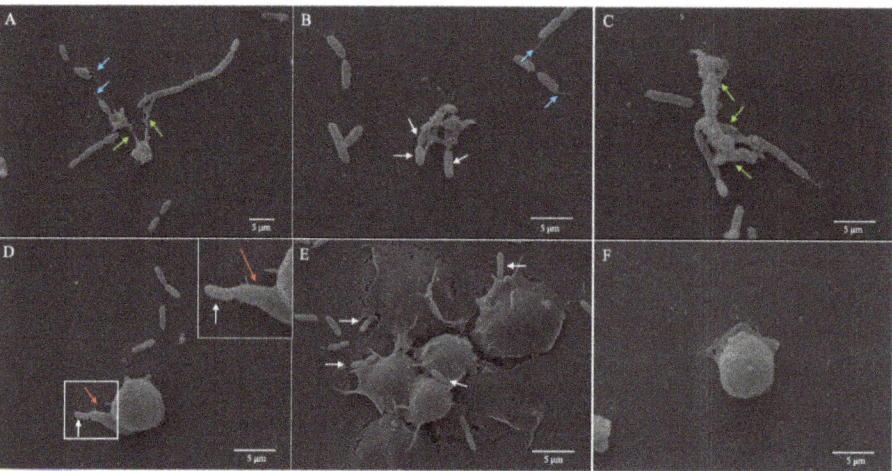

Figure 3. SEM images of extracellular traps formed by *Drosophila suzukii* plasmatocytes in response to *Pseudomonas entomophila*. The isolated plasmatocytes were incubated with *P. entomophila* (**A–E**) or PBS (control, **F**) at room temperature for 1 h. The plasmatocytes cast short spread extracellular traps (*spr*ETs) to entrap *P. entomophila* (**A**, green arrows). Filigree filaments (**A,B**, blue arrows) from disrupted extracellular DNA filaments also attached to *P. entomophila*. So-called aggregated extracellular traps (*agg*ETs) were observed when cells were challenged with *P. entomophila* (**B,C**), resulting in massive clusters of mesh fibers containing many immune cells (**C**, green arrows) and bacteria (**B**, white arrows). The formation of filopodia (**D**) was observed after further incubation, and *P. entomophila* was found stuck to these structures (**D,E**, white arrows). Scale bar = 5 μm.

To confirm that *D. suzukii* plasmatocytes cast extracellular traps, we stained the typical components of such structures in immunofluorescence assays. After challenging plasmatocytes with *P. entomophila* or 500 mg/mL LPS, the formation of extracellular traps was confirmed by the co-localization of extracellular DNA and histones (Figure 4). Interestingly, LPS induced short *spr*ETs (Figure 4, blue arrow) and diffuse extracellular traps (*diff*ETs), the latter characterized by nuclear expansion and thus cell expansion with histone redistribution (Figure 4, red arrows). We observed the same response to three different concentrations of LPS (100, 250 and 500 μg/mL). In contrast, *P. entomophila* induced *spr*ETs (Figure 4, blue arrows) and *agg*ETs (Figure 4, green arrows), both of which were shown to entrap the GFP⁺ bacteria (Figure 4, white arrows), confirming the SEM data.

The percentage of plasmatocytes that produced extracellular traps was calculated after coculture with *P. entomophila* or stimulation with LPS (Figure 5). Approximately 9% of plasmatocytes produced extracellular traps in response to *P. entomophila*, whereas only 3.6% produced extracellular traps in response to stimulation with LPS, although the difference was not statistically significant (Figure 5A). Additionally, different ETs were displayed when cells were stimulated after each condition (Figure 5B). In response to *P. entomophila*, 41% of the displayed ETs represented *spr*ETs, whereas 59% displayed *agg*ETs (Figure 5B). In addition, 77% of the LPS-stimulated plasmatocytes displayed *diff*ETs whereas 23% displayed *spr*ETs.

To confirm that the observed immunoreactive behavior was cast by *D. suzukii* plasmatocytes, plasmatocyte-specific anti-NimC1 antibody staining was used. Positive stained cells were the ones releasing extracellular traps (Figure 6, white asterisk). The *D. suzukii* plasmatocytes also engulfed *P. entomophila* by phagocytosis (white arrows). One hour after the challenge, 9.86% of the plasmatocytes were shown to engage in the phagocytosis of *P. entomophila* (Figure 7, orange arrow).

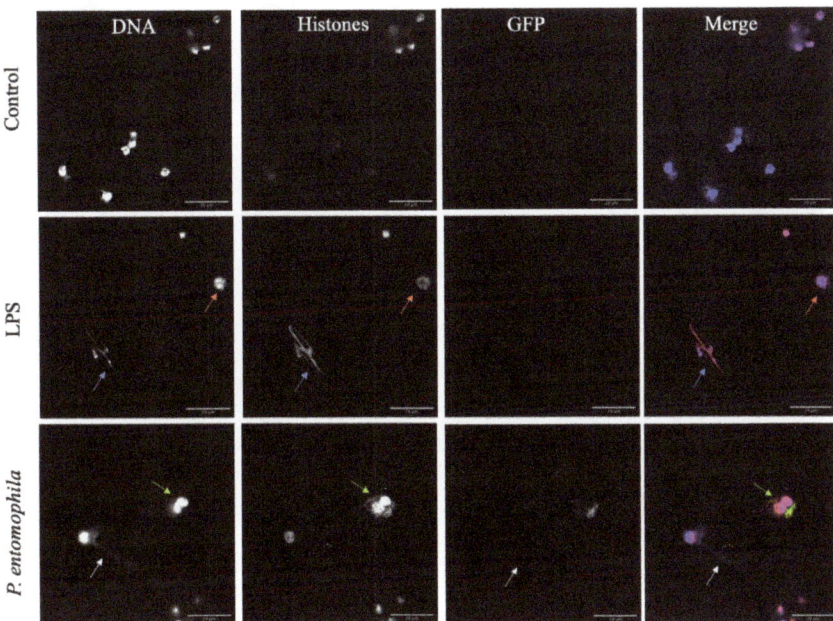

Figure 4. Characteristics of extracellular traps formed by *Drosophila suzukii* plasmatocytes in response to *Pseudomonas entomophila* and lipopolysaccharides (LPS). Isolated plasmatocytes were incubated with GFP+ *P. entomophila*, LPS or PBS as a control for 1 h before fixing with 4% PFA for 5 min at room temperature and staining with Hoechst (blue). Histones (H1, H2A, H2B, H3 and H4) were then detected with the monoclonal antibody MAB3422 followed by staining with the goat anti-mouse IgG Alexa Fluor 555 (red) and nuclear counterstaining with DAPI (blue). One hour after the challenge, two different phenotypes were observed. LPS induced spread extracellular traps (*spr*ETs, blue arrows), as well as diffuse extracellular traps (*diff*ETs, red arrows), whereas *P. entomophila* (white arrows) induced *spr*ETs (blue arrows) and aggregated extracellular traps (*agg*ETs, green arrows). Scale bar = 20 μm.

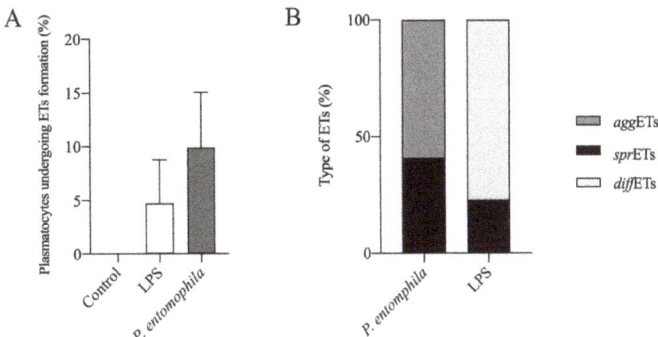

Figure 5. Quantification of extracellular traps induced by *P. entomophila* or LPS. (**A**) We compared the proportion of plasmatocytes that cast extracellular traps in response to GFP+ *P. entomophila* and LPS. *P. entomophila* induced higher ET formation than LPS when compared to control (no ET formation). (**B**) The three different ETs phenotypes were quantified and LPS induced *spr*ETs, as well as *diff*ETs (in greater percentage), whereas *P. entomophila* induced *spr*ETs and *agg*ETs, the latter in higher proportion.

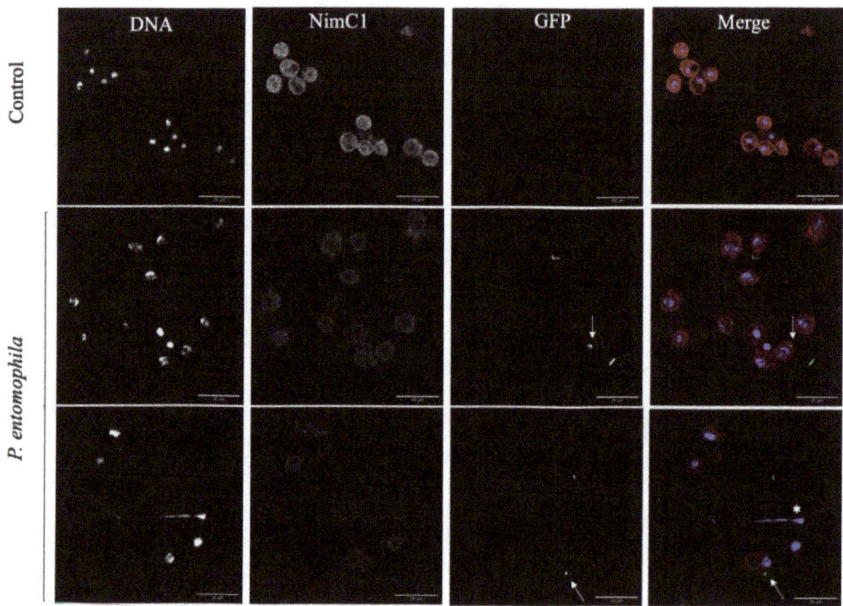

Figure 6. *Drosophila suzukii* plasmatocytes cast extracellular traps and engulf *Pseudomonas entomophila* by phagocytosis. Plasmatocytes were challenged with GFP+ *P. entomophila* and stained with the plasmatocyte-specific antibody anti-NimC1 to confirm their identify. We observed the formation of extracellular traps (white asterisk, lower row) but also the phagocytosis of *P. entomophila* (white arrows, middle and lower rows), indicating that plasmatocytes respond to the challenge by deploying multiple defense mechanisms. Scale bar = 20 µm.

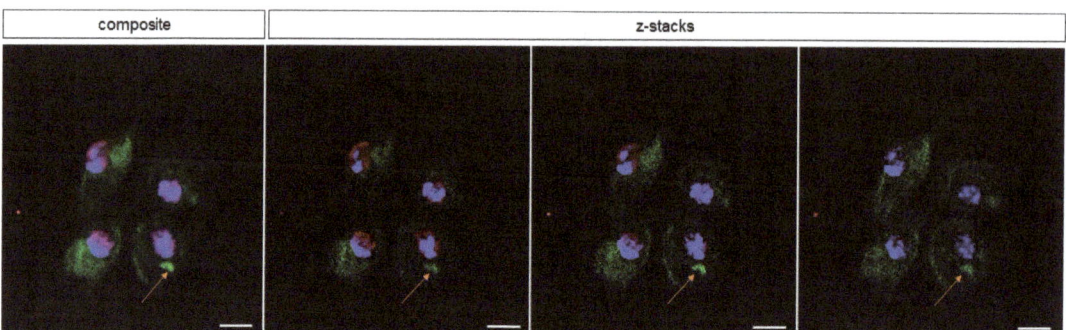

Figure 7. *Drosophila suzukii* plasmatocytes phagocyte *Pseudomonas entomophila*. After plasmatocytes were challenged with GFP+ *P. entomophila*, bacteria were observed intracellularly near to the nucleus of plasmatocytes (orange arrows), showing that plasmatocytes use multiple defense mechanisms, including phagocytosis. Nucleus was stained with DAPI (blue), histones in red and bacteria in green. Auto-fluorescence of the cell is observed. Scale bar = 10 µm.

In addition to phagocytosis and extracellular traps, we also observed the formation of filopodia as a third effector mechanism against pathogenic bacteria (Figure 3D, red arrow), followed by the adhesion of bacteria to these structures (Figure 8). Texas Red-X phalloidin staining (Figure 8, phalloidin) confirmed the actin-dependent formation filopodia in response to the bacteria and LPS, resulting in the presentation of rounded to slightly elongated plasmatocytes.

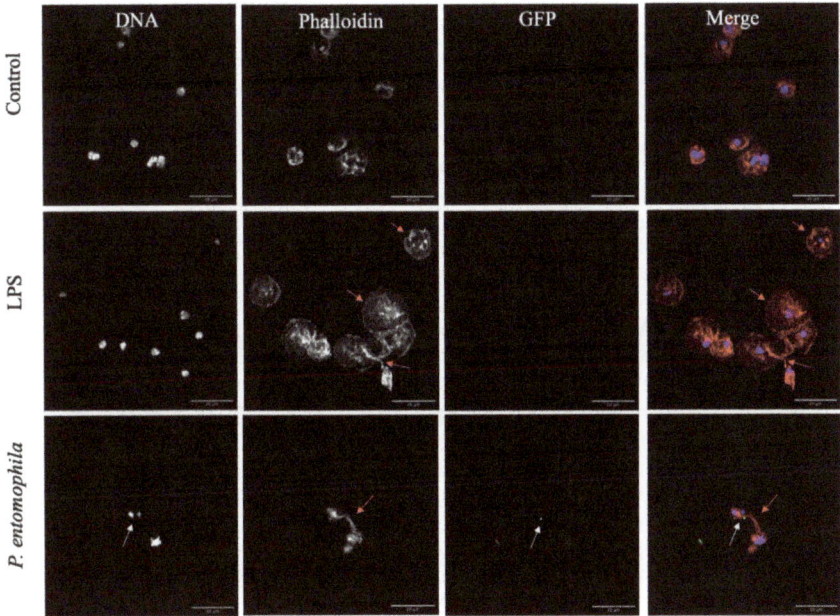

Figure 8. Formation of filopodia by *D. suzukii* plasmatocytes. Isolated plasmatocytes were incubated with GFP⁺ *P. entomophila*, 500 µg/mL LPS or PBS as a control for 1 h before fixing in 4% paraformaldehyde for 5 min at room temperature and staining for DNA with Hoechst (blue) and for actin with Texas Red-X phalloidin (Phalloidin, red). Filopodia (red arrows) formed in response to both LPS and *P. entomophila* (white arrows), resulting in the presentation of rounded to slightly elongated cells (arrow). Scale bar = 20 µm.

4. Discussion

In insects and other invertebrates, hemocytes are the first line of defense, eliminating pathogens upon first encounter in vivo and therefore fulfilling a similar role to professional phagocytes (PMNs, monocytes and macrophages) in mammals. We characterized the hemocyte population of the invasive pest insect *D. suzukii* to add to the understanding of diverse effector mechanisms as part of the early innate immune response, which has not been reported for other drosophilid species thus far. We observed phagocytosis and the formation of filopodia by *D. suzukii* plasmatocytes exposed to *P. entomophila* or LPS, but also the formation of extracellular traps (ETosis), highlighting the importance of this widespread cellular immune defense mechanism in eukaryotes [23,45]. ETosis has been reported in other insects [33,46], and also in other invertebrates, such as oysters [47,48], mussels [46] and slugs [29], and the mechanism appears highly conserved. The traps are composed of extracellular DNA decorated with nuclear histones (chromatin), combined with lactoferrin, pentraxin, myeloperoxidase, elastase, gelatinase and cathelicidin, among other antimicrobial molecules [22–24,26,40]. Interestingly, we observed the presence of multiple histones (H1, H2A/H2B, H3 and H4), whereas one recent study in the cockroach *Periplaneta americana* only identified H1/DNA complexes in extracellular traps [42], with only one study in slugs supporting our findings [29]. However, our results align with the mechanism of ETosis in mammals, where histones are one of the main components of extracellular traps both in vitro and in vivo [46]. The formation of extracellular traps by drosophilid hemocytes has not been reported before, and the absence of nucleic acid clots in the hemolymph of *D. melanogaster* was reported following a challenge with *Escherichia coli* JM109 [49]. The nature of the pathogenic stimulus may determine the mode of cellular defense. Here, we used *P. entomophila*, a bacterial pathogen that has already been shown to cause systemic infections that induce a range of immune responses in drosophilids [50,51]. The bacteria can be highly pathogenic when flies receive inoculum sizes sufficient to disrupt the gut epithelium and enter the hemolymph, which brings them into contact with hemocytes [50,51].

We characterized the morphology of *D. suzukii* hemocytes in detail and observed similar characteristics to the closely related fly *D. melanogaster* [13]. We were able to distinguish between lamellocytes, crystal cells and plasmatocytes using both morphological criteria and specific immunostaining, which allowed us to demonstrate the unique defense mechanisms of the plasmatocyte population. The revelation that such cells can form filopodia and extracellular traps in response to *P. entomophila* supports findings in other insects [42]. The initial detection of pathogenic bacteria is facilitated by the recognition of pathogen-associated molecular patterns (PAMPs) such as LPS. Our results suggest that PAMPs alone, which bind pathogen recognition receptors (PRRs) on the surface of plasmatocytes, are sufficient for inducing the formation of filopodia and the release of extracellular traps. Similar (dose-dependent) effects have been described in the cockroach *P. americana* [42] when hemocytes are stimulated with delipidated LPS. Naturally, hemocyte PRRs sense and respond differently to LPS or infections with live bacteria [52], highlighting the importance of adjusting the bacterial titer in order to study humoral and cellular immune responses. However, future studies should address the effect of delipidated LPS and/or other bacterial strains on the *D. suzukii* cellular response. The potential role of hemocyte "trained immunity" after a primary infection with *P. entomophila* is also an interesting topic because this form of innate immune memory has been well described in mammals and, despite the long-believed lack of "immune priming" capacities in invertebrates, more recent studies indicate its presence also in insects [53–56].

Interestingly, *D. suzukii* plasmatocytes-derived ETosis revealed up to three different types of extracellular traps, namely *spr*ETs, *agg*ETs and *diff*ETs, as previously described for other hosts and cells [29,43]. Exposure to bacteria or LPS induced the release of *spr*ETs, whereas *diff*ETs were only observed following a challenge with LPS. In addition, *agg*ETs were cast after *P. entomophila* stimulus. Neutrophils are known to discriminate between LPS and bacterial infection, releasing NETs that differ in structure and activity [57]. In mammals, it is likely that *spr*NETs and *diff*NETs are preliminary structures, whereas *agg*NETs are later and more mature forms [43]. Further experiments with longer exposure times would be necessary in determining whether a similar temporal profile exists in insects with the presence of even larger or a higher number of *agg*ETs. It would also be interesting to investigate whether insect *agg*ETs inhibit inflammation by degrading cytokines and chemokines as they do in mammals [44].

D. suzukii robust cellular immune responses might have facilitated its rapid worldwide spread by allowing it to overcome pathogen infections in newly colonized environments [55–57]. Such immunological diversity can help invasive species deal with unfamiliar pathogens [10–47,49–58], as recently shown for the invasive harlequin ladybird *Harmonia axyridis* [48,55–61]. We therefore propose that extracellular traps are a key component of the *D. suzukii* cellular innate immune response against pathogenic bacteria. The similarity between vertebrate and invertebrate cellular immunity highlights the evolutionary conservation of this ancient mechanism.

Author Contributions: Conceptualization, C.H., L.M.R.S., A.V., K.-Z.L., T.C. and S.T.; validation, C.H., L.M.R.S., A.V., K.-Z.L., T.C. and S.T.; investigation, C.H., L.M.R.S., D.P.-B., U.G., T.C. and S.T.; writing—original draft preparation, L.M.R.S., D.P.-B., T.C. and S.T.; writing—review and editing, C.H., L.M.R.S., A.V., K.-Z.L., A.T., T.C. and S.T.; funding acquisition A.V. All authors have read and agreed to the published version of the manuscript.

Funding: This work was funded by the excellence initiative of the Hessian Ministry of Science, Higher Education and the Arts (HMWK) supporting the LOEWE Centre for Insect Biotechnology and Bioresources.

Institutional Review Board Statement: Not applicable.

Informed Consent Statement: Not applicable.

Data Availability Statement: Not applicable.

Acknowledgments: We thank Anika Seipp (Institute of Anatomy and Cell Biology, JLU Giessen, Germany) for technical support with electron microscopy, and Henrike Schmidtberg for technical support with hemolymph extraction and processing. We also thank István Andó (Biological Research Centre, Szeged, Hungary) and Martin Speckmann (Justus Liebig University, Giessen, Germany) for the hemocyte-specific antibodies, and Richard M. Twyman for professional editing of the manuscript.

Conflicts of Interest: The authors declare no conflict of interest.

References

1. Calabria, G.; Máca, J.; Serra, L.; Pascual, M. First Records of the Potential Pest Species *Drosophila suzukii* (Diptera: Drosophilidae) in Europe. *J. Appl. Entomol.* **2012**, *136*, 139–147. [CrossRef]
2. Walsh, D.B.; Bolda, M.P.; Goodhue, R.E.; Dreves, A.J.; Lee, J.; Bruck, D.J.; Walton, V.M.; O'Neal, S.D.; Zalom, F.G. *Drosophila suzukii* (Diptera: Drosophilidae): Invasive Pest of Ripening Soft Fruit Expanding Its Geographic Range and Damage Potential. *J. Integr. Pest Manag.* **2011**, *2*, G1–G7. [CrossRef]
3. Andreazza, F.; Bernardi, D.; Dos Santos, R.S.S.; Garcia, F.R.M.; Oliveira, E.E.; Botton, M.; Nava, D.E. *Drosophila suzukii* in Southern Neotropical Region: Current Status and Future Perspectives. *Neotrop. Entomol.* **2017**, *46*, 591–605. [CrossRef] [PubMed]
4. Ørsted, I.V.; Ørsted, M. Species Distribution Models of the Spotted Wing Drosophila (*Drosophila suzukii*, Diptera: Drosophilidae) in Its Native and Invasive Range Reveal an Ecological Niche Shift. *J. Appl. Ecol.* **2019**, *56*, 423–435. [CrossRef]
5. Atallah, J.; Teixeira, L.; Salazar, R.; Zaragoza, G.; Kopp, A. The Making of a Pest: The Evolution of a Fruit-Penetrating Ovipositor in *Drosophila suzukii* and Related Species. *Proc. R. Soc. B Biol. Sci.* **2014**, *281*, 20132840. [CrossRef] [PubMed]
6. Tochen, S.; Dalton, D.T.; Wiman, N.; Hamm, C.; Shearer, P.W.; Walton, V.M. Temperature-Related Development and Population Parameters for *Drosophila suzukii* (Diptera: Drosophilidae) on Cherry and Blueberry. *Environ. Entomol.* **2014**, *43*, 501–510. [CrossRef] [PubMed]
7. Wiman, N.G.; Walton, V.M.; Dalton, D.T.; Anfora, G.; Burrack, H.J.; Chiu, J.C.; Daane, K.M.; Grassi, A.; Miller, B.; Tochen, S.; et al. Integrating Temperature-Dependent Life Table Data into a Matrix Projection Model for *Drosophila suzukii* Population Estimation. *PLoS ONE* **2014**, *9*, e106909. [CrossRef]
8. Kacsoh, B.Z.; Schlenke, T.A. High Hemocyte Load Is Associated with Increased Resistance against Parasitoids in *Drosophila suzukii*, a Relative of *D. melanogaster*. *PLoS ONE* **2012**, *7*, e34721. [CrossRef]
9. Poyet, M.; Havard, S.; Prevost, G.; Chabrerie, O.; Doury, G.; Gibert, P.; Eslin, P. Resistance of *Drosophila suzukii* to the Larval Parasitoids *Leptopilina heterotoma* and *Asobara japonica* Is Related to Haemocyte Load. *Physiol. Entomol.* **2013**, *38*, 45–53. [CrossRef]
10. Pech, L.L.; Strand, M.R. Granular Cells Are Required for Encapsulation of Foreign Targets by Insect Haemocytes. *J. Cell Sci.* **1996**, *109*, 2053–2060. [CrossRef]
11. Schmidt, O.; Theopold, U.; Strand, M. Innate Immunity and Its Evasion and Suppression by Hymenopteran Endoparasitoids. *BioEssays* **2001**, *23*, 344–351. [CrossRef]
12. Traver, D.; Zon, L.I. Walking the Walk: Migration and Other Common Themes in Blood and Vascular Development. *Cell* **2002**, *108*, 731–734. [CrossRef]
13. Banerjee, U.; Girard, J.R.; Goins, L.M.; Spratford, C.M. Drosophila as a Genetic Model for Hematopoiesis. *Genetics* **2019**, *211*, 367–417. [CrossRef]
14. Meister, M.; Lagueux, M. Drosophila Blood Cells. *Cell. Microbiol.* **2003**, *5*, 573–580. [CrossRef]
15. Lebestky, T.; Chang, T.; Hartenstein, V.; Banerjee, U. Specification of *Drosophila* Hematopoietic Lineage by Conserved Transcription Factors. *Science* **2000**, *288*, 146–149. [CrossRef] [PubMed]
16. Lavine, M.D.; Strand, M.R. Insect Hemocytes and Their Role in Immunity. *Insect Biochem. Mol. Biol.* **2002**, *32*, 1295–1309. [CrossRef]
17. Tepass, U.; Fessler, L.I.; Aziz, A.; Hartenstein, V. Embryonic Origin of Hemocytes and Their Relationship to Cell Death in *Drosophila*. *Development* **1994**, *120*, 1829–1837. [CrossRef] [PubMed]
18. Franc, N.C.; Heitzler, P.; Ezekowitz, R.A.B.; White, K. Requirement for Croquemort in Phagocytosis of Apoptotic Cells in *Drosophila*. *Science* **1999**, *284*, 1991–1994. [CrossRef] [PubMed]
19. Müller, U.; Vogel, P.; Alber, G.; Schaub, G.A. The Innate Immune System of Mammals and Insects. *Trends Innate Immun.* **2008**, *15*, 21–44. [CrossRef]
20. Franc, N.C.; Dimarcq, J.L.; Lagueux, M.; Hoffman, J.A.; Ezekowitz, R.A.B. Croquemort, A Novel *Drosophila* Hemocyte/Macrophage Receptor That Recognizes Apoptotic Cells. *Immunity* **1996**, *4*, 431–443. [CrossRef]
21. Villagra-Blanco, R.; Silva, L.M.R.; Conejeros, I.; Taubert, A.; Hermosilla, C. Pinniped- and Cetacean-Derived ETosis Contributes to Combating Emerging Apicomplexan Parasites (*Toxoplasma gondii*, *Neospora caninum*) Circulating in Marine Environments. *Biology* **2019**, *8*, 12. [CrossRef] [PubMed]
22. Neumann, A.; Brogden, G.; von Köckritz-Blickwede, M. Extracellular Traps: An Ancient Weapon of Multiple Kingdoms. *Biology* **2020**, *9*, 34. [CrossRef] [PubMed]

23. Nathan, C. Neutrophils and Immunity: Challenges and Opportunities. *Nat. Rev. Immunol.* **2006**, *6*, 173–182. [CrossRef] [PubMed]
24. Urban, C.F.; Ermert, D.; Schmid, M.; Abu-Abed, U.; Goosmann, C.; Nacken, W.; Brinkmann, V.; Jungblut, P.R.; Zychlinsky, A. Neutrophil Extracellular Traps Contain Calprotectin, a Cytosolic Protein Complex Involved in Host Defense against *Candida albicans*. *PLoS Pathog.* **2009**, *5*, e1000639. [CrossRef]
25. Parker, H.; Albrett, A.M.; Kettle, A.J.; Winterbourn, C.C. Myeloperoxidase Associated with Neutrophil Extracellular Traps Is Active and Mediates Bacterial Killing in the Presence of Hydrogen Peroxide. *J. Leukoc. Biol.* **2012**, *91*, 369–376. [CrossRef]
26. Webster, S.J.; Daigneault, M.; Bewley, M.A.; Preston, J.A.; Marriott, H.M.; Walmsley, S.R.; Read, R.C.; Whyte, M.K.B.; Dockrell, D.H. Distinct Cell Death Programs in Monocytes Regulate Innate Responses Following Challenge with Common Causes of Invasive Bacterial Disease. *J. Immunol.* **2010**, *185*, 2968–2979. [CrossRef]
27. Bartneck, M.; Keul, H.A.; Zwadlo-Klarwasser, G.; Groll, J. Phagocytosis Independent Extracellular Nanoparticle Clearance by Human Immune Cells. *Nano Lett.* **2010**, *10*, 59–63. [CrossRef]
28. Palić, D.; Ostojić, J.; Andreasen, C.B.; Roth, J.A. Fish Cast NETs: Neutrophil Extracellular Traps Are Released from Fish Neutrophils. *Dev. Comp. Immunol.* **2007**, *31*, 805–816. [CrossRef]
29. Lange, M.K.; Penagos-Tabares, F.; Muñoz-Caro, T.; Gärtner, U.; Mejer, H.; Schaper, R.; Hermosilla, C.; Taubert, A. Gastropod-Derived Haemocyte Extracellular Traps Entrap Metastrongyloid Larval Stages of *Angiostrongylus vasorum*, *Aelurostrongylus abstrusus* and *Troglostrongylus brevior*. *Parasites Vectors* **2017**, *10*, 50. [CrossRef]
30. Ng, T.H.; Chang, S.-H.; Wu, M.-H.; Wang, H.-C. Shrimp Hemocytes Release Extracellular Traps That Kill Bacteria. *Dev. Comp. Immunol.* **2013**, *41*, 644–651. [CrossRef]
31. Silva, L.M.R.; Muñoz-Caro, T.; Burgos, R.A.; Hidalgo, M.A.; Taubert, A.; Hermosilla, C. Far beyond Phagocytosis: Phagocyte-Derived Extracellular Traps Act Efficiently against Protozoan Parasites In Vitro and In Vivo. *Mediat. Inflamm.* **2016**, *2016*, 5898074. [CrossRef]
32. Altincicek, B.; Stötzel, S.; Wygrecka, M.; Preissner, K.T.; Vilcinskas, A. Host-Derived Extracellular Nucleic Acids Enhance Innate Immune Responses, Induce Coagulation, and Prolong Survival upon Infection in Insects. *J. Immunol.* **2008**, *181*, 2705–2712. [CrossRef] [PubMed]
33. Vodovar, N.; Vinals, M.; Liehl, P.; Basset, A.; Degrouard, J.; Spellman, P.; Boccard, F.; Lemaitre, B. *Drosophila* Host Defense after Oral Infection by an Entomopathogenic *Pseudomonas* Species. *Proc. Natl. Acad. Sci. USA* **2005**, *102*, 11414–11419. [CrossRef] [PubMed]
34. Merkling, S.H.; van Rij, R.P. Analysis of Resistance and Tolerance to Virus Infection in *Drosophila*. *Nat. Protoc.* **2015**, *10*, 1084–1097. [CrossRef] [PubMed]
35. Medd, N.C.; Fellous, S.; Waldron, F.M.; Xuéreb, A.; Nakai, M.; Cross, J.V.; Obbard, D.J. The Virome of *Drosophila suzukii*, an Invasive Pest of Soft Fruit. *Virus Evol.* **2018**, *4*, vey009. [CrossRef]
36. Tracy, C.; Krämer, H. Isolation and Infection of *Drosophila* Primary Hemocytes. *Bio-Protoc.* **2017**, *7*, e2300. [CrossRef]
37. Sandoz, P.A.; Tremblay, C.; Equis, S.; Pop, S.; Pollaro, L.; Cotte, Y.; van der Goot, F.G.; Frechin, M. Label Free 3D Analysis of Organelles in Living Cells by Refractive Index Shows Pre-Mitotic Organelle Spinning in Mammalian Stem Cells. *bioRxiv* **2018**, 407239. [CrossRef]
38. Velásquez, Z.D.; López-Osorio, S.; Mazurek, S.; Hermosilla, C.; Taubert, A. Eimeria Bovis Macromeront Formation Induces Glycolytic Responses and Mitochondrial Changes in Primary Host Endothelial Cells. *Front. Cell. Infect. Microbiol.* **2021**, *11*, 635. [CrossRef]
39. Larrazabal, C.; Hermosilla, C.; Taubert, A.; Conejeros, I. 3D Holotomographic Monitoring of Ca^{++} Dynamics during Ionophore-Induced *Neospora caninum* Tachyzoite Egress from Primary Bovine Host Endothelial Cells. *Parasitol. Res.* **2021**. [CrossRef]
40. Kurucz, E.; Váczi, B.; Márkus, R.; Laurinyecz, B.; Vilmos, P.; Zsámboki, J.; Csorba, K.; Gateff, E.; Hultmark, D.; Andó, I. Definition of *Drosophila* Hemocyte Subsets by Cell-Type Specific Antigens. *Acta Biol. Hung.* **2007**, *58*, 95–111. [CrossRef]
41. Mulet, M.; Gomila, M.; Lemaitre, B.; Lalucat, J.; García-Valdés, E. Taxonomic Characterisation of *Pseudomonas* Strain L48 and Formal Proposal of *Pseudomonas entomophila* Sp. Nov. *Syst. Appl. Microbiol.* **2012**, *35*, 145–149. [CrossRef] [PubMed]
42. Nascimento, M.T.C.; Silva, K.P.; Garcia, M.C.F.; Medeiros, M.N.; Machado, E.A.; Nascimento, S.B.; Saraiva, E.M. DNA Extracellular Traps Are Part of the Immune Repertoire of *Periplaneta americana*. *Dev. Comp. Immunol.* **2018**, *84*, 62–70. [CrossRef] [PubMed]
43. Muñoz-Caro, T.; Rubio, R.M.C.; Silva, L.M.R.; Magdowski, G.; Gärtner, U.; McNeilly, T.N.; Taubert, A.; Hermosilla, C. Leucocyte-Derived Extracellular Trap Formation Significantly Contributes to *Haemonchus contortus* Larval Entrapment. *Parasites Vectors* **2015**, *8*, 607. [CrossRef] [PubMed]
44. Schauer, C.; Janko, C.; Munoz, L.E.; Zhao, Y.; Kienhöfer, D.; Frey, B.; Lell, M.; Manger, B.; Rech, J.; Naschberger, E.; et al. Aggregated Neutrophil Extracellular Traps Limit Inflammation by Degrading Cytokines and Chemokines. *Nat. Med.* **2014**, *20*, 511–517. [CrossRef]
45. Hakkim, A.; Fuchs, T.A.; Martinez, N.E.; Hess, S.; Prinz, H.; Zychlinsky, A.; Waldmann, H. Activation of the Raf-MEK-ERK Pathway Is Required for Neutrophil Extracellular Trap Formation. *Nat. Chem. Biol.* **2011**, *7*, 75–77. [CrossRef]
46. Brinkmann, V.; Reichard, U.; Goosmann, C.; Fauler, B.; Uhlemann, Y.; Weiss, D.S.; Weinrauch, Y.; Zychlinsky, A. Neutrophil Extracellular Traps Kill Bacteria. *Science* **2004**, *303*, 1532–1535. [CrossRef]
47. Zhou, E.; Silva, L.; Conejeros, I.; Velásquez, Z.; Hirz, M.; Gärtner, U.; Jacquiet, P.; Taubert, A.; Hermosilla, C. *Besnoitia besnoiti* bradyzoite stages induce suicidal- and rapid vital-NETosis. *Parasitology* **2020**, *147*, 401–409. [CrossRef]

48. Beckert, A.; Wiesner, J.; Baumann, A.; Pöppel, A.-K.; Vogel, H.; Vilcinskas, A. Two C-Type Lysozymes Boost the Innate Immune System of the Invasive Ladybird *Harmonia axyridis*. *Dev. Comp. Immunol.* **2015**, *49*, 303–312. [CrossRef]
49. Bidla, G.; Lindgren, M.; Theopold, U.; Dushay, M.S. Hemolymph Coagulation and Phenoloxidase in *Drosophila* Larvae. *Dev. Comp. Immunol.* **2005**, *29*, 669–679. [CrossRef]
50. Hiebert, N.; Carrau, T.; Bartling, M.; Vilcinskas, A.; Lee, K.-Z. Identification of Entomopathogenic Bacteria Associated with the Invasive Pest *Drosophila suzukii* in Infested Areas of Germany. *J. Invertebr. Pathol.* **2020**, *173*, 107389. [CrossRef]
51. Dieppois, G.; Opota, O.; Lalucat, J.; Lemaitre, B. Pseudomonas entomophila: A Versatile Bacterium with Entomopathogenic Properties. In *Pseudomonas: New Aspects of Pseudomonas Biology*; Ramos, J.-L., Goldberg, J.B., Filloux, A., Eds.; Springer: Dordrecht, The Netherlands, 2015; Volume 7, pp. 25–49. ISBN 978-94-017-9555-5.
52. Johansson, K.C.; Metzendorf, C.; Söderhäll, K. Microarray Analysis of Immune Challenged Drosophila Hemocytes. *Exp. Cell Res.* **2005**, *305*, 145–155. [CrossRef]
53. Frangou, E.; Vassilopoulos, D.; Boletis, J.; Boumpas, D.T. An Emerging Role of Neutrophils and NETosis in Chronic Inflammation and Fibrosis in Systemic Lupus Erythematosus (SLE) and ANCA-Associated Vasculitides (AAV): Implications for the Pathogenesis and Treatment. *Autoimmun. Rev.* **2019**, *18*, 751–760. [CrossRef] [PubMed]
54. Mondotte, J.A.; Gausson, V.; Frangeul, L.; Blanc, H.; Lambrechts, L.; Saleh, M.-C. Immune Priming and Clearance of Orally Acquired RNA Viruses in *Drosophila*. *Nat. Microbiol.* **2018**, *3*, 1394–1403. [CrossRef] [PubMed]
55. Mondotte, J.A.; Gausson, V.; Frangeul, L.; Suzuki, Y.; Vazeille, M.; Mongelli, V.; Blanc, H.; Failloux, A.-B.; Saleh, M.-C. Evidence For Long-Lasting Transgenerational Antiviral Immunity in Insects. *Cell Rep.* **2020**, *33*, 108506. [CrossRef] [PubMed]
56. Cooper, D.; Eleftherianos, I. Memory and Specificity in the Insect Immune System: Current Perspectives and Future Challenges. *Front. Immunol.* **2017**, *8*, 539. [CrossRef]
57. Pieterse, E.; Rother, N.; Yanginlar, C.; Hilbrands, L.B.; van der Vlag, J. Neutrophils Discriminate between Lipopolysaccharides of Different Bacterial Sources and Selectively Release Neutrophil Extracellular Traps. *Front. Immunol.* **2016**, *7*, 484. [CrossRef]
58. Gegner, T.; Schmidtberg, H.; Vogel, H.; Vilcinskas, A. Population-Specific Expression of Antimicrobial Peptides Conferring Pathogen Resistance in the Invasive Ladybird *Harmonia axyridis*. *Sci. Rep.* **2018**, *8*, 3600. [CrossRef]
59. Vilcinskas, A.; Stoecker, K.; Schmidtberg, H.; Röhrich, C.R.; Vogel, H. Invasive Harlequin Ladybird Carries Biological Weapons against Native Competitors. *Science* **2013**, *340*, 862–863. [CrossRef]
60. Röhrich, C.R.; Ngwa, C.J.; Wiesner, J.; Schmidtberg, H.; Degenkolb, T.; Kollewe, C.; Fischer, R.; Pradel, G.; Vilcinskas, A. Harmonine, a Defence Compound from the Harlequin Ladybird, Inhibits Mycobacterial Growth and Demonstrates Multi-Stage Antimalarial Activity. *Biol. Lett.* **2012**, *8*, 308–311. [CrossRef]
61. Lee, K.A.; Klasing, K.C. A Role for Immunology in Invasion Biology. *Trends Ecol. Evol.* **2004**, *19*, 523–529. [CrossRef]

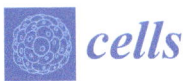

Article

The Endothelin Receptor Antagonist Macitentan Inhibits Human Cytomegalovirus Infection

Natalia Landázuri [1,2], Jennifer Gorwood [1,2], Ylva Terelius [3,†], Fredrik Öberg [3], Koon Chu Yaiw [1,2], Afsar Rahbar [1,2] and Cecilia Söderberg-Nauclér [1,2,*]

1. Microbial Pathogenesis Unit, Department of Medicine Solna, Karolinska Institutet, SE-171 76 Stockholm, Sweden; natalia.landazuri@disstockholm.se (N.L.); jennifer.gorwood@ki.se (J.G.); koon.chu.yaiw@ki.se (K.C.Y.); afsar.rahbar@ki.se (A.R.)
2. Division of Neurology, Karolinska University Hospital, SE-171 76 Stockholm, Sweden
3. Medivir AB, SE-141 22 Huddinge, Sweden; ylva.terelius@gmail.com (Y.T.); Fredrik.Oberg@medivir.com (F.Ö.)
* Correspondence: cecilia.naucler@ki.se
† Present address: ADMEYT AB, SE-179 62 Stenhamra, Sweden.

Abstract: Human cytomegalovirus (HCMV) infection is an important cause of morbidity and mortality in immunocompromised patients and a major etiological factor for congenital birth defects in newborns. Ganciclovir and its pro-drug valganciclovir are the preferred drugs in use today for prophylaxis and treatment of viremic patients. Due to long treatment times, patients are at risk for developing viral resistance to ganciclovir and to other drugs with a similar mechanism of action. We earlier found that the endothelin receptor B (ETBR) is upregulated during HCMV infection and that it plays an important role in the life cycle of this virus. Here, we tested the hypothesis that ETBR blockade could be used in the treatment of HCMV infection. As HCMV infection is specific to humans, we tested our hypothesis in human cell types that are relevant for HCMV pathogenesis; i.e., endothelial cells, epithelial cells and fibroblasts. We infected these cells with HCMV and treated them with the ETBR specific antagonist BQ788 or ETR antagonists that are approved by the FDA for treatment of pulmonary hypertension; macitentan, its metabolite ACT-132577, bosentan and ambrisentan, and as an anti-viral control, we used ganciclovir or letermovir. At concentrations expected to be relevant in vivo, macitentan, ACT-132577 and BQ788 effectively inhibited productive infection of HCMV. Of importance, macitentan also inhibited productive infection of a ganciclovir-resistant HCMV isolate. Our results suggest that binding or signaling through ETBR is crucial for viral replication, and that selected ETBR blockers inhibit HCMV infection.

Keywords: cytomegalovirus; endothelin receptor; repurposing

1. Introduction

Human cytomegalovirus (HCMV) is a ubiquitous, opportunistic double-stranded DNA virus of the herpesviridae family [1]. Depending on geographical location and socioeconomic status, 40% to >90% of the population is infected with HCMV [1]. After a primary HCMV infection, which is typically asymptomatic, the virus establishes lifelong latency and persistence. Latent HCMV has no obvious complications in otherwise healthy people. However, in immunocompromised individuals, such as AIDS patients and transplant patients, reactivation of HCMV can lead to significant morbidity and mortality [1]. HCMV establishes latency in myeloid lineage progenitor cells and can be transferred from donors to recipients of solid organ and bone marrow transplants [2,3]. The virus can be reactivated when monocytes differentiate into macrophages or dendritic cells by inflammatory stimuli [4–6], which may occur as a consequence of organ or stem cell graft rejection. Transplant recipients can hence acquire a primary infection from an HCMV-positive donor [2,3,7].

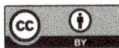

During acute infection, epithelial cells are major portal of entry and a main source of HCMV dissemination. HCMV is commonly excreted from epithelial cells and spreads to other individuals through saliva, urine, breast milk, and genital excretions [8]. Endothelial cells lining the vascular tree are also a primary source of HCMV entry and mediate viral spread to different organs during acute infection. Fibroblasts are easily infected with HCMV [9] and also represent target cells in widespread HCMV disease. In AIDS patients, HCMV infection of retinal epithelial cells is a major HCMV-driven complication causing retinitis, which can lead to blindness [10,11]. Moreover, HCMV infection is the most common etiological agent for congenital birth defects in newborns and is implicated in cardiovascular disease and cancer [12–14].

Patients at risk for HCMV-related complications are treated with antivirals either prophylactically for at least 3 months or as a pre-emptive therapy when frequent PCR monitoring shows evidence of HCMV replication in the patient [3]. Ganciclovir and its per oral pro-drug valganciclovir are long-standing first-line systemic drugs in use for prophylaxis and treatment of HCMV infections [15]. Ganciclovir, a deoxyguanosine analog, is phosphorylated once by the viral kinase encoded by UL97 and then twice by cellular kinases. The active form, ganciclovir triphosphate, is incorporated into the elongating DNA and inhibits the viral DNA polymerase encoded by the HCMV gene UL54 [15,16]. Mutations arising in the UL97 or UL54 genes often mediate resistance to ganciclovir [17,18].

Ganciclovir resistance may develop after treatment for more than 3–4 months, and necessitate the use of alternative drugs [3]. Extended treatment can also lead to myelo-suppression [19], a detrimental side effect for hematopoietic stem cell transplant patients or for patients treated with myelosuppressive drugs to prevent graft-versus-host disease. Ganciclovir is therefore not suitable for prophylactic use in this group of patients. Second-line drugs for systemic therapy also target the UL54 viral DNA polymerase. These include cidofovir, a nucleotide analog of cytidine, which only requires phosphorylation by cellular enzymes, and Foscavir, a pyrophosphate analog that prevents incorporation of dNTPs into the viral DNA polymerase [3]. Ganciclovir, cidofovir and Foscavir have similar mechanisms of action and cross-resistance has been reported [16,20]. Letermovir, which targets the viral terminase complex [21], was approved for HCMV prophylaxis and treatment in 2017 [22]. This was the first drug to be approved for HCMV treatment since 2003. Therefore, additional clinically approved drugs are needed that target other critical steps of HCMV infection, which can be used especially in patients infected with drug-resistant strains.

Previously, we found that HCMV infection upregulates the endothelin receptor type B (ETBR) at the transcriptional and protein levels in endothelial and smooth muscle cells [23], which raised the possibility that this receptor or the endothelin axis may play an important role during HCMV infection. In support of this hypothesis, we recently found that HCMV infection inhibits ET-1 transcript expression, and via downregulation of endothelin converting enzyme-1 (ECE-1) that cleaves the ET-1 precursor protein to mature ET-1, it also inhibits release of the ET-1 peptide [24]. ET-1 is the most common isoform peptide of endothelin and acts as a very potent vasoconstrictor. ET-1 provides its effect through binding to two G-protein-coupled receptor subtypes: ETAR and ETBR [25], which have opposite functions on vascular tone. Binding to both receptors on vascular smooth muscle cells leads to vasoconstriction, while binding to ETBR on endothelial cells leads to clearance of ET-1 and release of nitric oxide and prostacyclin, and consequent vasodilatation [25]. ETBR thus helps to clear endothelin-1 (ET-1) from the circulation.

ET-1 concentration is often elevated in patients with cardiovascular diseases, which can lead to vasoconstriction and hypertension [26]. Endothelin receptor (ETR) antagonists have been developed to treat pulmonary hypertension [27]. Three different ETR antagonists are today FDA-approved for the treatment of pulmonary hypertension: bosentan, macitentan, and ambrisentan [28–31]. Bosentan and macitentan target both ETAR and ETBR, while ambrisentan targets ETAR.

Here, we tested the hypothesis that an ETR antagonist could be repurposed to treat HCMV infections by testing their effects to prevent HCMV infection in clinically relevant cell types: endothelial cells, epithelial cells, and fibroblasts. We found that ETBR antagonists can inhibit HCMV infection in various cell types.

2. Materials and Methods

2.1. Materials

BQ788, ACT-132577, macitentan, and bosentan were from MedChemExpress LCC (MedChemExpress LCC, Princeton, NJ, USA). Ambrisentan was from Ark Pharm Inc. (Ark Pharm Inc., Microsoft Libertyville, IL, USA). Ganciclovir was from Hoffmann La Roche (Stockholm, Sweden). Human primary RPE-1 retinal pigment epithelial cells (a kind gift from Dr. Richard J. Stanton and Dr. Derrick Dargan, Medical Research Council Centre for Virology, UK [32,33]) were cultured in RPMI with 10% fetal bovine serum, penicillin (100 U/mL), and streptomycin (100 µg/mL). Human MRC5 fibroblasts (ATCC, US) were cultured in minimum essential medium with 10% fetal bovine serum, penicillin (100 U/mL), and streptomycin (100 µg/mL). Primary human umbilical vein endothelial cells (HUVECs) were harvested with collagenase as described [34] or purchased (Lonza, Basel, Switzerland) and cultured in endothelial cell growth medium (Lonza). All cells were cultured at 37 °C in 5% CO_2/95% air.

2.2. Cell Viability and Toxicity

Cells were plated on 96-well plates and treated the next day with BQ788, ACT-132577, macitentan, bosentan, ambrisentan, or ganciclovir (0–25 µM). Cell proliferation was evaluated with the CellTiter 96 AQueous Non-Radioactive Cell Proliferation Assay (Promega Biotech, Nacka, Sweden) according to the manufacturer's instructions.

2.3. Viral Infectivity

Cells were plated on chamber slides. The next day, cell monolayers were treated with the aforementioned chemical compounds and infected with HCMV strain VR1814 (titer of 2.5×10^6 pfu/mL) at multiplicity of infection (MOI) of 0.1 (or MOI of 2 when it's indicated in the text). The ganciclovir-resistant clinical isolate C17222 [35] was propagated in MRC5 fibroblasts. As this isolate is highly cell-associated, we infected HUVECs by exposing them to C17222 infected MRC5s at a HUVEC: infected MRC5 ratio of 100:1; 50:1 or 1:1, respectively. Infected cells were treated or not with 10 µM of ganciclovir, 10 µM of letermovir, 100 µM of BQ788 or 25 µM of macitentan, respectively. As a control, we verified that the infected MRC5 cells could no longer proliferate. Cells were immunostained with an antibody against HCMV immediate-early antigen (targeting exon 2 recognizing IE72, IE86 and IE55 [36], Argene, Biomerieux, Marcy l'Etoile, France) or an antibody against HCMV immediate-early antigen clone 6F8.2 (Merck, Darmstadt, Germany). Antibody binding was visualized with the anti-mouse ImmPRESS kit (Vector Laboratories, Peterborough, UK) or an anti-mouse antibody conjugated with AlexaFluor 488 (Invitrogen, Camarillo, CA, USA). The percentage of IE-positive cells was determined in at least three different images per well in duplicates of each experment. The t-test (two-tailed, unpaired) was conducted with Microsoft Excel 2011 (Microsoft, Redmond, WA, USA) or GraphPad Prism (versions 6 or 8, GraphPad Software, San Diego, CA, USA) and used for comparison between a treatment group and the control group, respectively. Differences were considered significant at p-values < 0.05.

2.4. Viral Output Assay

Cells were plated on 12- or 24-well plates. The next day, we treated the cells with the chemical compounds and infected them with HCMV VR1814 (at multiplicities of infection between 0.1 and 0.2). Three to four days later, the cells were washed with PBS, and the culture medium was replaced with drug-containing fresh medium. Seven days later, the supernatant was harvested. Since the virus produced by RPEs is strongly cell-associated, the cells were scraped and collected with the supernatant. The mixture was sonicated or freeze thawed, and cell debris was pelleted to harvest the supernatant that could contain infectious virus. As cells were incubated with the compounds for several days before collection of the virus-containing supernatant, the presence of active compounds was assumed to be minimal, if any. To account for any remaining active compounds and minimize their action, we diluted the collected supernatants 10-fold in fresh cell culture medium. MRC5 cells, plated on chamber slides, were exposed to the diluted supernatants for 1 or 2 days, fixed, and stained for HCMV-IE as described above. The percentage of IE-positive cells was determined in at least three images for each condition by manual counting. The EC50 for each compound-cell combination was determined in two independent experiments, using GraphPad Prism (versions 6 or 8, GraphPad Software, San Diego, CA, USA) and a non-linear fit of log[inhibitor] vs. response equation with three parameters, a standard slope (Hill Slope = -1.0) and a constraint of the bottom value greater than 0.0. The virus titer was measured by a standard TCID50 method [37] in MRC5 cells with minor modifications. Briefly, the cells were exposed for 5 days to a ten-fold dilution of virus inoculum from either the supernatants or cell-associated virions of HUVEC-infected VR1814 with or without treatment with 100 µM of BQ788 at the indicated time points (i.e. 5 hours after infection and at 3-, 5- and 7-dpi). The cytopathic effects were visualized by IE immunofluorescence staining and the TCID50/mL was calculated as previously described [37].

2.5. Plaque Formation Assay

Virus-containing supernatants collected from cells infected in the presence of chemical compounds (as described in the previous paragraph) were serially diluted and used to infect MRC5 cells. Two hours later, the cell culture medium was replaced with cell culture medium containing 0.5% methylcellulose. When plaques formed (10–14 days for HCMV), cells were fixed and stained with 70% methanol and 0.1% methylene blue. Plaques from wells where plaques were clearly distinguishable were counted and the titer of each supernatant was calculated.

2.6. Statistical Analysis

All analyses were performed using GraphPad Prism versions 6 or 8 (GraphPad Software, Inc., La Jolla, CA, USA). One-way ANOVA test followed by Dunnett's multiple comparisons test was used to assess the statistical significance between different variables. Data are presented as the mean ± standard error of the mean. $p < 0.05$ was considered as a statistically significant difference. ****; $p < 0.0001$ ***; $p < 0.001$; ** $p < 0.01$, *; $p < 0.05$. All experiments were performed with three independent repeats.

3. Results

3.1. ETR Antagonists Are Well Tolerated at Low Concentrations

We first assessed if macitentan, its metabolite ACT-132577, bosentan, ambrisentan, the ETBR-specific chemical compound BQ788, and ganciclovir affected cellular viability in HUVECs (human umbilical cord endothelial cells), MRC5 (human fibroblasts) and RPE-1 cells (human retinal pigment epithelial cells) (Figure 1A). After 7 days of treatment, the compounds did not affect cell viability at the expected peak serum concentration in patients reported in literature [38,39], considering that macitentan has a plasma protein binding capacity exceeding 99%. The most dramatic effect we observed was a reduced cell viability of approximately 30–35% in HUVECs and RPEs treated with the highest concentration of ACT-132577 (Figure 1B and Table 1).

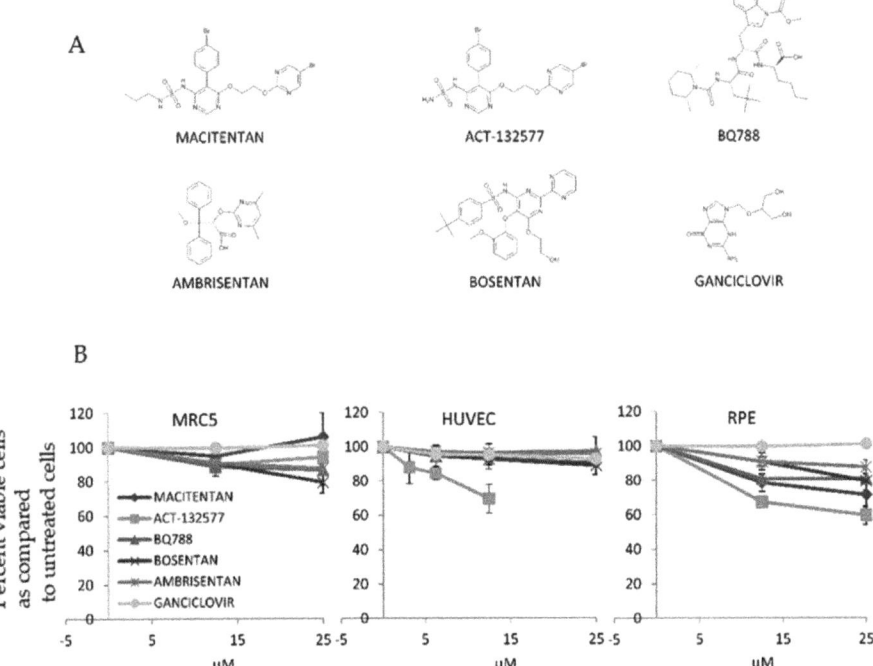

Figure 1. ETR antagonists are not toxic at low concentrations. HUVECs, MRC5, and RPE-1 cells were exposed to various concentrations of macitentan, ACT-132577, BQ788, ambrisentan, bosentan, or ganciclovir. (**A**) Chemical structures of the compounds. (**B**) Cells were treated with the compounds for 7 days, whereafter cell viability was quantified and normalized to untreated cells. ETR antagonists were not toxic for HUVECs, MRC5, and RPE-1 cells at low concentrations. Values are mean ± SD of triplicates.

Table 1. Treatment of HCMV infected MRC-5, HUVEC and RPE cells with ETR Antagonists or Ganciclovir at different concentrations and cellular viability was quantified.

	MRC5			HUVEC			RPE	
	Concentrations			Concentrations			Concentrations	
Compounds	12.5 µM	25.0 µM	3.2 µM	6.25 µM	12.5 µM	25.0 µM	12.5 µM	25.0 µM
Macitentan	ns	ns	-	ns	ns	ns	****	****
ACT-132577	ns	ns	*	***	****	-	****	****
BQ788	ns	ns	-	ns	ns	ns	****	****
Bosentan	*	****	-	ns	ns	*	ns	****
Ganciclovir	ns	ns	-	ns	ns	ns	ns	ns
Ambrisentan	**	*	-	ns	ns	ns	*	ns

Values are mean ± SD of triplicates. ns; not significant, -; not done. ****; $p < 0.0001$ ***; $p < 0.001$; ** $p < 0.01$, *; $p < 0.05$.

3.2. ETR Antagonists Prevent Production of Infectious HCMV

To assess the antiviral properties of the different ETR antagonists, we infected HUVECs, MRC5 and RPE-1 cells with HCMV (VR1814 strain) in the presence of macitentan (12.5 µM for HUVEC and 25 µM for RPE-1 and MRC5), ACT-132577 (6.25 µM for HUVEC and 12.5 µM for RPE-1 and MRC5), BQ788 (25 µM), or bosentan (25 µM) and quantified infected cells by their expression of the HCMV IE protein. We did not observe a reduction in the number of IE-positive cells on day 1 after infection (Figure 2A). On day 5, the cell-to-cell spread of the virus appeared to be inhibited by some of the compounds as judged from a reduced formation of IE-positive foci. The IE foci formed in the presence of macitentan, ACT-132577 and BQ788 were visibly smaller than those formed in control or bosentan-treated cells (Figure 2B). This implied that ETR antagonists prevented viral replication or spread.

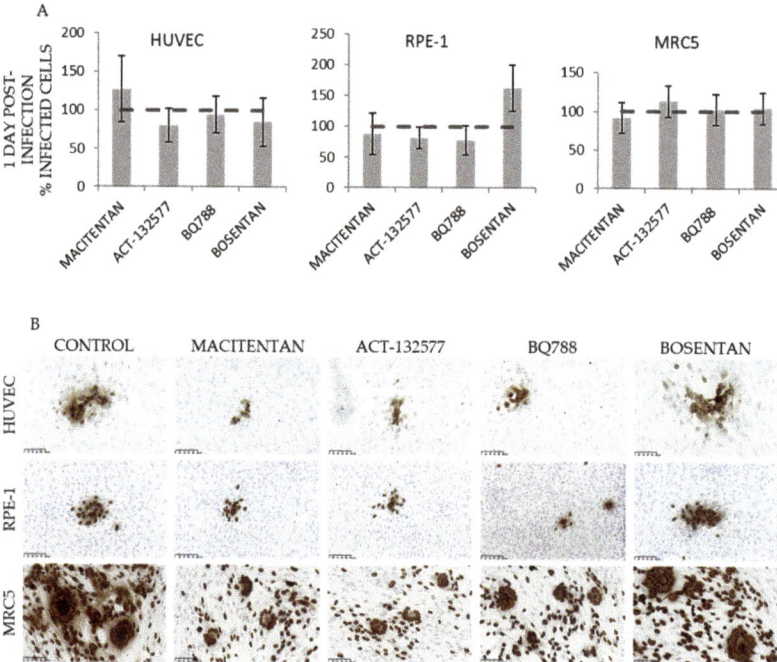

Figure 2. ETR antagonists prevent virion production. HUVECs, RPE-1 and MRC5 cells were treated with macitentan (12.5 μM for HUVEC, 25 μM for RPE and MRC5), ACT-132577 (6.25 μM for HUVEC, 12.5 μM for RPE and MRC5), BQ788 (25 μM), or bosentan (25 μM) and simultaneously exposed to HCMV. Infectivity was assessed by immunostaining for IE. (**A**) Number of IE-positive cells on day 1 post-infection normalized to infected, non-treated cells. (**B**) Representative images of HCMV-driven foci on day 5 after infection. Broken line corresponds to the level of IE expression in infected cells not treated with drugs. Scale bar 100 μM.

3.3. ETR Antagonists Inhibit HCMV Replictaion by Post Entry Mechanisms

To determine whether blockade of ETR prior to virus entry was necessary to inhibit viral replication, we pretreated HUVECs with ETR antagonists for 1 h before infection with HCMV. As a control, we exposed cells to the virus for 1 h to allow binding and entry of viral particles [40,41] before we added the antagonists to the culture medium. Seven days later, virus-containing supernatants were harvested and used to infect MRC5 fibroblasts (Figure 3A). At one day post infection and before new virions could be produced [42], the percentage of IE-positive MRC5 cells was similar regardless of whether cells had been treated with ETR blockers before or after infection, indicating that the ETR blockers inhibited, to a great extent, post-entry steps of HCMV infection (Figure 3B,C).

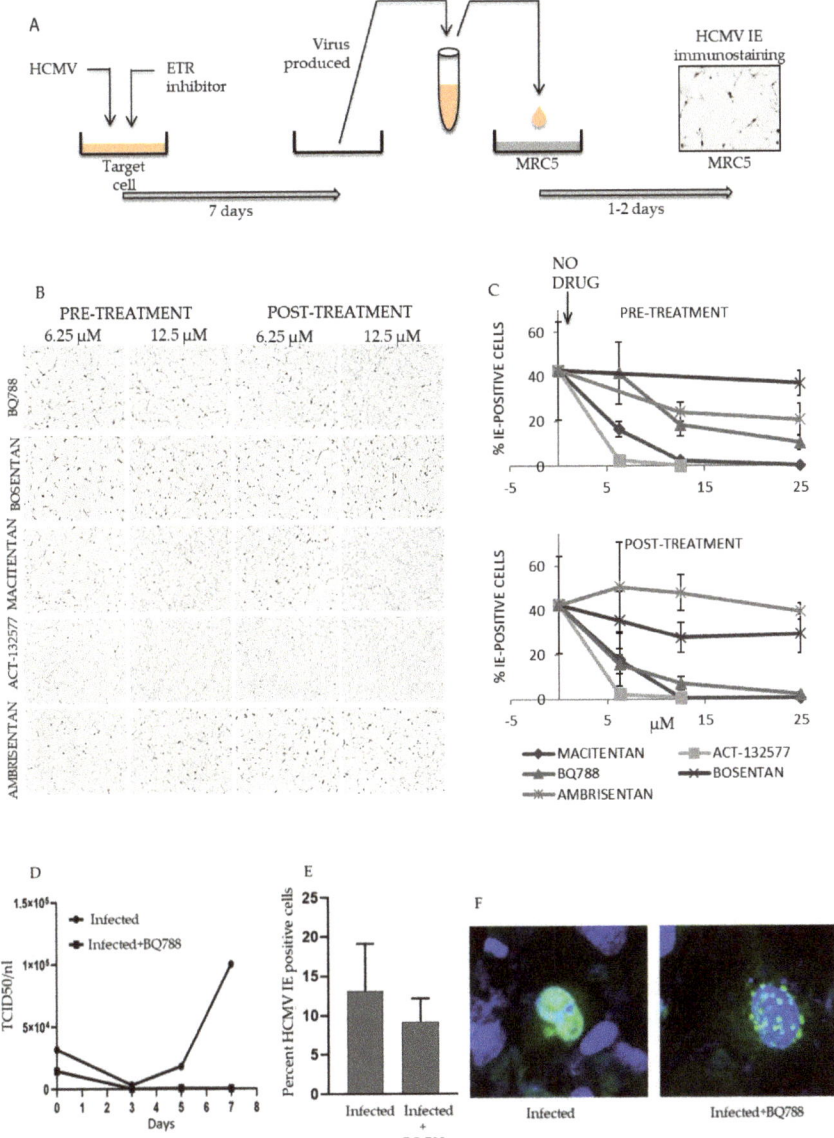

Figure 3. ETR antagonists prevent virus production. HUVECs were treated with ETR antagonists for 1 h before (pretreatment) or after (post-treatment) exposure to HCMV. (**A–C**) At seven days post infection, the virus-containing supernatant was harvested and used to infect MRC5 cells. (**A**) Schematic diagram of the experimental procedure. (**B**) Representative images of infected MRC5 fibroblasts 1 day after infection. The brown stain corresponds to IE immunoreactivity. (**C**) Percentage of IE-positive MRC5 cells after 1 day post infection after exposure to supernatant from 7-day infected HUVECs. The arrow indicates data points with no drug (0 μM). (**D**) TCID50/mL was measured in MRC-5 cells. Cells were exposed for 5 days to either supernatants or HUVECs infected with VR1814 (MOI of 2) and treated or not with 100 μM of BQ788 and were collected at 5 h after infection (0-dpi), 3-, 5- and 7-dpi. (**E**) Percentage of positive IE stained cells in HUVECs exposed to C17222 infected MRC-5 cells with ratio 1:50 ($p = 0.058$). (**F**) Representative images of infected and infected and treated with BQ788 at 100 μM with confocal microscopy (×20 magnification). The nuclei are stained with DAPI (blue) and an IE specific antibody (green). Values are mean ± SD of at least triplicate images.

At concentrations as low as 6–12 μM of macitentan and its metabolite ACT-132577, dual ETAR and ETBR antagonists, we did not detect any measurable levels of viral production (Figure 3C and Table 2). BQ788, an ETBR-specific antagonist, inhibited viral production by 80% at 12 μM (Figure 3C) and completely at 100 μM (Figure 3D). Ambrisentan, and ETAR-specific antagonist, did not affect viral output (Figure 3C and Table 2), which suggests that the ETAR is not essential for HCMV replication. However, the dual ETAR-ETBR antagonist bosentan also failed to inhibit viral replication (Table 2). The ETBR binding site for bosentan may hence differ from that of macitentan and BQ788. Bosentan either does not interfere with the binding of HCMV proteins to this receptor, or the drug does not affect post entry effects of HCMV involving ETBR signaling.

Table 2. Pre and post treatment of HCMV infected HUVECs with Ambrisentan, and ETAR- antagonists at different concentrations.

	PRE-TREATMENT			POST-TREATMENT		
Compounds	6.25 μM	12.5 μM	25 μM	6.25 μM	12.5 μM	25.0 μM
Macitentan	*	***	***	*	****	****
ACT-132577	***	***	***	***	****	****
BQ788	ns	ns	**	*	***	***
Bosentan	ns	***	ns	ns	ns	ns
Ambrisentan	***	ns	ns	ns	ns	ns

ns; no significance, -; not done. ****; $p < 0.0001$ ***; $p < 0.001$; ** $p < 0.01$, *; $p < 0.05$.

3.4. HCMV Infection Is Inhibited at Low Concentrations of ETR Antagonists in HUVECs, MRC5 and RPE-1 Cells

Next, we treated HUVECs, MRC5 and RPE-1 cells with macitentan, ACT-132577, BQ788, ambrisentan or ganciclovir, and thereafter infected them with HCMV. Seven days later, we collected the virus-containing supernatants (HUVECs and MRC5 fibroblasts) or virus-containing cell lysates (RPE-1 cells) and used them to infect MRC5 cells (Figure 3A). We judged viral output from the percentage of IE-expressing cells one day after infection (Figure 4A, Table 3). We also titered the virus-containing supernatants and lysates with a plaque assay (Figure 4B). Ambrisentan did not inhibit virus production in HUVECs or in MRC5 cells and was the least effective inhibitor in RPE-1 cells. BQ788 was the most efficient compound that inhibited virus production in MRC5 and RPE-1 cells and at 25 μM, it essentially blocked virus production in all cell types. Interestingly, we observed that the number of IE positive cells only trended to be reduced (Figure 3E), but the IE staining pattern was completely different in BQ788 treated cells (Figure 3F), which suggest that ETBR signaling is linked to regulation of HCMV IE expression and possibly to control of HCMV replication. At 12.5 μM, macitentan and ACT-132577 reduced virus production by 98–100% in HUVECs, respectively.

Table 3. HCMV infected HUVECs, MRC5 and RPE were treated with different concentrations of ETR antagonists or Ganciclovir and viral output was calculated from the percentage of IE-expressing cells one day after infection. These results were obtained from data in Figure 4.

Viral output from different cell lines as determined by IE-positive staining in MRC5 cells						
	HUVEC					
Compounds	0.8 μM	1.6 μM	3.0 μM	6.25 μM	12.5 μM	25.0 μM
Macitentan	ns	ns	ns	****	****	****
ACT-132577	ns	ns	****	****	****	****

Table 3. Cont.

Viral output from different cell lines as determined by IE-positive staining in MRC5 cells						
BQ788	-	ns	ns	*	***	****
Ambrisentan	-	-	-	-	-	ns
Ganciclovir	ns	****	****	****	****	****
MRC5						
Compounds	0.8 µM	1.6 µM	3.0 µM	6.3 µM	12.5 µM	25.0 µM
Macitentan	-	-	-	ns	**	**
ACT-132577	-	-	-	ns	****	ns
BQ788	-	-	ns	*	****	****
Ambrisentan	-	-	-	-	-	ns
Ganciclovir	****	****	****	****	****	****
RPE						
Compounds	0.8 µM	3.0 µM	6.3 µM	12.5 µM	25.0 µM	
Macitentan	-	-	ns	ns	***	
ACT-132577	-	-	ns	ns	**	
BQ788	-	ns	-	***	****	
Ambrisentan	-	-	-	ns	*	
Ganciclovir	****	****	-	-	-	
Viral output from different cells lines as determined by plaque formation in MRC5 cells						
HUVEC						
Compounds	1.6 µM	3.0 µM	6.25 µM	12.5 µM	25.0 µM	
Macitentan	-	****	****	****	****	
ACT-132577	****	****	****	****	****	
BQ788	****	****	****	****	****	
Ambrisentan	ns	****	****	****	****	
Ganciclovir	****	****	****	****	****	
MRC5						
Compounds	1.6 µM	3.0 µM	6.3 µM	12.5 µM	25.0 µM	
Macitentan	-	-	-	ns	ns	
ACT-132577	-	-	-	ns	ns	
BQ788	-	ns	ns	*	**	
Ambrisentan	-	-	-	-	ns	
Ganciclovir	-	****	****	****	****	
RPE						
Compounds	1.6 µM	3.0 µM	6.3 µM	12.5 µM	25.0 µM	
Macitentan	-	-	-	ns	ns	
ACT-132577	-	ns	ns	ns	-	
BQ788	-	ns	ns	***	****	
Ambrisentan	-	-	-	ns	ns	
Ganciclovir	****	****	****	****	****	

ns; no significance. ****; $p < 0.0001$ ***; $p < 0.001$; ** $p < 0.01$, *; $p < 0.05$.

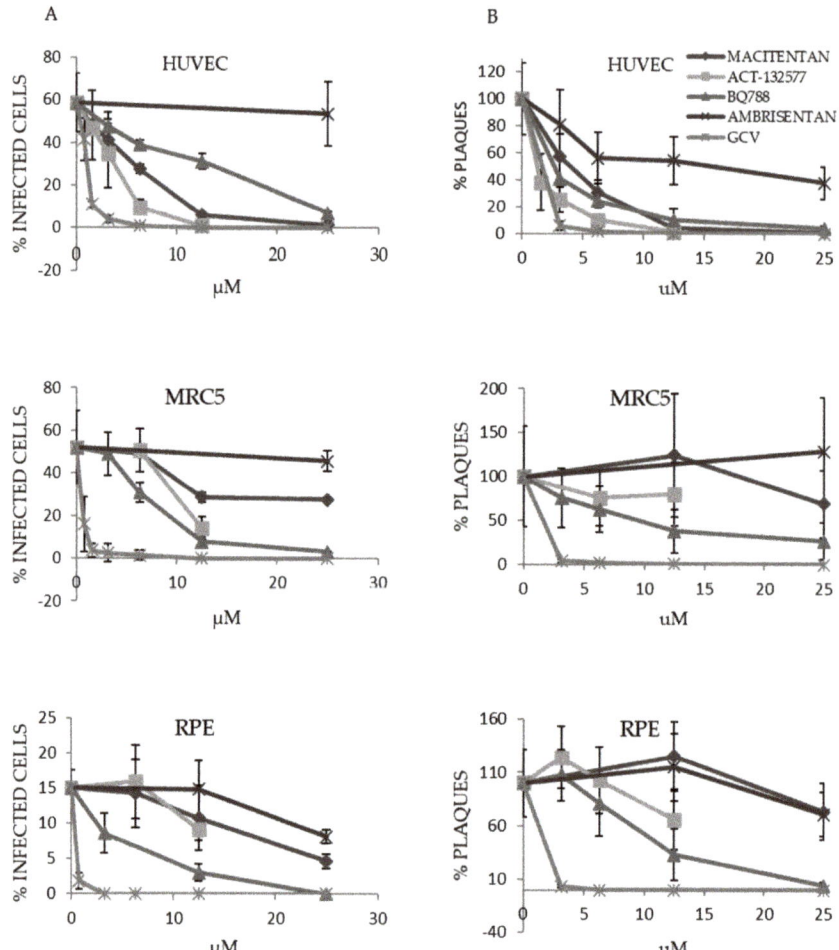

Figure 4. ETR antagonists at low concentrations inhibit production of HCMV in various cell types. HUVECs, MRC5 and RPE-1 cells were treated with low concentrations of ETR antagonists or ganciclovir (GCV) and exposed to HCMV. Seven days later, the virus-containing supernatant was collected or, in the case of RPEs, viral particles were extracted from cells by sonication. The harvested virus containing supernatant was used to infect MRC5 cells. (**A**) The percentage of IE-positive MRC5 cells was determined one day after infection. (**B**) The harvested virus was subjected to serial dilution and titered by a plaque assay in MRC5 cells. Two hours after infection, the supernatant was replaced with methylcellulose-containing medium. At 14 days post infection, the number of plaques formed was quantified from wells where plaques were easy to distinguish, and the titers were calculated. Values are presented as percentage of control without drugs (mean ± SD).

3.5. Macitentan, Its Metabolite ATC-132577 and BQ788 Inhibit Infection of a Ganciclovir-Resistant HCMV Strain

To determine whether ETR antagonists could be used as an alternative therapy for ganciclovir-resistant HCMV infections, we treated HUVECs with ETR antagonists and exposed them to MRC5s that were infected with a ganciclovir-resistant HCMV clinical isolate (C17222). This HCMV strain contained the viral UL97 kinase amino acid changes A594V and L595S, which confers ganciclovir resistance [35]. The C17222 virus is highly cell associated, wherefore we used infected MRC-5 cells to infect HUVECs. At the same time, we treated cells with 10 µM of ganciclovir, 10 µM of letermovir, 100 µM of BQ788 or 25 µM of Macitentan, respectively. Three days after infection, we assessed the level of IE expression in HCMV infected cells by immunostaining. We found that macitentan, its metabolite ATC-132577 and BQ788 decreased IE positive cells by 60 to 67% (Figure 5A,B,D) and by 42% with letermovir (5D) compared to controls in cultures infected with the ganciclovir-resistant HCMV isolate. We observed significantly less IE-positive foci in HUVECs treated with ETR antagonists (Figure 5C) or letermovir (Figure 5D), while ganciclovir, as expected, did not affect infection with this ganciclovir-resistant HCMV strain (Table 4).

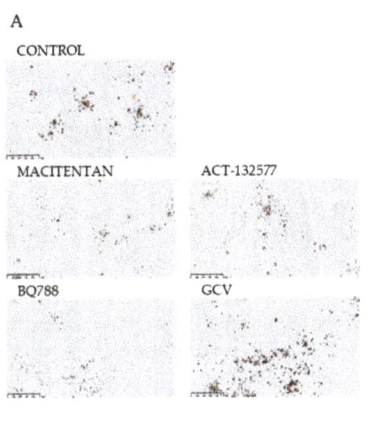
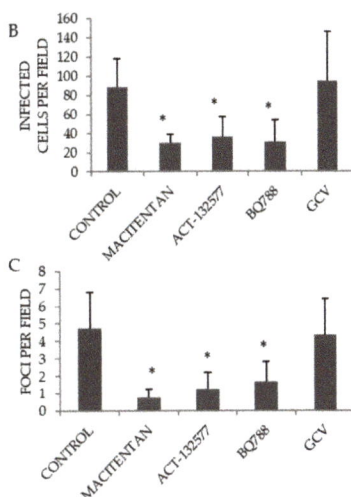
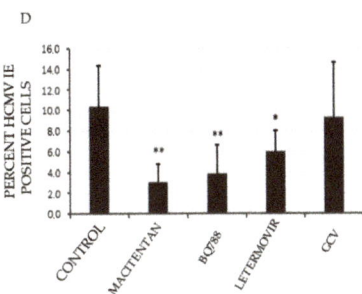

Figure 5. Decreased HCMV-IE positive cells in cultures treated with macitentan, its metabolite ATC-132577 and BQ788. HUVECs were treated with ETR antagonists (12.5 µM) and exposed to MRC5s infected with the ganciclovir-resistant HCMV clinical isolate C17222. Seven days later, IE expression was assessed by immunostaining. (**A**) Representative images. Brown stain corresponds to IE immunoreactivity and represent HCMV positive cells. (**B**) The number of IE-immunopositive cells per field of view was quantified. (**C**) The number of IE-positive foci (comprising more than 3 IE-positive cells) per field of view was quantified. (**D**) HUVEC cells were infected by exposing them to C17222 infected MRC5s (HUVEC: infected MRC5 ratio of 1:1) and treated or not with 10 µM of ganciclovir, 10 µM of letermovir, 100 µM of BQ788 or 25 µM of macitentan. At seven days post infection, the virus-containing cells were harvested and used to infect MRC5 cells. Percentage of positive IE stained cells was measured at 3 dpi. Values are mean ± SD of at least triplicate images. Asterisks (*) denote a statistically significant difference with respect to the control ((*) p-value < 0.05 and (**) a p-value < 0.01).

Table 4. EC$_{50}$ for inhibition of infectious viral production.

Compound	HUVEC		RPE-1		MRC5	
	EC$_{50}$ (µM)	R^2	EC$_{50}$ (µM)	R^2	EC$_{50}$ (µM)	R^2
Macitentan	0.05	0.66	17.30	0.60	20.49	0.33
	4.32	0.81	9.90	0.63	23.95	0.55
ACT-132577	1.01	0.66	29.16	0.28	5.66	0.59
	2.75	0.78	9.58	0.50	12.26	0.44
BQ-788	3.61	0.66	3.32	0.90	1.66	0.91
	10.07	0.80	9.90	0.58	6.08	0.72
Ganciclovir	0.49	0.80	0.09	0.97	0.22	0.88
	0.68	0.87	0.66	0.83	0.24	0.86

Two EC 50 values for each cell-drug combination derived from two independent experiments.

4. Discussion

This study shows that the FDA-approved drug macitentan, its metabolite ACT-132577, and the ETBR-specific antagonist BQ788 are highly effective to inhibit HCMV replication and spread in different human cell types. Macitentan also inhibited infection with a ganciclovir-resistant strain, which is generally very difficult to treat and lacks good treatment options for patients. The effect of macitentan on infection with a ganciclovir-resistant HCMV strain was similar or slightly better than the most recently approved antiviral drug against HCMV; letermovir. Therefore, macitentan may serve as a novel drug with potential efficacy in the treatment of HCMV infections including those infected with a ganciclovir-resistant strain.

The most common cell types infected during acute HCMV disease are macrophages, endothelial cells and epithelial cells. These cell types are relevant during both acute and late phases of infection due to their role in viral dissemination and pathogenesis. The choice of HUVECs, MRC5 and RPE-1 cells also allowed us to compare the outcome of ETR blockade on cells with different modes of viral entry. Specific glycoprotein complexes that are present in the virus envelope bind to particular receptors on target cells, which determine, at least in part, cellular viral tropism [43]. Entry can occur through fusion of the virion with the cellular plasma membrane in a pH-independent manner, as in fibroblasts [44], or through a pH-dependent receptor-mediated endocytosis, which occurs in monocyte/macrophages, endothelial and epithelial cells [9,40,45,46].

HCMV infection is initiated by tethering of the virus to heparin sulphate proteoglycans. The gM/gN heterodimer and the gB protein bind to heparin, whereafter the virus docks to more stable virus receptor interactions before fusion and release of viral components to the cytoplasm takes place. This can occur either at the plasma membrane or after receptor mediated endocytosis, which is followed by intracellular fusion of the viral envelope with the endosome. Several different receptors including platelet-derived growth factor receptor-α (PDGFR-α) [47], integrins (especially subtype αVβ3) [48,49], epidermal growth factor receptor (EGFR) [50], CD13 [51], Neuropilin-2 [52], CD147 [53] and OR14I1 [54] have been shown to mediate entry into different cell types. Two glycoprotein complexes appear to be the main viral components mediating virus cellular tropism. The gH/gL/gO trimer engages PDGFR-α [55] and mediates infection into fibroblasts by initiating fusion at the plasma membrane, but this protein complex does not support HCMV entry into monocytes, endothelial or epithelial cells [56]. In contrast, HCMV enters monocyte/macrophages, endothelial and epithelial cells by an interaction between the gH/gL/UL128/UL130/UL131A pentamer complex and specific receptors on these cell types that mediate receptor mediated endocytosis [52–54]. The pentamer complex receptor was difficult to identify, but recent studies suggest that Neuropilin-2 [52], OR14I1 [54] or CD147 [53] can serve as receptors for the pentamer complex.

The pentamer also activates EGFR, and pharmacological inhibition of EGFR signaling hampers translocation of the viral DNA to the nucleus in CD34+ cells. This led to the hypothesis that EGFR activation is involved in pentamer dependent virus entry into myeloid lineage cells [57]. In this context, it is interesting to note that endothelin activation of ETBR transactivates EGFR [58]. Thus, if HCMV interacts with ETBR, this may also result in EGFR activation. Furthermore, when HCMV attaches to target cells, it also elicits a potent cellular interferon-like response, which results in activation of downstream growth factor-like receptor tyrosine kinase (RTK) and integrin pathways [49,59]. Both EGFR and PDGFR, in conjunction with αvβ3 integrins, activate downstream signaling via PI3K/Akt, phospholipase Cγ and focal adhesion kinase [47–50] and trigger endosome formation and virus uptake. In monocytes, engagement of the viral pentamer complex with an unidentified cellular receptor results in engagement of integrins, src and paxillin, which is followed by activation of an actin and dynamin process that also promotes endocytosis of the viral particle for later intracellular fusion and capsid release [60]. EGFR and downstream PI3K signaling are also important to mediate infection that leads to establishment of latency in CD34+ cells [57]. Thus, an interaction between HCMV and its receptors will result in activation of intracellular signaling pathways that are critical for both latent infection and efficient virus production.

In the present study, we provide evidence that macitentan, its metabolite ATC-132577 and BQ788, all targeting ETBR and prevent HCMV infection. Although it cannot be excluded that binding to ETBR is relevant for HCMV entry, ETBR appears to mediate post-entry cellular activation that is necessary for productive HCMV infection, perhaps by controlling IE expression. With an MOI = 1, we observed very little, if any, inhibition of BQ788 in infected MRC5, which suggests post-entry effects of this drug in this cell type at a low MOI (unpublished data). It is possible that ETBR-mediated cellular signaling triggers transcription of viral or cellular genes that favors completion of the viral life cycle. We provide evidence that the expression pattern of IE is completely different in BQ788 treated infected cells, which suggest that ETBR signaling is connected with regulation of IE expression that could have a profound effect on virus replication. It is also possible that interactions between HCMV proteins and ETBR take place in intracellular compartments or that the interaction between HCMV and ETBR leads to activation of intracellular mechanisms of crucial relevance for HCMV replication. As ETBR inhibitors could also affect HCMV replication after infection, common signaling pathways activated by binding of HCMV to receptors on fibroblasts, endothelial and epithelial cells may be similar to those induced by ETBR ligand interaction. HCMVs ability to activate intracellular signaling pathways is however complex and still poorly understood in the context of promoting HCMV replication.

Today, clinical management of HCMV infections is dependent on effective anti-viral therapies, and multiple options for antiviral therapy of HCMV infections in patients are therefore warranted. An emerging problem of acyclovir- and ganciclovir-resistant strains has fueled the development of new anti-virals. Letermovir, which is the latest approved antiviral drug against HCMV acts on ganciclovir-resistant strains. We found that macitentan compared equal or slightly better than letermovir at tested concentrations to inhibit HCMV infection in vitro, wherefore this drug may provide one additional option for treatment of patients infected with ganciclovir-resistant HCMV strains. Whether or not letermovir or ETR antagonist-resistant HCMV strains could emerge under long term culture or during treatment in patients, is unknown and will require evaluation in future studies.

In addition to an important role of antiviral compounds to combat HCMV infections, immunotherapy strategies have been evaluated for treatment of HCMV disease in transplant patients and for HCMV-positive glioblastoma. HCMV vaccines are also under evaluation for congenitial infections. Development of vaccines have been hampered by the lack of knowledge of the mechanisms of entry into monocyte/macrophages, endothelial cells and epithelial cells, as these cells serve as primary virus targets in early infections.

This knowledge has increased in recent years, and our results presented here demonstrate that targeting ETBR is an additional potential new therapeutic option for HCMV infected patients, even for those infected with ganciclovir-resistant strains. Findings from our study suggest that binding or signaling through ETBR is essential for the replication and spread of HCMV. Thus, we provide proof-of-concept evidence that an FDA-approved drug for treatment of PAH may be possible to repurpose for prevention and treatment of HCMV infections. We have observed that inhibition of ETBR fails to inhibit murine or rat CMV infection in mouse or rat cells, respectively, making our study not amenable for testing in common laboratory in vivo models (unpublished results). We have therefore based our conclusions on results obtained from clinically relevant cell types as in vivo preclinical models are unavailable, owing to the selective tropism of HCMV for human cells. Whether our in vitro results mirror any clinical significance remains to be proven in future clinical trials.

5. Conclusions

We demonstrate that an FDA approved ETBR inhibitor can prevent HCMV infection in vitro in clinically relevant cell types. This discovery is relevant as novel therapeutic options for HCMV are needed. Ganciclovir-resistant strains are on the rise, and ganciclovir has myelosuppressive effects that are highly undesirable in immunocompromised stem cell transplant recipients. Letermovir, which targets the viral terminase complex [21] was approved for HCMV prophylaxis and treatment in 2017 [22]. We found that macitentan compared equal or slightly better than letermovir to inhibit HCMV infection in vitro with a ganciclovir-resistant strain. Other investigational drugs that target other viral mechanisms have been tested with variable results [15]. Brincidofovir, which also inhibits the HCMV DNA polymerase, failed in a phase III study evaluating its prophylactic effect in stem cell transplant patients [61]. Maribavir failed to show an effect as a prophylactic drug, but is under evaluation for pre-emptive treatment and treatment of established HCMV disease (NCT 02927067 and NCT02931539). Additional preclinical and early clinical trials are therefore warranted to assess the possibility of repurposing macitentan to treat HCMV infections.

6. Patents

A patent application for the use of ETBR inhibitors in the treatment of HCMV infections was filed, but was later dropped.

Author Contributions: Conceptualization, N.L., K.C.Y. and C.S.-N.; methodology, N.L.,Y.T., F.Ö. and C.S.-N.; validation, N.L., Y.T. and F.Ö.; formal analysis, N.L.; investigation, N.L.; J.G. and K.C.Y. resources, C.S.-N.; data curation, N.L., J.G. and A.R.; writing—original draft preparation, N.L. and C.S.-N.; writing—review and editing, C.S.-N., A.R., Y.T., K.C.Y. and F.Ö.; J.G. visualization, N.L. and J.G.; supervision, C.S.-N.; project administration, A.R.; funding acquisition, C.S.-N. All authors have read and agreed to the published version of the manuscript.

Funding: This research was funded by VINNOVA, through the BIO-X program "New opportunities for existing drugs" (Sweden) and by Medivir AB (Sweden) that acted as the industrial partner in this project. Funding from Swedish Medical Research Council (VR2019-01736), Erling-Persson Family Foundation, Sten A Olsson Foundation, BILTEMA Foundation, Jochnick Family Foundation, The Cancer Foundation in Sweden (5044-B05-01XAB), Stockholm County Council also supported the project.

Institutional Review Board Statement: Not applicable.

Informed Consent Statement: Not applicable.

Data Availability Statement: The datasets generated during the present study are not publicly available, but are available from the corresponding author upon reasonable request.

Acknowledgments: We thank Shunwen Chou (Oregon Health and Science University, Portland, Oregon, (unpublished results) USA) for kindly providing the ganciclovir-resistant HCMV clinical isolate. We thank Richard Bethell for comments and suggestions, and Susana Ayesa Alvarez for comments and suggestions for chemistry input during this work. We thank Belghis Davoudi for help with scanning of slides and Anna Ridderstad Wollberg for guidance and fruitful discussions.

Conflicts of Interest: The authors declare no conflict of interest.

References

1. Boppana, S.B.; Britt, W.J. *Synopsis of Clinical Aspects of Human Cytomegalovirus Diseases*; Reddehase, M.J., Ed.; Caister Academic Press: Poole, UK, 2013; pp. 1–25.
2. Ariza-Heredia, E.J.; Nesher, L.; Chemaly, R.F. Cytomegalovirus diseases after hematopoietic stem cell transplantation: A mini-review. *Cancer Lett.* **2014**, *342*, 1–8. [CrossRef]
3. Eid, A.J.; Razonable, R.R. New developments in the management of cytomegalovirus infection after solid organ transplantation. *Drugs* **2010**, *70*, 965–981. [CrossRef] [PubMed]
4. Söderberg-Nauclér, C.; Fish, K.N.; Nelson, J.A. Reactivation of latent human cytomegalovirus by allogeneic stimulation of blood cells from healthy donors. *Cell* **1997**, *91*, 119–126. [CrossRef]
5. Söderberg-Nauclér, C.; Fish, K.N.; Nelson, J.A. Interferon-gamma and tumor necrosis factor-alpha specifically induce formation of cytomegalovirus-permissive monocyte-derived macrophages that are refractory to the antiviral activity of these cytokines. *J. Clin. Investig.* **1997**, *100*, 3154–3163. [CrossRef] [PubMed]
6. Reeves, M.; Sissons, P.; Sinclair, J. Reactivation of human cytomegalovirus in dendritic cells. *Discov. Med.* **2005**, *5*, 170–174. [PubMed]
7. Einsele, H.; Mielke, S.; Grigoleit, G.U. Diagnosis and treatment of cytomegalovirus 2013. *Curr. Opin. Hematol.* **2014**, *21*, 470–475. [CrossRef]
8. Twite, N.; Andrei, G.; Kummert, C.; Donner, C.; Perez-Morga, D.; De Vos, R.; Snoeck, R.; Marchant, A. Sequestration of human cytomegalovirus by human renal and mammary epithelial cells. *Virology* **2014**, *460-461*, 55–65. [CrossRef]
9. Sinzger, C.; Grefte, A.; Plachter, B.; Gouw, A.; The, T.; Jahn, G. Fibroblasts, epithelial cells, endothelial cells and smooth muscle cells are major targets of human cytomegalovirus infection in lung and gastrointestinal tissues. *J. Gen. Virol.* **1995**, *76*, 741–750. [CrossRef] [PubMed]
10. Jabs, D.A.; Enger, C.; Dunn, J.P.; Forman, M. Cytomegalovirus retinitis and viral resistance: Ganciclovir resistance. CMV Retinitis and Viral Resistance Study Group. *J. Infect. Dis.* **1998**, *177*, 770–773. [CrossRef] [PubMed]
11. Scholz, M.; Doerr, H.W.; Cinatl, J. Human cytomegalovirus retinitis: Pathogenicity, immune evasion and persistence. *Trends Microbiol.* **2003**, *11*, 171–178. [CrossRef]
12. Popovic, M.; Smiljanic, K.; Dobutovic, B.; Syrovets, T.; Simmet, T.; Isenovic, E.R. Human cytomegalovirus infection and atherothrombosis. *J. Thromb Thrombolysis* **2012**, *33*, 160–172. [CrossRef] [PubMed]
13. Hamilton, S.T.; van Zuylen, W.; Shand, A.; Scott, G.M.; Naing, Z.; Hall, B.; Craig, M.E.; Rawlinson, W.D. Prevention of congenital cytomegalovirus complications by maternal and neonatal treatments: A systematic review. *Rev. Med. Virol.* **2014**, *24*, 420–433. [CrossRef]
14. Johnsen, J.I.; Baryawno, N.; Söderberg-Nauclér, C. Is human cytomegalovirus a target in cancer therapy? *Oncotarget* **2011**, *2*, 1329–1338. [CrossRef]
15. Mercorelli, B.; Lembo, D.; Palu, G.; Loregian, A. Early inhibitors of human cytomegalovirus: State-of-art and therapeutic perspectives. *Pharmacol. Ther.* **2011**, *131*, 309–329. [CrossRef]
16. Gilbert, C.; Boivin, G. Human cytomegalovirus resistance to antiviral drugs. *Antimicrob. Agents Chemother.* **2005**, *49*, 873–883. [CrossRef] [PubMed]
17. Foulongne, V.; Turriere, C.; Diafouka, F.; Abraham, B.; Lastere, S.; Segondy, M. Ganciclovir resistance mutations in UL97 and UL54 genes of Human cytomegalovirus isolates resistant to ganciclovir. *Acta Virol.* **2004**, *48*, 51–55.
18. Smith, I.L.; Cherrington, J.M.; Jiles, R.E.; Fuller, M.D.; Freeman, W.R.; Spector, S.A. High-level resistance of cytomegalovirus to ganciclovir is associated with alterations in both the UL97 and DNA polymerase genes. *J. Infect. Dis.* **1997**, *176*, 69–77. [CrossRef] [PubMed]
19. Torres-Madriz, G.; Boucher, H.W. Immunocompromised hosts: Perspectives in the treatment and prophylaxis of cytomegalovirus disease in solid-organ transplant recipients. *Clin. Infect. Dis.* **2008**, *47*, 702–711. [CrossRef] [PubMed]
20. Erice, A. Resistance of human cytomegalovirus to antiviral drugs. *Clin. Microbiol. Rev.* **1999**, *12*, 286–297. [CrossRef]
21. Melendez, D.P.; Razonable, R.R. Letermovir and inhibitors of the terminase complex: A promising new class of investigational antiviral drugs against human cytomegalovirus. *Infect. Drug Resist.* **2015**, *8*, 269–277. [CrossRef] [PubMed]
22. Imlay, H.N.; Kaul, D.R. Letermovir and Maribavir for the Treatment and Prevention of Cytomegalovirus Infection in Solid Organ and Stem Cell Transplant Recipients. *Clin. Infect. Dis.* **2020**. [CrossRef]
23. Yaiw, K.-C.; Mohammad, A.-A.; Costa, H.; Taher, C.; Badrnya, S.; Assinger, A.; Wilhelmi, V.; Ananthaseshan, S.; Estekizadeh, A.; Davoudi, B.; et al. Human Cytomegalovirus Up-Regulates Endothelin Receptor Type B: Implication for Vasculopathies? *Open Forum. Infect. Dis.* **2015**, *2*, ofv155. [CrossRef] [PubMed]

24. Yaiw, K.C.; Mohammad, A.A.; Taher, C.; Cui, H.L.; Costa, H.; Kostopoulou, O.N.; Jung, M.; Assinger, A.; Wilhelmi, V.; Yang, J.; et al. Human Cytomegalovirus Reduces Endothelin-1 Expression in Both Endothelial and Vascular Smooth Muscle Cells. *Microorganisms* **2021**, *9*, 1137. [CrossRef] [PubMed]
25. Dupuis, J.; Hoeper, M.M. Endothelin receptor antagonists in pulmonary arterial hypertension. *Eur. Respir. J.* **2008**, *31*, 407–415. [CrossRef] [PubMed]
26. Luscher, T.F.; Barton, M. Endothelins and endothelin receptor antagonists: Therapeutic considerations for a novel class of cardiovascular drugs. *Circulation* **2000**, *102*, 2434–2440. [CrossRef]
27. Hoeper, M.M.; McLaughlin, V.V.; Dalaan, A.M.; Satoh, T.; Galie, N. Treatment of pulmonary hypertension. *Lancet Respir Med.* **2016**, *4*, 323–336. [CrossRef]
28. Enderby, C.Y.; Burger, C. Medical treatment update on pulmonary arterial hypertension. *Ther. Adv. Chronic. Dis.* **2015**, *6*, 264–272. [CrossRef]
29. Zebadua, R.; Hernandez-Perez, A.P.; Garcia, A.; Zayas, N.; Sandoval, J.; Lopez, J.; Pulido, T. Macitentan in the treatment of pulmonary arterial hypertension. *Future Cardiol.* **2021**, *17*, 49–58. [CrossRef]
30. Savale, L.; Magnier, R.; Le Pavec, J.; Jais, X.; Montani, D.; O'Callaghan, D.S.; Humbert, M.; Dingemanse, J.; Simonneau, G.; Sitbon, O. Efficacy, safety and pharmacokinetics of bosentan in portopulmonary hypertension. *Eur. Respir. J.* **2013**, *41*, 96–103. [CrossRef] [PubMed]
31. Kingman, M.; Ruggiero, R.; Torres, F. Ambrisentan, an endothelin receptor type A-selective endothelin receptor antagonist, for the treatment of pulmonary arterial hypertension. *Expert Opin. Pharmacother.* **2009**, *10*, 1847–1858. [CrossRef]
32. Murrell, I.; Bedford, C.; Ladell, K.; Miners, K.L.; Price, D.A.; Tomasec, P.; Wilkinson, G.W.G.; Stanton, R.J. The pentameric complex drives immunologically covert cell-cell transmission of wild-type human cytomegalovirus. *Proc. Natl. Acad. Sci. USA* **2017**, *114*, 6104–6109. [CrossRef] [PubMed]
33. Miceli, M.V.; Newsome, D.A.; Novak, L.C.; Beuerman, R.W. Cytomegalovirus replication in cultured human retinal pigment epithelial cells. *Curr. Eye Res.* **1989**, *8*, 835–839. [CrossRef] [PubMed]
34. Cooke, B.M.; Usami, S.; Perry, I.; Nash, G.B. A simplified method for culture of endothelial cells and analysis of adhesion of blood cells under conditions of flow. *Microvasc. Res.* **1993**, *45*, 33–45. [CrossRef] [PubMed]
35. Rosen, H.R.; Benner, K.G.; Flora, K.D.; Rabkin, J.M.; Orloff, S.L.; Olyaei, A.; Chou, S. Development of ganciclovir resistance during treatment of primary cytomegalovirus infection after liver transplantation. *Transplantation* **1997**, *63*, 476–478. [CrossRef] [PubMed]
36. Awasthi, S.; Isler, J.A.; Alwine, J.C. Analysis of splice variants of the immediate-early 1 region of human cytomegalovirus. *J. Virol.* **2004**, *78*, 8191–8200. [CrossRef] [PubMed]
37. Reed, L.J.; Muench, H. A simple method of estimating fifty per cent endpoints. *Am. J. Epidemiol.* **1938**, *27*, 493–497. [CrossRef]
38. Sidharta, P.N.; Treiber, A.; Dingemanse, J. Clinical pharmacokinetics and pharmacodynamics of the endothelin receptor antagonist macitentan. *Clin. Pharmacokinet* **2015**, *54*, 457–471. [CrossRef] [PubMed]
39. Weber, C.; Gasser, R.; Hopfgartner, G. Absorption, excretion, and metabolism of the endothelin receptor antagonist bosentan in healthy male subjects. *Drug Metab. Dispos.* **1999**, *27*, 810–815. [PubMed]
40. Bodaghi, B.; Slobbe-van Drunen, M.E.; Topilko, A.; Perret, E.; Vossen, R.C.; van Dam-Mieras, M.C.; Zipeto, D.; Virelizier, J.L.; LeHoang, P.; Bruggeman, C.A.; et al. Entry of human cytomegalovirus into retinal pigment epithelial and endothelial cells by endocytosis. *Investig. Ophthalmol. Vis. Sci.* **1999**, *40*, 2598–2607.
41. Topilko, A.; Michelson, S. Hyperimmediate entry of human cytomegalovirus virions and dense bodies into human fibroblasts. *Res. Virol.* **1994**, *145*, 75–82. [CrossRef]
42. Detrick, B.; Rhame, J.; Wang, Y.; Nagineni, C.N.; Hooks, J.J. Cytomegalovirus replication in human retinal pigment epithelial cells. Altered expression of viral early proteins. *Investig. Ophthalmol. Vis. Sci.* **1996**, *37*, 814–825.
43. Vanarsdall, A.L.; Johnson, D.C. Human cytomegalovirus entry into cells. *Curr. Opin. Virol.* **2012**, *2*, 37–42. [CrossRef] [PubMed]
44. Compton, T.; Nepomuceno, R.R.; Nowlin, D.M. Human cytomegalovirus penetrates host cells by pH-independent fusion at the cell surface. *Virology* **1992**, *191*, 387–395. [CrossRef]
45. Dankner, W.M.; McCutchan, J.A.; Richman, D.D.; Hirata, K.; Spector, S.A. Localization of human cytomegalovirus in peripheral blood leukocytes by in situ hybridization. *J. Infect. Dis.* **1990**, *161*, 31–36. [CrossRef]
46. Jarvis, M.A.; Nelson, J.A. Human cytomegalovirus tropism for endothelial cells: Not all endothelial cells are created equal. *J. Virol.* **2007**, *81*, 2095–2101. [CrossRef] [PubMed]
47. Soroceanu, L.; Akhavan, A.; Cobbs, C.S. Platelet-derived growth factor-alpha receptor activation is required for human cytomegalovirus infection. *Nature* **2008**, *455*, 391–395. [CrossRef]
48. Wang, X.; Huang, D.Y.; Huong, S.M.; Huang, E.S. Integrin alphavbeta3 is a coreceptor for human cytomegalovirus. *Nat. Med.* **2005**, *11*, 515–521. [CrossRef]
49. Feire, A.L.; Koss, H.; Compton, T. Cellular integrins function as entry receptors for human cytomegalovirus via a highly conserved disintegrin-like domain. *Proc. Natl. Acad. Sci. USA* **2004**, *101*, 15470–15475. [CrossRef]
50. Wang, X.; Huong, S.M.; Chiu, M.L.; Raab-Traub, N.; Huang, E.S. Epidermal growth factor receptor is a cellular receptor for human cytomegalovirus. *Nature* **2003**, *424*, 456–461. [CrossRef] [PubMed]
51. Söderberg, C.; Giugni, T.D.; Zaia, J.A.; Larsson, S.; Wahlberg, J.M.; Moller, E. CD13 (human aminopeptidase N) mediates human cytomegalovirus infection. *J. Virol.* **1993**, *67*, 6576–6585. [CrossRef]

52. Martinez-Martin, N.; Marcandalli, J.; Huang, C.S.; Arthur, C.P.; Perotti, M.; Foglierini, M.; Ho, H.; Dosey, A.M.; Shriver, S.; Payandeh, J.; et al. An Unbiased Screen for Human Cytomegalovirus Identifies Neuropilin-2 as a Central Viral Receptor. *Cell* **2018**, *174*, 1158–1171.e19. [CrossRef] [PubMed]
53. Vanarsdall, A.L.; Pritchard, S.R.; Wisner, T.W.; Liu, J.; Jardetzky, T.S.; Johnson, D.C. CD147 Promotes Entry of Pentamer-Expressing Human Cytomegalovirus into Epithelial and Endothelial Cells. *mBio* **2018**, *9*. [CrossRef] [PubMed]
54. E, X.; Meraner, P.; Lu, P.; Perreira, J.M.; Aker, A.M.; McDougall, W.M.; Zhuge, R.; Chan, G.C.; Gerstein, R.M.; Caposio, P.; et al. OR14I1 is a receptor for the human cytomegalovirus pentameric complex and defines viral epithelial cell tropism. *Proc. Natl. Acad. Sci. USA* **2019**, *116*, 7043–7052. [CrossRef] [PubMed]
55. Kabanova, A.; Marcandalli, J.; Zhou, T.; Bianchi, S.; Baxa, U.; Tsybovsky, Y.; Lilleri, D.; Silacci-Fregni, C.; Foglierini, M.; Fernandez-Rodriguez, B.M.; et al. Platelet-derived growth factor-alpha receptor is the cellular receptor for human cytomegalovirus gHgLgO trimer. *Nat. Microbiol.* **2016**, *1*, 16082. [CrossRef]
56. Vanarsdall, A.L.; Howard, P.W.; Wisner, T.W.; Johnson, D.C. Human Cytomegalovirus gH/gL Forms a Stable Complex with the Fusion Protein gB in Virions. *PLoS Pathog.* **2016**, *12*, e1005564. [CrossRef] [PubMed]
57. Kim, J.H.; Collins-McMillen, D.; Buehler, J.C.; Goodrum, F.D.; Yurochko, A.D. Human Cytomegalovirus Requires Epidermal Growth Factor Receptor Signaling To Enter and Initiate the Early Steps in the Establishment of Latency in CD34+ Human Progenitor Cells. *J. Virol.* **2017**, *91*. [CrossRef]
58. Moody, T.W.; Ramos-Alvarez, I.; Moreno, P.; Mantey, S.A.; Ridnour, L.; Wink, D.; Jensen, R.T. Endothelin causes transactivation of the EGFR and HER2 in non-small cell lung cancer cells. *Peptides* **2017**, *90*, 90–99. [CrossRef]
59. Compton, T. Receptors and immune sensors: The complex entry path of human cytomegalovirus. *Trends Cell Biol.* **2004**, *14*, 5–8. [CrossRef]
60. Nogalski, M.T.; Chan, G.C.; Stevenson, E.V.; Collins-McMillen, D.K.; Yurochko, A.D. The HCMV gH/gL/UL128-131 complex triggers the specific cellular activation required for efficient viral internalization into target monocytes. *PLoS Pathog* **2013**, *9*, e1003463. [CrossRef]
61. Alvarez-Cardona, J.J.; Whited, L.K.; Chemaly, R.F. Brincidofovir: Understanding its unique profile and potential role against adenovirus and other viral infections. *Future Microbiol.* **2020**, *15*, 389–400. [CrossRef]

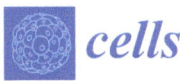

Article

Albumin Might Attenuate Bacteria-Induced Damage on Kupffer Cells for Patients with Chronic Liver Disease

Hao Lin [1], Yuhui Fan [1], Andreas Wieser [2,3,4], Jiang Zhang [5], Ivonne Regel [1], Hanno Nieß [6], Julia Mayerle [1], Alexander L. Gerbes [1] and Christian J. Steib [1,*]

[1] Liver Center Munich, Department of Medicine II, University Hospital, 81377 Munich, Germany; Hao.Lin@med.uni-muenchen.de (H.L.); fyhmed@yeah.net (Y.F.); Ivonne.Regel@med.uni-muenchen.de (I.R.); Julia.Mayerle@med.uni-muenchen.de (J.M.); Gerbes@med.uni-muenchen.de (A.L.G.)
[2] Max von Pettenkofer Institute, Faculty of Medicine, Medical Microbiology and Hospital Epidemiology, 80336 Munich, Germany; wieser@mvp.lmu.de
[3] Division of Infectious Diseases and Tropical Medicine, University Hospital, 80802 Munich, Germany
[4] German Center for Infection Research (DZIF), Partner Site Munich, 80802 Munich, Germany
[5] Liver Transplantation Center, Department of Liver Surgery, Ren Ji Hospital, School of Medicine, Shanghai Jiao Tong University, Shanghai 200127, China; zhangjiang@renji.com
[6] Biobank of the Department of General, Visceral and Transplant Surgery, University Hospital, 80802 Munich, Germany; Hanno.Niess@med.uni-muenchen.de
* Correspondence: Christian.Steib@med.uni-muenchen.de; Tel.: +49-89-4400-72298; Fax: +49-89-4400-75299

Citation: Lin, H.; Fan, Y.; Wieser, A.; Zhang, J.; Regel, I.; Nieß, H.; Mayerle, J.; Gerbes, A.L.; Steib, C.J. Albumin Might Attenuate Bacteria-Induced Damage on Kupffer Cells for Patients with Chronic Liver Disease. *Cells* **2021**, *10*, 2298. https://doi.org/10.3390/cells10092298

Academic Editors: Silvia Fischer and Alexander E. Kalyuzhny

Received: 2 August 2021
Accepted: 1 September 2021
Published: 3 September 2021

Publisher's Note: MDPI stays neutral with regard to jurisdictional claims in published maps and institutional affiliations.

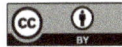

Copyright: © 2021 by the authors. Licensee MDPI, Basel, Switzerland. This article is an open access article distributed under the terms and conditions of the Creative Commons Attribution (CC BY) license (https://creativecommons.org/licenses/by/4.0/).

Abstract: Chronic liver diseases (CLDs) are complex diseases that cause long-term inflammation and infection, which in turn accelerate their development. The usage of albumin in patients with CLDs has been debated for years. Human serum albumin (HSA) plays a key role in immunomodulation during the process of CLDs. The correlation between albumin and C-reactive protein (CRP) in CLD patients was analyzed by linear regression with the Pearson statistic. The damage of THP-1 and primary cells was evaluated by measuring the lactate dehydrogenase (LDH) in the supernatant. Immunofluorescence staining was performed to determine underlying pathways in Kupffer cells (KCs). Albumin negatively correlated with infection in patients with CLDs. In vitro experiments with THP-1 cells and KCs showed that albumin reduced LDH release after stimulation with bacterial products, while no differences in hepatic stellate cells (HSCs) and sinusoidal endothelial cells (SECs) were detected. Moreover, immunofluorescence staining revealed an increase of p-ERK and p-NF-kB p65 density after albumin treatment of KCs stimulated by bacterial products. In conclusion, albumin could assist CLD patients in alleviating inflammation caused by bacterial products and might be beneficial to patients with CLDs by securing KCs from bacteria-induced damage, providing a compelling rationale for albumin therapy in patients with CLDs.

Keywords: hepatic non-parenchymal cells; albumin; chronic liver diseases; bacteria

1. Introduction

Chronic liver diseases (CLDs) are a long-term pathological process involving continuous destruction and regeneration of liver parenchyma that leads to cirrhosis at its most advanced stage. The mechanism of the progression of CLDs is complicated and remains unsettled, but unceasing inflammation and bacterial infections may play an important role in this process [1,2]. Spontaneous bacterial peritonitis (SBP) is one of the most common infections during CLDs [3]. Gram-negative aerobic or facultative aerobic organisms such as *Klebsiella pneumoniae* (*K. pneumoniae*), *Escherichia coli* (*E. coli*), *Pseudomonas aeruginosa* (*P. aeruginosa*) and *Enterobacter cloacae* (*E. cloacae*) are the most common cause of SBP patients; other common organisms include the Gram-positive species *Enterococcus faecium* (*E. faecium*), *Streptococcus pneumoniae* (*S. peneumoniae*) and *Staphylococcus aureus* (*S. aureus*) [4].

Kupffer cells (KCs) are resident liver macrophages as well as the largest population of innate immune cells in the liver [5]. The major function of KCs is to scavenge and phagocyte cell debris, small particles, protein complexes and senescent red blood cells through an interplay with pattern recognition receptors. In addition, gut-derived toxic materials including pathogens from the intestinal flora and endotoxic lipopolysaccharide (LPS) are removed by KCs [5–7]. Thus, KCs play an essential role in maintaining the homeostasis to protect the host and in prompting immunogenic and tolerogenic immune responses.

Human serum albumin (HSA) is a crucial plasma protein often administered in the therapies of patients with CLDs. However, there still are debates on the benefit of albumin in patients with cirrhosis over the long term. Notably, a recent clinical trial presented that the long-term albumin administration to patients with cirrhosis reduced systemic inflammation [8] and the cumulative incidence of complications of cirrhosis, including SBP and non-SBP bacterial infections [9,10]. Among the reasons of benefits of albumin in patients with cirrhosis, expander function depending on its known oncotic properties is well known, although it is now irrefutably clear that the immunomodulatory function of albumin turns to be more important during the therapies for liver cirrhosis [11–13]. HSA is capable of binding inflammatory factors and mediators including LPS, lipoteichoic acid and peptidoglycan, which are the surface components of Gram-negative and Gram-positive bacteria capable of activating the innate immune system through Toll-like receptor 2/4 (TLR 2/4) and initiating inflammation [12–15]. Albumin preconditioning abrogated the LPS-mediated inflammation through the Nuclear Factor-κB (NF-κB) activation [16] and enhanced monocyte interleukin-6 (IL-6) gene expression via the extracellular signal-regulated kinase (ERK) and NF-κB pathways [17]. Albumin can modulate innate immune responses to sepsis and cirrhosis-associated prostaglandin E2-mediated immune dysfunction following albumin infusion [18]. Nevertheless, the role of albumin on KCs, the first barrier against bacteria and a vital role in bacteria-induced immune responses, has not been investigated.

Hence, our study underscores a protective role of albumin in patients with CLDs and in KCs stimulated by the bacterial products, suggesting that albumin therapies aim to not only improve plasma osmolality for patients with CLDs but benefit KCs in reducing the damage from microbial products, providing a convincing rationale for albumin application in patients with CLDs.

2. Materials and Method

2.1. Study Cohort

From July 2016 to March 2019, 138 outpatients or consecutive hospitalized patients with CLDs were obtained to be included in this study. The types of CLDs included in this study are: chronic viral hepatitis B ($n = 26$), autoimmune hepatitis ($n = 21$), chronic viral hepatitis C ($n = 18$), liver cirrhosis ($n = 33$, including 29 hepatitis-induced, 3 alcohol-induced and 1 Alagille syndrome-induced), primary sclerosing cholangitis ($n = 8$), primary biliary cholangitis ($n = 6$), steatosis hepatitis ($n = 5$), nonalcoholic steatohepatitis (NASH, $n = 4$), alcoholic liver disease ($n = 3$), cryptogenic cirrhosis ($n = 3$), cystic liver disease ($n = 2$), Budd–Chiari Syndrome ($n = 2$), hemochromatosis ($n = 2$), liver adenoma ($n = 2$), M. Wilson disease ($n = 1$), sarcoidosis ($n = 1$) and toxic liver disease ($n = 1$). The study protocol was approved by the ethics committee of the Faculty of Medicine at the Ludwig-Maximilians University (LMU) (approval number 17-756), and patients provided written informed consent. All indicators were measured by the clinical chemistry laboratory of the university hospital of LMU using an automatic analyzer (cobas®8000 modular analyzer series, Roche, Switzerland) and standardized operating procedures according to the manual. A score was calculated using the following formula: MELD Score = $10 \times (0.957 \times \ln(\text{Creatinine}) + 0.378 \times \ln(\text{Bilirubin}) + 1.12 \times \ln(\text{INR}) + 0.643)$.

2.2. Human Tissue Specimens

Double-coded liver tissue samples and corresponding data used in this study were provided by the Biobank of the Department of General, Visceral and Transplant Surgery of LMU. This Biobank operates under the administration of the Human Tissue and Cell Research (HTCR) Foundation. The framework of HTCR Foundation [19], which includes obtaining written informed consent from all donors, has been approved by the ethics committee of the Faculty of Medicine at the LMU (approval number 025-12) as well as the Bavarian State Medical Association (approval number 11142) in Germany. A total of 10 human liver tissues were included in our experiments and were from patients with liver metastasis.

2.3. Primary Hepatic Non-Parenchymal Cells Isolation and Culture

Liver tissues were preserved in RPMI 1640 medium (Gibco, Karlsruhe, Germany) on ice immediately after surgical removal, and cells were isolated within 6 h. Nycodenz (Axis Shield, Rodelokka, Norway) gradients density centrifugation was performed to isolate primary liver KCs and hepatic stellate cells (HSCs). In brief, liver samples were cut into 1–5 mm thick slices and rinsed by phosphate-buffered saline (PBS). The tissue slices were digested with 15 mg/mL pronase (Sigma, St. Louis, USA) at 37 °C for 20 min. After two times of 80 μm and 60 μm nylon mesh filtration, the tissue solution was mixed with Nycodenz solution (16.7% for KCs and 28.7% for HSCs) and centrifuged ($1400\times g$, 20 min) without the brake, dividing into three layers. We collected the middle layer and interfaces. To isolate sinusoidal endothelial cells (SECs), CD146 MicroBeads (Miltenyi Biotec, Teterow, Germany) and a magnetically activated cell sorting system were employed to filtrate the tissue digestive solution instead of Nycodenz. Cells were seeded in multiple well plates and cultured at 37 °C in 5% CO_2 in RPMI 1640 with 10% fetal calf serum (FCS, PAN, Aidenbach, Germany) and 1% Penicillin-Streptomycin (Sigma, St. Louis, MO, USA). Detailed procedures were described previously [20–22].

2.4. Cell Culture and Treatment

The THP-1 cell line (American Type Culture Collection, reference number TIB-202™) was a gift from Prof. Peter Nelson. Cells were cultured at 37 °C in 5% CO_2 in RPMI 1640 with 10% FCS and 1% Penicillin–Streptomycin. To differentiate THP-1 into adherent macrophages, 20 ng/mL phorbol myristate acetate (PMA) was used to treat cells in a complete medium for 48 h. The medium was changed into a serum-free medium before the stimulation of bacterial products. Cells were treated with albumin at the same time with (peri-treatment) or 24 h before (pre-treatment) the stimulation of bacterial products. The supernatant was harvested after 24 h of the microbial isolate stimulation.

2.5. Bacterial Products Isolation and Stimulation

Bacterial strains including *K. pneumoniae, E. coli* and *E. cloacae, P. aeruginosa, E. faecium, S. peneumoniae* and *S. aureus* were isolated from patients with SBP (different groups of patients from the study cohort). The isolates were cultured on Columbia 5% sheep blood media (Becton Dickinson, Heidelberg, Germany) at 37 °C under aeration. Bacterial colonies were taken off the solid media with caution not to include any parts of the media. The bacterial pellet was resuspended in phosphate-buffered saline (PBS pH 7.4) by pipetting up and down and vortex mixing. Cells were washed in PBS three times to remove any residual media or debris. After the last washing steps, the bacterial cell mass was resuspended in PBS buffer and sterilized using heat inactivation [23]. Bacterial inactivation was confirmed twice by plating the heat-inactivated extracts on media and cultivating them for 48 h at 37 °C. Bacterial product solutions were measured for protein content in serial dilutions (Bradford) and were subsequently divided into aliquots and stored frozen until use. The bacterial products solutions were diluted to various concentrations (1, 8, 16 μg/mL) with serum-free medium and then were used to stimulate cells at different concentrations with or without HSA.

2.6. Evaluation of Cell Damage

The lactate dehydrogenase (LDH) was used to assess the cell damage of THP-1 and primary cells. LDH catalyzes the reversible conversion of lactate to pyruvate with the reduction of NAD+ to NADH. Thus, the production of NADH was employed to determine the LDH activity indirectly, which was measured by the absorbance value at 365 nm [20,24,25]. 5% Triton-X-100, which is inducing cell damage, was applied as a positive control.

2.7. Immunofluorescence Staining

Cells were fixed with 4% paraformaldehyde for 10 min (Roth, Karlsruhe, Germany), then they were blocked in 10% donkey serum for 30 min, and were permeabilized with 0.1–0.5% Triton X-100 in PBS for 10 min [26]. Subsequently, cells were incubated with the primary antibodies (1:250 p-ERK and 1:1000 p-NF-kB p65, Cell Signaling Technology) overnight at 4 °C and fluorescent-labeled secondary antibodies at room temperature for 1 h the next day. The images were captured by immunofluorescence microscopy (Leica, Germany).

2.8. Statistical Analyses

Results are presented as mean ± standard deviation (SD) or median and interquartile range (IQR). Normality of data distribution was tested by Kolmogorov–Smirnov Z test (Table 1). Statistical comparisons by using the unpaired two-tailed Student's t-test and Mann–Whitney U test were performed. Correlations between variables were calculated using linear regression with the Pearson statistic. A p-value less than 0.05 was considered significant. SPSS was used for data analysis.

Table 1. Normality test of laboratory parameters.

Characteristic	All (N)	K-S Test	p-Value
Age (years)	53.45 + 14.66 (138)	0.642	0.804
NaCl (mmol/L)	137.8 + 3.63 (138)	1.699	0.006
KCl (mmol/L)	4.3 + 0.47 (138)	1.079	0.195
Zinc (mmol/L)	67.83 + 20.87 (138)	0.782	0.573
CRP (mg/dL)	0.98 + 1.86 (106)	3.177	<0.001
Leukocytes (G/L)	6.38 + 2.34 (137)	1.191	0.117
Bilirubin (mg/dL)	2.55 + 4.71 (138)	3.717	<0.001
GOT (U/L)	116.19 + 426.89 (132)	4.757	<0.001
GPT (U/L)	154.49 + 673.88 (138)	5.071	<0.001
Gamma-GT (U/L)	106.31 + 130.97 (138)	2.699	<0.001
LDH (U/L)	247.17 + 160.85 (71)	2.226	<0.001
INR	2.22 + 0.39 (138)	2.595	<0.001
Creatinine (mg/dL)	1.07 + 0.86 (138)	3.635	<0.001
MELD Score	10.79 + 6.7 (138)	2.787	<0.001

K-S test: Kolmogorov–Smirnov Z test. Data are expressed as mean ± SD.

3. Results

3.1. Albumin Negatively Correlated with Infection in Patients with CLDs

All 138 patients with CLDs were divided into two groups according to their HSA levels: the normal albumin group (≥3.5 g/dL) and the low albumin group (<3.5 g/dL). Table 2 displayed that CLD patients with lower albumin had higher bilirubin, aspartate aminotransferase (GOT), Gamma-GT, LDH, international normalized ratio (INR), and creatinine, C-reactive protein (CRP), MELD Score, while NaCl, KCl and Zinc serum levels were remarkably lower. Pearson correlation analysis and linear regression were performed to investigate the association between these indicators and albumin levels. As exhibited in Table 3 and Figure 1, high serum albumin levels correlated with a low concentration of CRP in patients with CLDs showing an r value of 0.565 ($p < 0.001$). Which indicated that patients with CLDs with high serum albumin had less infection. In addition, the levels of NaCl, KCl and Zinc positively correlated with albumin levels in patients with CLDs while bilirubin, GOT, Gamma-GT, LDH, INR, and creatinine had a negative correlation with albumin levels (Table 3 and Figure S1).

Table 2. Characteristic analysis based on different albumin concentrations.

Characteristic	Normal Albumin (n)	Low Albumin (n)	p-Value
	N = 99	N = 39	
Age (years)	52.92 + 15.49 (99)	54.80 + 12.40 (39)	0.501 [a]
Sex (Male/Female)	42/57	23/16	/
NaCl (mmol/L)	138(139–140) (99)	135(133–138) (39)	<0.001 [b]
KCl (mmol/L)	4.45 + 0.38 (99)	3.40 + 0.43 (39)	<0.001 [a]
Zinc (mmol/L)	75.96 + 17.14 (99)	47.15 + 14.15 (39)	<0.001 [a]
CRP (mg/dL)	0.10(0.10–0.30) (67)	1.30(0.60–2.00) (39)	<0.001 [b]
Leukocytes (G/L)	6.54 ± 2.24 (98)	5.97 + 2.55 (39)	0.195 [a]
Bilirubin (mg/dL)	0.70(0.50–1.10) (99)	2.9(2.3–10.5) (39)	<0.001 [b]
GOT (U/L)	29.00(25.00–39.00) (99)	73.00(42.00–118.00) (35)	<0.001 [b]
GPT (U/L)	30.00(21.00–49.00) (99)	33.00(19.00–93.00) (39)	0.192 [b]
Gamma-GT (U/L)	37.00(22.00–98.00) (98)	147.00(55.00–202.00) (39)	<0.001 [b]
LDH (U/L)	197.50(166.50–234.75)	238.00(195.50–316.00) (28)	0.003 [b]
INR	1.00(0.90–1.10) (99)	1.40(1.20–1.60) (39)	<0.001 [b]
Creatinine (mg/dL)	0.80(0.90 + 1.00) (99)	1.20(0.90–1.40) (39)	<0.001 [b]
MELD Score	7.00(6.00–8.00) (99)	17.00(13.00–22.00) (39)	<0.001 [b]

Data are expressed as mean ± SD or median and interquartile range (IQR); [a] Student's t-test.; [b] Mann–Whitney U test.

Table 3. Correlation between characteristic and different albumin concentrations.

Characteristic	Normal Albumin		Low Albumin		All	
	R	p-Value	R	p-Value	R	p-Value
Age (years)	−0.358	<0.001	−0.0101	0.541	−0.189	0.026
NaCl (mmol/L)	0.084	0.408	0.635	<0.001	0.637	<0.001
KCl (mmol/L)	0.145	0.152	0.037	0.823	0.504	<0.001
Zinc (mmol/L)	0.466	<0.001	0.460	0.003	0.716	<0.001
CRP (mg/dL)	−0.409	0.001	−0.308	0.056	−0.565	<0.001
Leukocytes (G/L)	0.090	0.376	−0.238	0.145	0.092	0.286
Bilirubin (mg/dL)	−0.273	0.006	−0.067	0.686	−0.495	<0.001
GOT (U/L)	−0.217	0.032	0.132	0.450	−0.221	0.011
GPT (U/L)	−0.115	0.258	0.102	0.538	−0.077	0.375
Gamma-GT (U/L)	−0.299	0.003	0.102	0.537	−0.344	<0.001
LDH (U/L)	−0.128	0.43	−0.103	0.949	−0.316	0.009
INR	−0.204	0.043	−0.395	0.013	−0.604	<0.001
Creatinine (mg/dL)	−0.42	0.68	−0.080	0.627	−0.293	<0.001
MELD Score	−0.337	0.001	−0.227	0.165	−0.022	0.828

R and p values were obtained using the Pearson correlation test.

The CRP levels were negatively correlated with albumin levels in patients with CLDs (r = −0.565, p < 0.001).

3.2. Albumin Reduces the Cell Damage Caused by a Bacterial Infection in THP-1 Cells

It is well-known that a CRP test could be used to monitor conditions that cause inflammation, including bacterial infections, fungal infections and inflammatory bowel diseases. CLD patients would most likely have SBP during the development of CLDs, and the most common reasons for SBP are bacterial invasions [3,4]. Besides this, the sensitivity and specificity of CRP are high enough to evaluate the condition of bacterial infection in patients with CLDs [27]. Together, the increase of CRP levels in CLD patients are mainly attributed to the bacterial infection in our study; therefore, we used bacterial products to stimulate THP-1 and primary cells in the subsequent experiments. Our previous publication indicated that Zinc protects KCs from microbial infection [28]. As shown in

Table 3 and Figure S1, the concentration of albumin had a strong positive correlation with Zinc levels in patients with CLDs (r = 0.752, $p < 0.001$). In this study, we postulated that albumin protects macrophages from the damage of bacterial infection. Instead of KCs, we selected the macrophage cell line THP-1 to perform in vitro validation experiments, because the amounts of KCs from human liver specimens were limited. First, we optimized the concentration of bacterial products that causes LDH release, as a marker for cell damage. We treated THP-1 cells with different concentrations of bacterial products and demonstrated increased LDH levels when using 8 and 16 μg/mL of bacterial isolates (Figure 2A) Next, we tested the cell damage caused by 8 bacterial strains associated with CLDs including regular Gram-negative and Gram-positive bacteria, such as *K. pneumoniae, E. coli* and *E. cloacae, P. aeruginosa, E. faecium, S. pneumoniae* and *S. aureus*. Figure 2B showed that all of the eight most ubiquitous bacteria in CLDs can cause considerable increases in LDH levels when THP-1 cells were treated with 8 μg/mL of the bacterial products.

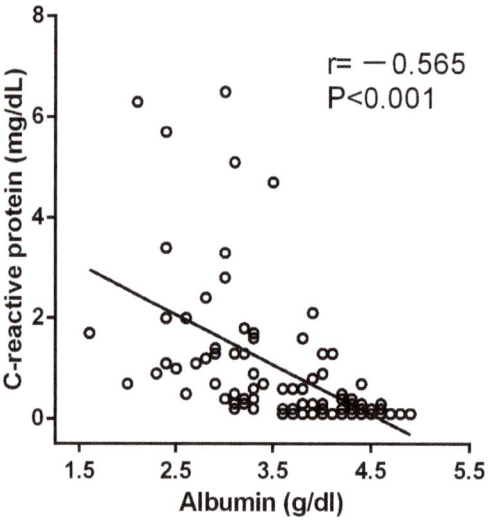

Figure 1. The correlation between albumin and CRP.

Moreover, we analyzed whether albumin might show toxic effects on THP-1 macrophages when treated with increasing concentrations. Notably, in a range from 0.01–0.4 mg/mL, albumin treatment of THP-1 cells did not result in a meaningful increase of LDH levels. To investigate if albumin protects macrophages from bacterial damage, we treated THP-1 cells with 8 μg/mL bacterial products of four bacteria strains including *E. coli TOP10* and *E. cloacae* (Gram-negative bacteria strains) and *S. pneumoniae* and *S. aureus* (Gram-positive bacteria strains) in combination with 0.4 mg/mL albumin. Therefore, THP-1 cells either were treated with albumin 24h before (pre-treatment) or at the same time (peri-treatment) with microbial stimulation. Our data demonstrated, consistent with our previous results, that bacterial products increased LDH release in THP-1 cells compared to the control group ($^\#\,p < 0.05$, Figure 2D). Furthermore, both the pre-treatment and peri-treatment of albumin significantly decreased LDH release in four bacterial product groups compared to no-albumin (blank) treatment (* $p < 0.05$, Figure 2D). These results demonstrated that albumin protected THP-1 cells from bacteria-associated damage, irrespective of the pre-treatment or peri-treatment conditions with albumin.

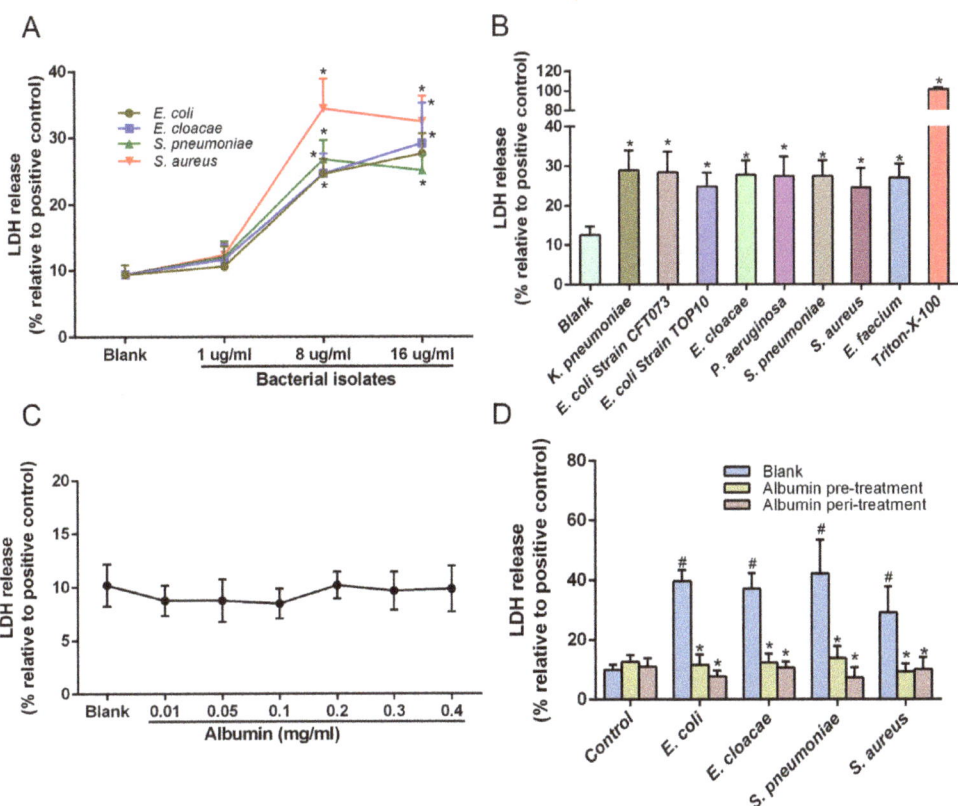

Figure 2. Effects of albumin on the injury induced by bacteria in THP-1. (**A**) The cell damage caused by bacteria products at various concentrations. (**B**) Measurement of the cell damage caused by bacterial components (8 μg/mL) isolated from indicated bacteria strain from patients with CLDs. (**C**) Toxic measurement of different doses of albumin in THP-1. (**D**) Effects of albumin treatment (0.4 mg/mL) on THP-1 stimulated with bacterial isolates (8 μg/mL). All LDH data are normalized to a positive control (5% Triton-X-100). The 5% Triton-X-100 was set as a positive control in all LDH measurement assays. Data expressed as means ± SD, * $p < 0.05$ vs. blank treatment in their own group, # $p < 0.05$ vs. blank treatment in the control group, $n = 6$ in each group from three independent experiments.

3.3. Albumin Safeguards KCs, Rather Than HSCs and SECs from Bacteria-Induced Cell Damage

To investigate whether albumin has identical effects on primary hepatic non-parenchymal cells as it was shown above for the THP-1 cell line, KCs, HSCs and SECs isolated from human liver specimens were examined. Like the THP-1 cells, primary KCs, HSCs and SECs were treated with albumin and stimulated by bacterial products. LDH was measured to assess cell damage. Albumin treatment of KCs remarkably reduced LDH release caused by bacterial isolates in both pre-and peri-treatment conditions. Interestingly, for HSCs, the bacterial products notably increased LDH levels (# $p < 0.05$); however, no significant changes in LDH levels were found after albumin treatment (Figure 3B). In addition, bacterial product stimulation and albumin treatment did not induce any notable changes in LDH levels in SECs (Figure 3C). From these findings, we conclude that albumin has a protective role on KCs preventing KC damage during a bacterial invasion in CLD patients.

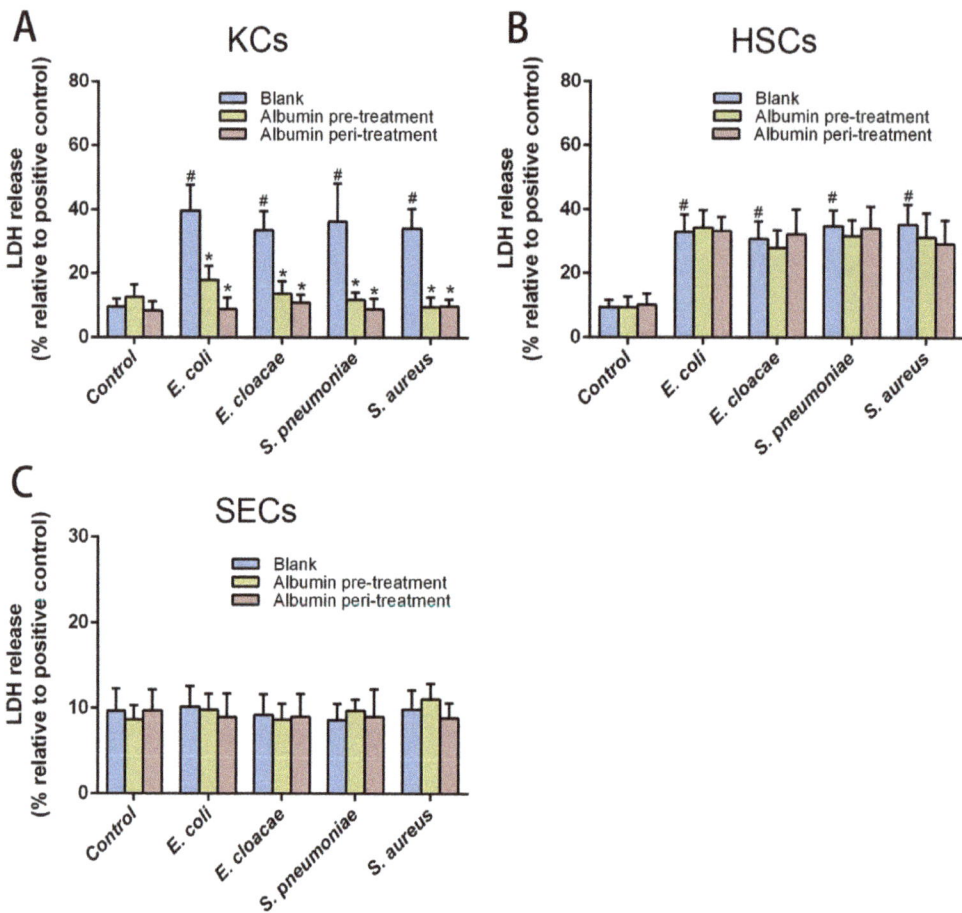

Figure 3. Different effects of albumin on different hepatic non-parenchymal cells. (**A**) Effects of albumin (0.4 mg/mL) on the cell damage induced by bacterial products (8 μg/mL) for KCs. No significant effects of albumin on HSCs (**B**) and SECs (**C**) were found in both pre-treatment and peri-treatment. Data expressed as means ± SD, * $p < 0.05$ vs. blank treatment in their own group, # $p < 0.05$ vs. blank treatment in the control group, $n = 6$ in each group from three independent experiments with a total of three different human livers.

3.4. ERK and NF-kB Pathways Were Involved in the Protective Effects of Albumin

ERK and NF-kB pathways are the most important pathways participating in the TLR/MyD88/IRAK4 axis that is activated by Gram-positive and Gram-negative bacteria in livers [29–31]. To determine the activation of the ERK and NF-kB pathway in KCs, we performed immunofluorescence staining of phosphor-ERK (p-ERK) and phosphor-NF-kB (p-NF-kB) under control, *E. coli* and *E. coli* plus albumin treatment. The results showed that albumin intensifies the staining density of p-ERK and p-NF-kB compared to the control group and *E. coli* group in KCs (Figure 4). These findings provided preliminary evidence of the involvement of ERK and the NF-kB pathway in the process of albumin protection on liver macrophages.

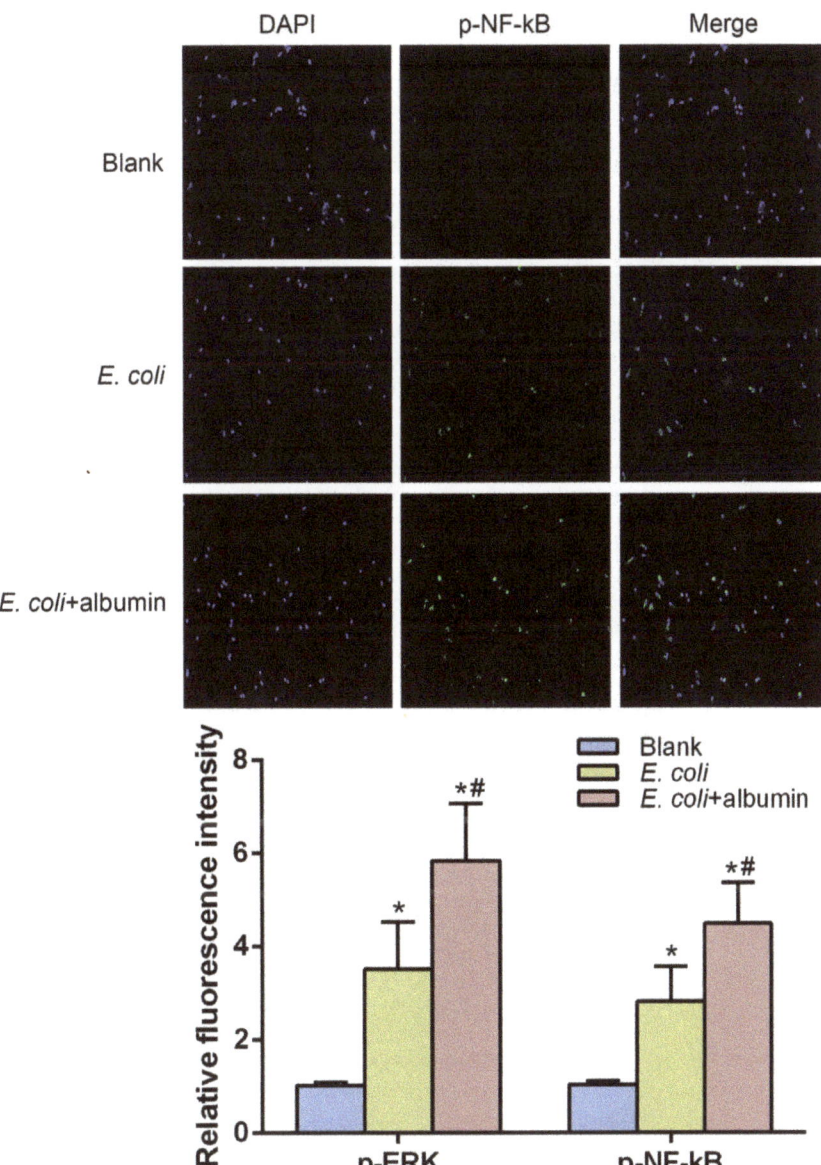

Figure 4. The potential mechanism of the protective effects of albumin in KCs. Immunofluorescence labeling of p-ERK and p-NF-kB protein (green) of KCs treated with albumin and *E. coli*. The nuclei were stained with 4′-6-diamidino-2-phenylindole (blue). Scale bars, 100μm. The relative fluorescence intensity compared with DAPI intensity in the staining experiments was measured. Data expressed as means ± SD, * $p < 0.05$ vs. blank group, # $p < 0.05$ vs. *E. coli* group, $n = 6$ in each group from three independent experiments with a total of three different human livers.

4. Discussion

In the present study, we described for the first time the beneficial effects of albumin reducing the damage of KCs caused by bacteria infections. Albumin is applied regularly to improve osmotic pressure for patients with cirrhosis, but there is only little information on further functions of albumin. This study highlighted the relationship of albumin and inflammation after bacteria invasion in patients with CLDs, the immune-related role of albumin in patients with CLDs, and its underlying mechanism. Novel findings in this study were: (1) In patients with CLDs, albumin levels were found to be inversely correlated to CRP levels, a marker for infection. (2) Albumin protects KCs against bacterial-induced cell injury, but no effects were observed in HSCs. (3) The ERK and NF-kB pathway may be involved in the protective effects of albumin treatment in KCs.

In patients with CLDs, the clinical benefits of albumin therapy have been debated for years. Several reports have failed to show any favorable effect on the administration of albumin in CLDs except for delaying the onset of renal failure [32,33]. Nevertheless, the wide range of potential benefits of albumin administration, such as anti-inflammatory activity, antioxidant function, immunomodulation and the transportation of many endogenous and exogenous substances, still need to be further investigated [34]. Recently, there were some important clinical trials conducted to supply more convincing evidence of the benefits of albumin administration in patients with CLDs. The data indicated that long-term albumin supplementation to patients with cirrhosis and ascites improved survival, lowered hospitalizations and prevented complications [8,9,35]. In our present study, we found that patients with lower albumin levels had more severe inflammation (Figure 1), suggesting that albumin eased the inflammation in patients with CLDs and participated in decreasing the immune responses due to the bacterial invasion. Albumin has the ability to bind and inactivate many inflammatory mediators, such as pathogen-associated molecular patterns, reactive oxygen species, bioactive lipid metabolites and nitric oxide, which could be the underlying reason for improving the inflammation for patients with CLDs with normal albumin.

The immunomodulatory function of albumin has been increasingly studied recently. Decreased serum albumin in patients with cirrhosis binds fewer prostaglandin E2 (PGE2) resulting in increased bioavailability of PGE2, which dampens the macrophage response to LPS [18], indicating that albumin may promote immune functions in some ways. KCs are one of the most important immune cells participating in the immune reaction. To explore the relative mechanism of albumin on reducing the inflammation presented in Figure 1, we treated KCs with albumin in our study. Another study showed no positive changes under the administration of albumin on patients with cirrhosis [36], even though there were three clinical trials to prove the benefit of albumin on patients with CLDs referred above. Interestingly, a loading dose of albumin administration in the other three studies has been considered to be the reason behind this difference [12], which means that the concentration of albumin administration is critical to show its advantages. In addition, it has previously been observed that 0.4 mg/mL albumin could improve PGE2-mediated immunosuppression [18]. Taken together, 0.4 mg/mL albumin was used in our cell experiments. KC isolation from the human liver is a tricky technique, and the number of cells was limited. THP-1 is a human monocytic cell line obtained from a patient with acute monocytic leukemia, and the cells differentiated with PMA are commonly utilized as a model for human macrophage function and biology [36]. Therefore, we used them rather than KCs to measure the damage from different strains and various concentrations of bacterial products. Our results presented that 8 μg/mL and 16 μg/mL of bacterial product stimulation had a significant injury on THP-1 cells (Figure 2A). Bacterial products of all tested strains damaged THP-1 cells regardless of Gram-negative or Gram-positive bacteria (Figure 2B), whereas albumin with increasing concentrations had no toxic effects on cells (Figure 2C).

Next, we treated KCs and THP-1 with albumin to examine its protective effects on primary macrophages. Our data showed that albumin treatment before and during the stimulation with bacterial products protected KCs and THP-1 from injury by microbial isolates (Figures 2D and 3A), which might be caused by the capability of albumin to bind inflammatory factors as mentioned above. Another possible explanation for this is that the albumin might strengthen the phagocytosis of KCs, and increase the albumin levels inside cells, and this might have a synergistic effect on the protection of KCs. Besides, we confirmed our previous conclusion that microbial isolates did damage to KCs and HSCs rather than SECs (Figure 3B,C) [28]. However, one unanticipated finding was that albumin treatment had no notable protective effects on HSCs (Figure 3B). The receptor of polymerized albumin was found on macrophages [37] and its role for endocytosis of albumin has been described [38]. Similarly, stellate cells can actively take up albumin from extracellular sources [39]. Nonetheless, the phagocytosis of macrophages is stronger than stellate cells, which might be a possible mechanism behind this unexpected result.

Taken together, we initially had speculated that patients with CLDs with normal albumin could inactive inflammatory factors and bacterial products. Furthermore, it allows KCs to function normally and facilitate an immune response to foreign bacteria. We hypothesized that at the beginning of immune responses, CLD patients with normal albumin might have more intense inflammation and higher CRP for a short time (acute inflammation responses) due to the response of a healthy immune system, then finally return to normal with the development of the effective immune responses maintained by the protective effect of albumin on KCs, which can explain the relationship between our CRP data in patients with CLDs in Figure 1 and the cell damage assay in Figures 2D and 3A. Thus, we conjectured that the protective effect of albumin on KCs might confer some benefits of diminishing the inflammation in patients with CLDs.

Our previous publication revealed that Zinc protects KCs from this damage caused by bacterial isolates [28]. Considering similar protective effects of Zinc and albumin, we hypothesized that a potential interacting mechanism of these effects might exist. Bacteria or bacterial products stimulate TLRs which are the essential molecules involved in bacteria-induced inflammation in macrophages. Activation of TLRs triggers ERK and NF-κB signaling pathways, which are critical for a normal immune response [29,30]. A previous study demonstrated that albumin treatment produces a dose-dependent increase in pro-inflammatory gene expression (acute inflammation responses) in vitro through activation of ERK and NF-κB pathways [40–43]. Thus, we speculated that the protective effects of albumin on liver macrophages are dependent on the ERK and NF-kB pathways. An amplifying effect of albumin on the activation of the ERK and NF-kB pathways caused by bacteria products was observed compared to the *E. coli* stimulation (Figure 4). Together, our findings provided possible mechanisms for the effect of albumin and aided in understanding the therapeutic benefits of albumin on patients with CLDs.

In conclusion, our results revealed that albumin might help patients with CLDs to better overcome the effects caused by bacterial infection and defend KCs from the injury caused by bacteria in patients with CLDs (Figure 5), implying immunomodulatory-related benefits of albumin administration on patients with CLDs. Thus, we conjectured that albumin supplementation might mitigate bacterial infection in patients with CLDs.

Bacteria raised higher CRP levels in patients with CLDs with low albumin than CLD patients with high albumin. HSCs and SECs instead of SECs could be demolished by bacteria. However, albumin could protect KCs rather than HSCs from the cell damage caused by bacteria.

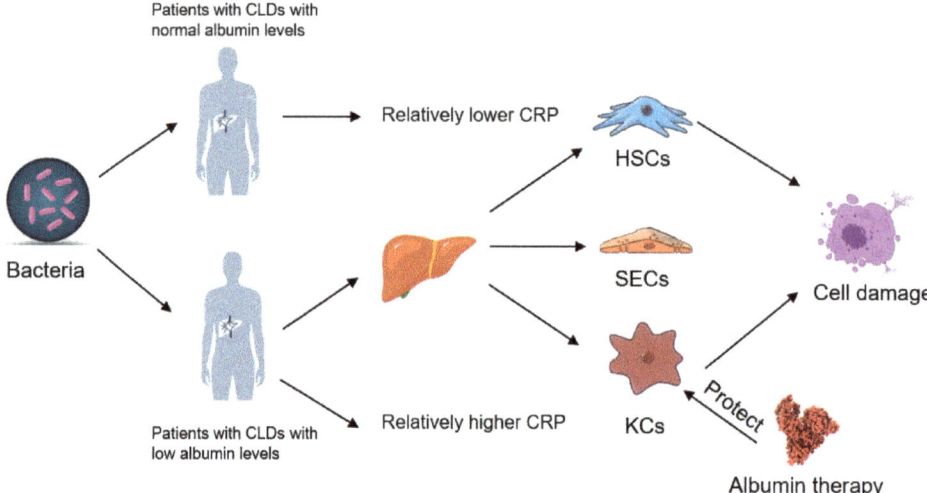

Figure 5. A proposed role of albumin in patients with CLDs and different hepatic non-parenchymal cells.

Supplementary Materials: The following are available online at https://www.mdpi.com/article/10.3390/cells10092298/s1, Figure S1: Correlation between albumin and various clinical characteristics.

Author Contributions: H.L., A.W., J.Z. and C.J.S. conceived and designed the experiments; H.L., Y.F. and J.Z. performed the experiments; H.L., Y.F. and C.J.S. analyzed the data; A.W., I.R., H.N., J.M., A.L.G. and C.J.S. contributed reagents/materials/analysis tools; J.Z., A.W. and C.J.S. wrote the manuscript; I.R., A.L.G. and C.J.S. provided guidance for the research. All authors have read and agreed to the published version of the manuscript.

Funding: This study was supported by the Deutsche Forschungsgemeinschaft under Grant Numbers DFG STE 1022/2-3 and DFG STE 1022/4-1, and the Human Tissue and Cell Research Foundation, a non-profit foundation regulated by German civil law, which facilitates research with human tissue through the provision of an ethical and legal framework for prospective sample collection.

Institutional Review Board Statement: The framework of HTCR Foundation has been approved by the ethics committee of the Faculty of Medicine at the LMU (approval number 025-12) as well as the Bavarian State Medical Association (approval number 11142) in Germany.

Informed Consent Statement: Written informed consent has been obtained from the patient(s) to publish this paper.

Data Availability Statement: The data presented in this study are available on request from the corresponding author.

Acknowledgments: The authors thank Elisabeth-Ingrid Liß for her excellent technical assistance.

Conflicts of Interest: The authors declare no conflict of interest.

References

1. Acharya, C.; Dharel, N.; Sterling, R.K. Chronic liver disease in the human immunodeficiency virus patient. *Clin. Liver Dis.* **2015**, *19*, 1–22. [CrossRef]
2. Fernández, J.; Acevedo, J.; Wiest, R.; Gustot, T.; Amoros, A.; Deulofeu, C.; Reverter, E.; Martínez, J.; Saliba, F.; Jalan, R.; et al. Bacterial and fungal infections in acute-on-chronic liver failure: Prevalence, characteristics and impact on prognosis. *Gut* **2018**, *67*, 1870–1880. [CrossRef]
3. Bernsmeier, C.; Triantafyllou, E.; Brenig, R.; Lebosse, F.J.; Singanayagam, A.; Patel, V.C.; Pop, O.T.; Khamri, W.; Nathwani, R.; Tidswell, R.; et al. CD14(+) CD15(−) HLA-DR(−) myeloid-derived suppressor cells impair antimicrobial responses in patients with acute-on-chronic liver failure. *Gut* **2018**, *67*, 1155–1167. [CrossRef]
4. Gravito-Soares, M.; Gravito-Soares, E.; Lopes, S.; Ribeiro, G.; Figueiredo, P. Spontaneous fungal peritonitis: A rare but severe complication of liver cirrhosis. *Eur. J. Gastroenterol. Hepatol.* **2017**, *29*, 1010–1016. [CrossRef] [PubMed]

5. Vollmar, B.; Menger, M.D. The hepatic microcirculation: Mechanistic contributions and therapeutic targets in liver injury and repair. *Physiol. Rev.* **2009**, *89*, 1269–1339. [CrossRef] [PubMed]
6. Bilzer, M.; Roggel, F.; Gerbes, A.L. Role of Kupffer cells in host defense and liver disease. *Liver Int. Off. J. Int. Assoc. Study Liver* **2006**, *26*, 1175–1186. [CrossRef] [PubMed]
7. Kolios, G.; Valatas, V.; Kouroumalis, E. Role of Kupffer cells in the pathogenesis of liver disease. *World J. Gastroenterol.* **2006**, *12*, 7413–7420. [CrossRef] [PubMed]
8. Fernandez, J.; Claria, J.; Amoros, A.; Aguilar, F.; Castro, M.; Casulleras, M.; Acevedo, J.; Duran-Guell, M.; Nunez, L.; Costa, M.; et al. Effects of Albumin Treatment on Systemic and Portal Hemodynamics and Systemic Inflammation in Patients With Decompensated Cirrhosis. *Gastroenterology* **2019**, *157*, 149–162. [CrossRef] [PubMed]
9. Caraceni, P.; Riggio, O.; Angeli, P.; Alessandria, C.; Neri, S.; Foschi, F.G.; Levantesi, F.; Airoldi, A.; Boccia, S.; Svegliati-Baroni, G.; et al. Long-term albumin administration in decompensated cirrhosis (ANSWER): An open-label randomised trial. *Lancet* **2018**, *391*, 2417–2429. [CrossRef]
10. Sort, P.; Navasa, M.; Arroyo, V.; Aldeguer, X.; Planas, R.; Ruiz-del-Arbol, L.; Castells, L.; Vargas, V.; Soriano, G.; Guevara, M.; et al. Effect of intravenous albumin on renal impairment and mortality in patients with cirrhosis and spontaneous bacterial peritonitis. *N. Engl. J. Med.* **1999**, *341*, 403–409. [CrossRef]
11. Spinella, R.; Sawhney, R.; Jalan, R. Albumin in chronic liver disease: Structure, functions and therapeutic implications. *Hepatol. Int.* **2016**, *10*, 124–132. [CrossRef]
12. Bernardi, M.; Angeli, P.; Claria, J.; Moreau, R.; Gines, P.; Jalan, R.; Caraceni, P.; Fernandez, J.; Gerbes, A.L.; O'Brien, A.J.; et al. Albumin in decompensated cirrhosis: New concepts and perspectives. *Gut* **2020**, *69*, 1127–1138. [CrossRef]
13. Arroyo, V.; García-Martinez, R.; Salvatella, X. Human serum albumin, systemic inflammation, and cirrhosis. *J. Hepatol.* **2014**, *61*, 396–407. [CrossRef] [PubMed]
14. Jürgens, G.; Müller, M.; Garidel, P.; Koch, M.H.; Nakakubo, H.; Blume, A.; Brandenburg, K. Investigation into the interaction of recombinant human serum albumin with Re-lipopolysaccharide and lipid A. *J. Endotoxin Res.* **2002**, *8*, 115–126. [CrossRef] [PubMed]
15. Fukui, H. Relation of endotoxin, endotoxin binding proteins and macrophages to severe alcoholic liver injury and multiple organ failure. *Alcohol. Clin. Exp. Res.* **2005**, *29*, 172s–179s. [CrossRef]
16. Wheeler, D.S.; Giuliano, J.S., Jr.; Lahni, P.M.; Denenberg, A.; Wong, H.R.; Zingarelli, B. The immunomodulatory effects of albumin in vitro and in vivo. *Adv. Pharm. Sci.* **2011**, *2011*, 691928. [CrossRef]
17. Shen, C.Y.; Wu, C.H.; Lu, C.H.; Kuo, Y.M.; Li, K.J.; Hsieh, S.C.; Yu, C.L. Advanced Glycation End Products of Bovine Serum Albumin Suppressed Th1/Th2 Cytokine but Enhanced Monocyte IL-6 Gene Expression via MAPK-ERK and MyD88 Transduced NF-κB p50 Signaling Pathways. *Molecules* **2019**, *24*, 2461. [CrossRef] [PubMed]
18. O'Brien, A.J.; Fullerton, J.N.; Massey, K.A.; Auld, G.; Sewell, G.; James, S.; Newson, J.; Karra, E.; Winstanley, A.; Alazawi, W.; et al. Immunosuppression in acutely decompensated cirrhosis is mediated by prostaglandin E2. *Nat. Med.* **2014**, *20*, 518–523. [CrossRef] [PubMed]
19. Thasler, W.E.; Weiss, T.S.; Schillhorn, K.; Stoll, P.T.; Irrgang, B.; Jauch, K.W. Charitable State-Controlled Foundation Human Tissue and Cell Research: Ethic and Legal Aspects in the Supply of Surgically Removed Human Tissue For Research in the Academic and Commercial Sector in Germany. *Cell Tissue Bank.* **2003**, *4*, 49–56. [CrossRef] [PubMed]
20. Steib, C.J.; Bilzer, M.; Op den Winkel, M.; Pfeiler, S.; Hartmann, A.C.; Hennenberg, M.; Göke, B.; Gerbes, A.L. Treatment with the leukotriene inhibitor montelukast for 10 days attenuates portal hypertension in rat liver cirrhosis. *Hepatology* **2010**, *51*, 2086–2096. [CrossRef]
21. Steib, C.J.; Gmelin, L.; Pfeiler, S.; Schewe, J.; Brand, S.; Göke, B.; Gerbes, A.L. Functional relevance of the cannabinoid receptor 2—Heme oxygenase pathway: A novel target for the attenuation of portal hypertension. *Life Sci.* **2013**, *93*, 543–551. [CrossRef]
22. Kegel, V.; Deharde, D.; Pfeiffer, E.; Zeilinger, K.; Seehofer, D.; Damm, G. Protocol for Isolation of Primary Human Hepatocytes and Corresponding Major Populations of Non-parenchymal Liver Cells. *J. Vis. Exp. JoVE* **2016**, *109*, e53069. [CrossRef]
23. Wieser, A.; Romann, E.; Magistro, G.; Hoffmann, C.; Nörenberg, D.; Weinert, K.; Schubert, S. A multiepitope subunit vaccine conveys protection against extraintestinal pathogenic Escherichia coli in mice. *Infect. Immun.* **2010**, *78*, 3432–3442. [CrossRef] [PubMed]
24. Steib, C.J.; Hartmann, A.C.; Von Hesler, C.; Benesic, A.; Hennenberg, M.; Bilzer, M.; Gerbes, A.L. Intraperitoneal LPS amplifies portal hypertension in rat liver fibrosis. *Lab. Investig.* **2010**, *90*, 1024–1032. [CrossRef] [PubMed]
25. Op den Winkel, M.; Gmelin, L.; Schewe, J.; Leistner, N.; Bilzer, M.; Göke, B.; Gerbes, A.L.; Steib, C.J. Role of cysteinyl-leukotrienes for portal pressure regulation and liver damage in cholestatic rat livers. *Lab. Investig.* **2013**, *93*, 1288–1294. [CrossRef] [PubMed]
26. Lin, H.; Weng, J.; Mei, H.; Zhuang, M.; Xiao, X.; Du, F.; Lin, L.; Wu, J.; Chen, Z.; Huang, Y.; et al. 5-Lipoxygenase promotes epithelial-mesenchymal transition through the ERK signaling pathway in gastric cancer. *J. Gastroenterol. Hepatol.* **2020**, *36*, 455–466. [CrossRef] [PubMed]
27. Lin, K.H.; Wang, F.L.; Wu, M.S.; Jiang, B.Y.; Kao, W.L.; Chao, H.Y.; Wu, J.Y.; Lee, C.C. Serum procalcitonin and C-reactive protein levels as markers of bacterial infection in patients with liver cirrhosis: A systematic review and meta-analysis. *Diagn. Microbiol. Infect. Dis.* **2014**, *80*, 72–78. [CrossRef] [PubMed]

28. Zhang, J.; Wieser, A.; Lin, H.; Fan, Y.; Li, H.; Schiergens, T.S.; Mayerle, J.; Gerbes, A.L.; Steib, C.J. Pretreatment with zinc protects Kupffer cells following administration of microbial products. *Biomed. Pharmacother. Biomed. Pharmacother.* **2020**, *127*, 110208. [CrossRef] [PubMed]
29. Kawai, T.; Akira, S. The role of pattern-recognition receptors in innate immunity: Update on Toll-like receptors. *Nat. Immunol.* **2010**, *11*, 373–384. [CrossRef]
30. Arthur, J.S.; Ley, S.C. Mitogen-activated protein kinases in innate immunity. *Nat. Rev. Immunol.* **2013**, *13*, 679–692. [CrossRef]
31. Cohen, P. The TLR and IL-1 signalling network at a glance. *J. Cell Sci.* **2014**, *127*, 2383–2390. [CrossRef] [PubMed]
32. Thévenot, T.; Bureau, C.; Oberti, F.; Anty, R.; Louvet, A.; Plessier, A.; Rudler, M.; Heurgué-Berlot, A.; Rosa, I.; Talbodec, N.; et al. Effect of albumin in cirrhotic patients with infection other than spontaneous bacterial peritonitis. A randomized trial. *J. Hepatol.* **2015**, *62*, 822–830. [CrossRef]
33. Pulimood, T.B.; Park, G.R. Debate: Albumin administration should be avoided in the critically ill. *Crit. Care* **2000**, *4*, 151–155. [CrossRef] [PubMed]
34. Merli, M.; Lucidi, C.; Lattanzi, B.; Riggio, O. Albumin infusion in cirrhotic patients with infections other than spontaneous bacterial peritonitis: End of the story? *J. Hepatol.* **2015**, *63*, 767–768. [CrossRef]
35. Di Pascoli, M.; Fasolato, S.; Piano, S.; Bolognesi, M.; Angeli, P. Long-term administration of human albumin improves survival in patients with cirrhosis and refractory ascites. *Liver Int. Off. J. Int. Assoc. Study Liver* **2019**, *39*, 98–105. [CrossRef] [PubMed]
36. Tsuchiya, S.; Yamabe, M.; Yamaguchi, Y.; Kobayashi, Y.; Konno, T.; Tada, K. Establishment and characterization of a human acute monocytic leukemia cell line (THP-1). *Int. J. Cancer* **1980**, *26*, 171–176. [CrossRef] [PubMed]
37. Thung, S.N.; Gerber, M.A. Presence of receptors for polymerized albumin in HBsAg-containing hepatocytes and hepatoma cell line. *Hepatology* **1981**, *1*, 132–136. [CrossRef]
38. Yoshioka, T.; Yamamoto, K.; Kobashi, H.; Tomita, M.; Tsuji, T. Receptor-mediated endocytosis of chemically modified albumins by sinusoidal endothelial cells and Kupffer cells in rat and human liver. *Liver* **1994**, *14*, 129–137. [CrossRef] [PubMed]
39. Beljaars, L.; Olinga, P.; Molema, G.; de Bleser, P.; Geerts, A.; Groothuis, G.M.; Meijer, D.K.; Poelstra, K. Characteristics of the hepatic stellate cell-selective carrier mannose 6-phosphate modified albumin (M6P(28)-HSA). *Liver* **2001**, *21*, 320–328. [CrossRef]
40. Drumm, K.; Gassner, B.; Silbernagl, S.; Gekle, M. Albumin in the mg/l-range activates NF-kappaB in renal proximal tubule-derived cell lines via tyrosine kinases and protein kinase C. *Eur. J. Med Res.* **2001**, *6*, 247–258.
41. Tang, S.; Leung, J.C.; Abe, K.; Chan, K.W.; Chan, L.Y.; Chan, T.M.; Lai, K.N. Albumin stimulates interleukin-8 expression in proximal tubular epithelial cells in vitro and in vivo. *J. Clin. Investig.* **2003**, *111*, 515–527. [CrossRef] [PubMed]
42. Poteser, M.; Wakabayashi, I. Serum albumin induces iNOS expression and NO production in RAW 267.4 macrophages. *Br. J. Pharmacol.* **2004**, *143*, 143–151. [CrossRef] [PubMed]
43. Ralay Ranaivo, H.; Patel, F.; Wainwright, M.S. Albumin activates the canonical TGF receptor-smad signaling pathway but this is not required for activation of astrocytes. *Exp. Neurol.* **2010**, *226*, 310–319. [CrossRef] [PubMed]

MDPI
St. Alban-Anlage 66
4052 Basel
Switzerland
Tel. +41 61 683 77 34
Fax +41 61 302 89 18
www.mdpi.com

Cells Editorial Office
E-mail: cells@mdpi.com
www.mdpi.com/journal/cells

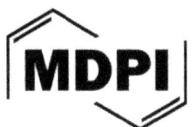